Applied Medical Statistics Using SAS

Applied Medical Statistics Using SAS

Geoff Der

Brian S. Everitt

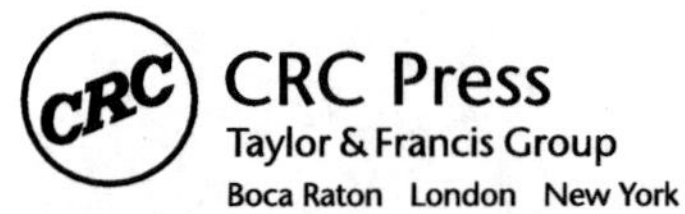

CRC Press
Taylor & Francis Group
Boca Raton   London   New York

CRC Press is an imprint of the
Taylor & Francis Group, an **informa** business

A CHAPMAN & HALL BOOK

CRC Press
Taylor & Francis Group
6000 Broken Sound Parkway NW, Suite 300
Boca Raton, FL 33487-2742

© 2013 by Taylor & Francis Group, LLC
CRC Press is an imprint of Taylor & Francis Group, an Informa business

No claim to original U.S. Government works

Printed in the United States of America on acid-free paper
Version Date: 20120813

International Standard Book Number: 978-1-4398-6797-6 (Hardback)

Visit the Taylor & Francis Web site at
http://www.taylorandfrancis.com

and the CRC Press Web site at
http://www.crcpress.com

Contents

Preface

In 2006 our book, *Statistical Analysis of Medical Data Using SAS,* was published and in 2010 we started to work on a second edition. But as work began, the number of new topics that we thought it would be valuable to include started to increase, to the point that we thought a new book was needed rather than a relatively light revision of the earlier book. The result is *Applied Medical Statistics Using SAS.* In this book, more attention has been given to the planning stage of medical studies in the sense that several chapters now contain details of sample size estimation. In addition, various methods of randomisation that might be employed for clinical trials are illustrated. Several completely new chapters cover topics that have become of great importance in the twenty-first century—for example, Bayesian methods and multiple imputation.

To save the book from becoming overly long, we have omitted the multivariate analysis chapters found in *Statistical Analysis of Medical Data Using SAS.* And, again with the aim of limiting the size of the book, larger data sets are given only in an abbreviated form; in many cases, the output has been edited to include only the most relevant sections. However, all complete data sets, all the SAS code, and complete outputs can be found on the website, http://support.sas.com/amsus.

The book is based on version 9.3 of SAS—the latest at press time. A major change in SAS since the previous book is that the output delivery system (ODS) has come of age. The power and flexibility of SAS for manipulating data prior to analysis is now equally matched at the other end of the process by its facilities for publishing the results. This is reflected in the book in that all tables and graphs are presented exactly as generated by SAS using ODS tables and graphs and the new graphics procedures.

We hope this new book will prove to be of use to many medical statisticians and to medical researchers in general who use SAS in their work.

Brian Everitt and Geoff Der
London and Glasgow

The Authors

Geoff Der works as a consulting statistician at the Medical Research Council's Social and Public Health Sciences Unit in Glasgow. He advises research staff in the unit on study design and statistical analysis and also conducts his own research.

Brian Everitt is professor emeritus, King's College, London, having retired 7 years ago. He is the author of more than 60 books on statistics. In retirement, he still finds some time to write about statistics, although it has to fit into a busy schedule that includes playing tennis, learning new pieces on the guitar, walking, reading, and working out at the gym.

1

An Introduction to SAS

1.1 Introduction

SAS, originally an acronym for Statistical Analysis System, comprises a broad range of software modules that can be added to the basic system, known as BASE SAS. Here our focus is on the SAS/STAT module in addition to the main features of the base system. Where we use any features of SAS that require additional modules, this will be indicated in the text. As of version 9.3 of SAS, there are sufficient graphical capabilities in the BASE and STAT modules that the SAS/GRAPH module will not be needed by most users.

Although there are graphical user interfaces to SAS, we will use SAS programs. This is the most common way of using SAS and the one which most users want to learn.

The SAS system is available for a wide range of different computers and operating systems and the way in which SAS programs are entered and run differs somewhat according to the computing environment. We describe the Microsoft Windows interface, as this is by far the most popular, although other windowing environments, such as X-windows, are quite similar.

At the time of writing, the latest version of SAS is version 9.3 and all the examples have used version 9.3 running under Microsoft Windows XP.

1.2 User Interface

Figure 1.1 shows the SAS user interface. At the top are the SAS title bar, the menu bar, and the tool bar with the command bar at its left end. The buttons of the tool bar change, depending on which window is active. The command bar allows less frequently used commands to be typed in. At the bottom, the status line comprises a message area with the current directory and editor cursor position at the right. Double clicking on the current directory allows it to be changed. Above the status line is a series of tabs, which allow a window to be selected when it is hidden behind other windows.

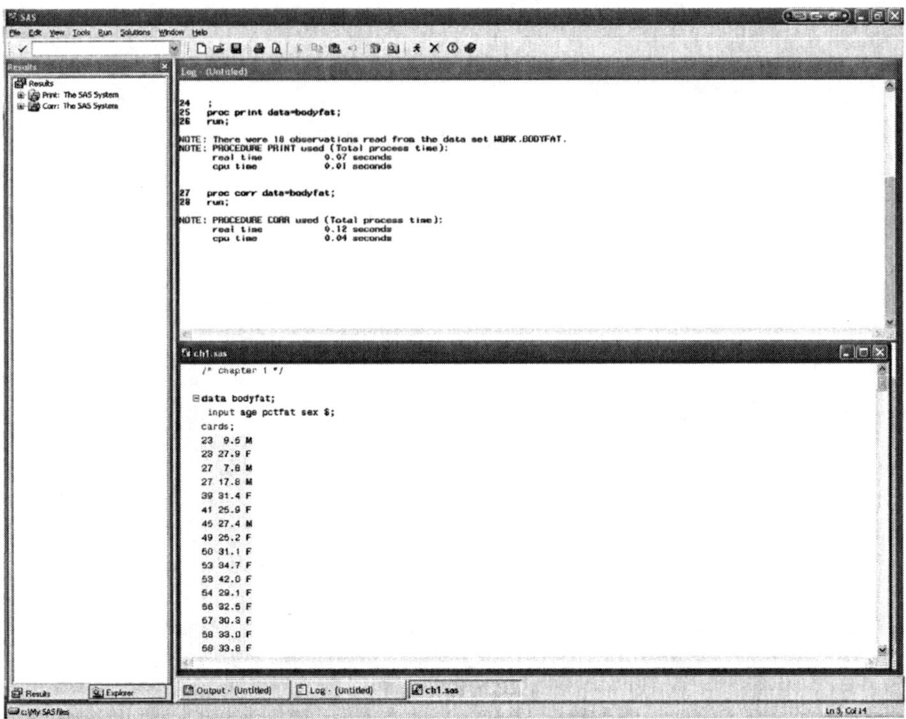

FIGURE 1.1
SAS version 9.3 running under Windows XP.

When SAS is started, there are five main windows open: the editor, log, output, results, and explorer windows. In Figure 1.1, the editor, log, and results windows are visible. The explorer window is hidden behind the results window and the output window is hidden behind the program editor and log windows.

If any of these windows has been closed, it can be reopened using the view menu.

The purpose of the main windows is described in the following subsections.

1.2.1 Editor Window

The editor window is for typing in programs, editing them, and running them.* The editor is essentially a built-in text editor specifically

---

* SAS has two editors: the current default version, referred to as the enhanced editor, and an older version, known as the program editor. The program editor has been retained for reasons of compatibility but is not recommended. Here we describe the enhanced editor and may refer to it simply as 'the editor'. If SAS starts up using the program editor rather than the enhanced editor, then from the Tools menu select Options; Preferences, then the Edit tab, and select the use Enhanced Editor box. The enhanced editor can be recognised by the + in its icon.

tailored to the SAS language, with additional facilities for running SAS programs.

The program currently in the editor window may be run by choosing the Submit option from the Run menu. The Run menu is specific to the editor window and will not be available if another window is the active window. Submitting a program may remove it from the editor window (but see below to disable this). If so, it can be retrieved by choosing Recall Last Submit from the Run menu.

It is possible to run part of the program in the editor window by selecting the text and then choosing Submit from the Run menu. With this method, the submitted text is not cleared from the editor window.

Other ways of submitting programs are the F3 key, the Running Man icon, and right-click followed by submit all or submit selection.

The Options submenu within Tools allows the editor to be configured. When the enhanced editor window is the active window (View; Enhanced Editor will ensure that it is), Tools; Options; Enhanced Editor will open a window similar to that in Figure 1.2. This shows the setup we recommend—in particular, that the options for collapsible code sections and automatic indentation are selected and that clear text on submit is not.

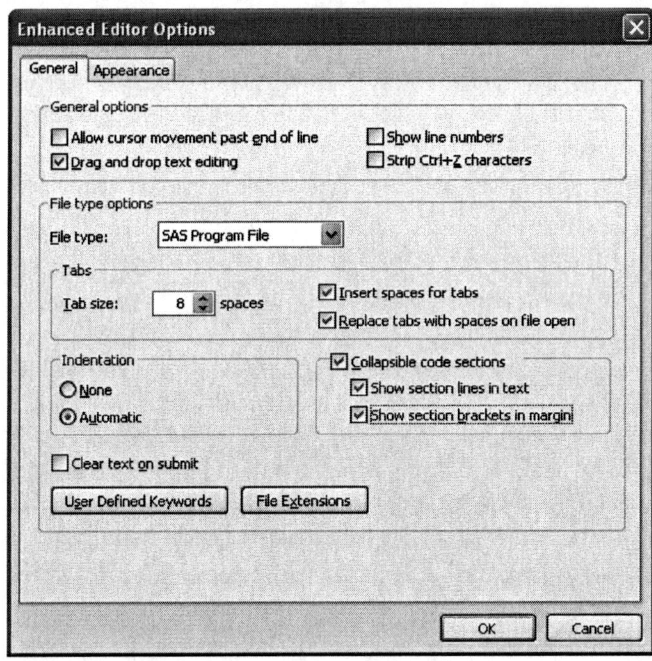

FIGURE 1.2
The enhanced editor options window with recommended options set.

When a SAS program is run, two types of output are generated: the log and the procedure output, and they are displayed in the log and output windows.

1.2.2 Log Window

The log window is the main source of feedback to the user about the program or statements that have been submitted. It shows the statements themselves, together with information about the execution of the program in the form of notes, warnings, and error messages. Although it is tempting to assume that if some output is generated, the program has 'worked', this is by no means always the case. It is a good discipline to check the log every time. Whilst error messages and warnings obviously demand attention, the notes can also be important. For example, when a SAS data set is created, a note in the log gives the number of observations and variables which the data set contains and, if these are not as anticipated, there may be an error in the program.

The `Clear all` option in the `Edit` menu, or the `New` button on the toolbar, will empty the window. This is useful if a program has been run several times as errors were being corrected.

1.2.3 Output Window

This window shows the textual output of any procedures, if the 'listing' form of output has been enabled. It is here that the results of any statistical analyses are shown.[*]

The output window works in tandem with the results window. The entire contents of the window can be cleared in the same way as the log window or sections can be deleted via the results window.

1.2.4 Results Window

This provides a graphical index to the various procedure results, including the contents of the output window, and any output in other formats, such as rich text format (rtf) or HTML, that may have been generated. It is useful for navigating around large amounts of output. Double clicking on a section of output opens the appropriate window with that section of the output visible. Right clicking on a procedure, or section of output, allows further options depending on the output format being used. For listing output that portion of the output can be viewed, printed, deleted, or saved to file.

1.2.5 Explorer Window

This performs much the same functions as the Windows explorer, but with the added advantage of being able to view the contents of SAS data sets or

---

[*] In SAS 9.3 listing output is disabled by default. See the following section.

a list of the variables they contain (right click, Open and right click, View Columns, respectively).

1.2.6 Results Viewer Window

The output delivery system (described in detail below) allows results to be produced in alternative formats. When this is enabled, a results viewer window will open to display the formatted results. In version 9.3 of SAS, the default setup is to produce HTML output and open a results viewer window to display it.

1.2.7 Options for Displaying Procedure Results

There are two main ways of displaying procedure output: listing format in the output window and HTML format in the results viewer window. The default is to produce HTML output. The main advantage of this is that all output appears in one window, including the graphs. Whereas with listing output, the graphs are not displayed by default, but double-clicking on a graph in the results window which will display it in a separate window outside SAS. The disadvantage of the default HTML format is that there is less control over individual sections of output. With listing output, individual sections of output and graphs can be deleted, saved, or printed. The ability to delete individual sections of output is often useful. The choice is a matter of personal preference.

However, we believe it is simpler while learning SAS to switch off HTML output and work with listing output. This is done via the tools menu, selecting Options, Preferences and then clicking on the Results tab. Figure 1.3 shows the resulting window and the necessary settings, with Create HTML, View results as they are generated, and Use ODS Graphics all deselected and Create listing selected. The default settings are the converse, with all options selected except Create listing.

1.2.8 Help and Documentation

The Help menu tends to become more useful as experience of SAS is gained, although there may be access to some tutorial materials, if they have been licensed from SAS. There are also links to the main SAS website and the customer support website.

Context-sensitive help can be invoked with the F1 key. Within the editor, when the cursor is positioned over the name of a SAS procedure, the F1 key brings up the help for that procedure.

Pdf files of the documentation are available online at http://support.sas. com/documentation/onlinedoc/.

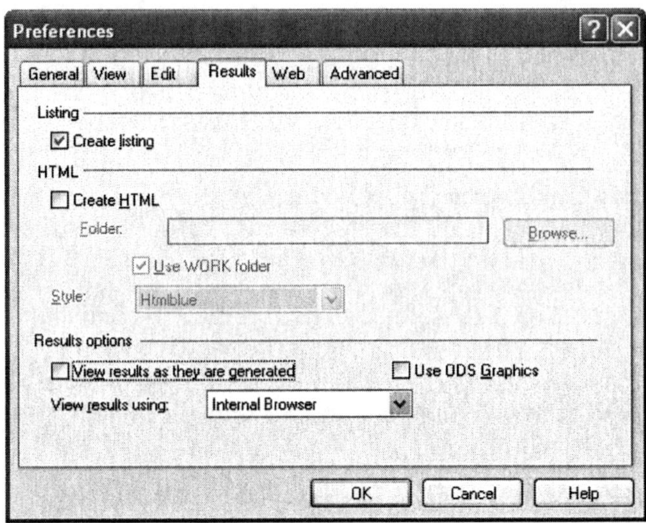

FIGURE 1.3
Setting the results options in the preferences window.

Note, though, that some of these are very large, so they can take time to open or download.

1.3 SAS Programs

SAS programs are made up of a sequence of statements that specify how data are to be processed and analysed. The statements specify operations to be performed on the data or instructions about the analysis and are grouped together into blocks, referred to as 'steps'. There are two types of program steps: data steps and proc (procedure) steps. A data step is used to prepare data for analysis. It creates a SAS data set and may reorganise the data and modify them in the process. A proc step is used to perform a particular type of analysis, or statistical test, on the data in a SAS data set.

A simple program might consist of a data step to read in some raw data followed by a series of proc steps analysing that data. If, in the course of the analysis, the data need to be modified, a second data step would be used to do this. Although the emphasis of this book is on the statistical analysis, one of the great strengths of SAS is the power and flexibility it gives the user to perform the data manipulation that is so often a large part of the overall task of analysing data.

Learning to use the SAS language is largely a question of learning the statements that are needed to do the analysis required and of knowing how to structure them into steps. There are a few general principles that are useful to know.

Most SAS statements begin with a keyword that identifies the type of statement. (The most important exception is the assignment statement, which begins with a variable name.) The enhanced editor recognises keywords as they are typed and changes their colour to blue. If a word remains red, this indicates a problem. The word may have been mistyped or is invalid for some other reason.

All SAS statements must end with a semicolon.

The most common mistake for new users is to omit the semicolon and the effect of this is to combine two statements into one. However, it may not be obvious that a semicolon has been omitted before the program is run, as the combined statement will typically begin with a valid keyword. Usually, the combined statement will be invalid and there will be an error message in the SAS log when the program is submitted. Sometimes it will still be a valid statement, albeit one that has unintended results.

Although statements may occupy more than one line and there may be more than one statement per line, keeping to one statement per line, as far as possible, helps to avoid errors and to identify those that do occur.

SAS statements fall into four broad categories according to where in a program they can be used:

- Data step statements
- Proc step statements
- Statements that can be used in both data and proc steps
- Global statements, which apply to all following steps

Since the functions of the data and proc steps are so different, it is perhaps not surprising that many statements are only applicable to one type of step.

1.3.1 Program Steps

Data and proc steps begin with a `data` or `proc` statement, respectively, and end at the next `data` or `proc` statement or the next `run` statement. When a data step has the data included within it, the step ends after the data. Understanding where steps begin and end is important because SAS programs are executed in whole steps. If an incomplete step is submitted, it will not run. The statements that were submitted will be listed in the log, but SAS will appear to have stopped at that point without explanation. In fact, SAS will simply be waiting for the step to be completed before running it. For this reason it is good practice to mark the end of each step explicitly by inserting a `run` statement, and it is especially important to include one as the last statement in the program.

The enhanced editor offers several visual indicators of the beginning and end of steps. The `data`, `proc`, and `run` keywords are colour coded in navy blue, rather than the standard blue used for other keywords. If the enhanced editor options for collapsible code sections have been selected as shown in Figure 1.2, each data and proc step will be separated by lines in the text and indicated by brackets in the margin. This gives the appearance of enclosing each data and proc step in its own box.

Data step statements must be within the relevant data step—that is, after the `data` statement and before the end of the step. Likewise, proc step statements must be within the proc step.

Global statements may be placed anywhere. If they are placed within a step, they will apply to that step and all subsequent steps until reset. A simple example of a global statement is the `title` statement, which defines a title for procedure output and graphs. The title is then used until changed or reset.

1.3.2 Variable Names and Data Set Names

In writing a SAS program, names must be given to variables and data sets. These may contain letters, numbers, and underline characters, and they may be up to 32 characters long but cannot begin with a number. (Prior to version 7 of SAS, the maximum length was eight characters.) Variable names may be in upper or lower case, or a mixture, but differences in case are ignored: `Height`, `height`, and `HEIGHT` would all refer to the same variable.[*]

1.3.3 Variable Lists

When a list of variable names is needed in a SAS program, an abbreviated form can often be used. A variable list of the form `sex -- weight` refers to the variables `sex` and `weight` and all the variables positioned between them in the data set. A second form of variable list may be used where a set of variables have names of the form `score1`, `score2`,... `score10`. That is, there are 10 variables with the root, `score`, in common and ending in the digits 1 to 10. In this case, they can be referred to by the variable list `score1-score10` and do *not* need to be contiguous in the data set.

Before looking at the SAS language in more detail, the short example shown in Table 1.1 can be used to illustrate some of the preceding material. The data are adapted from Table 17 of *A Handbook of Small Data Sets* (SDSs) and show the age, sex, and percentage body fat for 18 subjects. The program consists of three steps: a data step followed by two proc steps. Submitting this program results in the log and procedure output shown in Table 1.2 and Table 1.3.

---

[*] However, the first form that SAS encounters is the one that will be used in procedure output.

TABLE 1.1

A Simple SAS Program

```
data bodyfat;
  input age pctfat sex $;
cards;
23     9.5    M
23    27.9    F
27     7.8    M
27    17.8    M
39    31.4    F
41    25.9    F
45    27.4    M
49    25.2    F
50    31.1    F
53    34.7    F
53    42.0    F
54    29.1    F
56    32.5    F
57    30.3    F
58    33.0    F
58    33.8    F
60    41.1    F
61    34.5    F
;
proc print data=bodyfat;
run;
proc corr data=bodyfat;
run;
```

TABLE 1.2

SAS Log after Submitting the Program in Table 1.1

```
27 data bodyfat;
28  input age pctfat sex $;
29 cards;

NOTE: The data set WORK.BODYFAT has 18 observations and 3 variables.
NOTE: DATA statement used (Total process time):
      real time           0.00 seconds
      cpu time            0.00 seconds

48 ;
49 proc print data=bodyfat;
50 run;

NOTE: There were 18 observations read from the data set WORK.BODYFAT.
NOTE: PROCEDURE PRINT used (Total process time):
      real time           0.00 seconds
      cpu time            0.00 seconds
```

(*Continued*)

TABLE 1.2 (*Continued*)

SAS Log after Submitting the Program in Table 1.1

```
51 proc corr data=bodyfat;
52 run;

NOTE: PROCEDURE CORR used (Total process time):
      real time          0.01 seconds
      cpu time           0.01 seconds
```

TABLE 1.3

Procedure Output of the Program in Table 1.1

```
                Obs      age      pctfat     sex

                  1       23        9.5        M
                  2       23       27.9        F
                  3       27        7.8        M
                  4       27       17.8        M
                  5       39       31.4        F
                  6       41       25.9        F
                  7       45       27.4        M
                  8       49       25.2        F
                  9       50       31.1        F
                 10       53       34.7        F
                 11       53       42.0        F
                 12       54       29.1        F
                 13       56       32.5        F
                 14       57       30.3        F
                 15       58       33.0        F
                 16       58       33.8        F
                 17       60       41.1        F
                 18       61       34.5        F


                      The CORR Procedure

                2 Variables:    age    pctfat


                      Simple Statistics

Variable     N      Mean      Std Dev       Sum        Minimum     Maximum

age         18   46.33333    13.21764   834.00000    23.00000    61.00000
pctfat      18   28.61111     9.14439   515.00000     7.80000    42.00000


          Pearson Correlation Coefficients, N = 18
             Prob > |r| under H0: Rho=0


                          age        pctfat

          age          1.00000      0.79209
                                    <.0001


          pctfat       0.79209      1.00000
                                    <.0001
```

From the log we can see that the program has been split into steps and each step run separately. Notes on how the step ran follow the statements that comprise the step and, in the case of the data step, show that the `bodyfat` data set contains the correct number of observations and variables.[*]

1.4 Reading Data—The Data Step

Before data can be analysed in SAS, they need to be read into a SAS data set. Creating a SAS data set for subsequent analysis is the primary function of the data step. The data may be 'raw' data or come from a previously created SAS data set. A data step is also used to manipulate or reorganise the data. This can range from relatively simple operations, like transforming variables, to more complex restructuring of the data. In many practical situations, organising and preprocessing the data take up a large proportion of the overall time and effort. The power and flexibility of SAS for such data manipulation are two of its great strengths.

We begin by describing how to create SAS data sets from raw data and store them on disk before turning to data manipulation. Each of the subsequent chapters includes the data step used to prepare the data for analysis and several of them illustrate features not described in this chapter.

1.4.1 Creating SAS Data Sets from Raw Data[†]

Table 1.4 shows some hypothetical data on members of a slimming club, giving the membership number, team, starting weight and current weight. The following data step could be used to create a SAS data set:

```
data SlimmingClub;
   infile 'c:\amsus\data\slimmingclub.dat';
   input idno team $ startweight weightnow;
run;
```

1.4.2 Data Statement

The `data` statement often takes the simple form where it merely names the data set being created—in this case, `SlimmingClub`.

---

[*] The reason the log refers to the SAS data set as 'WORK.BODYFAT' rather than simply 'bodyfat' will be explained later.

[†] A 'raw' data file may also be referred to as a text file, or ASCII file. Such files only include the printable characters plus tabs, spaces, and end-of-line characters. The files produced by database programs, spreadsheets, and word processors are not normally raw data, although such programs usually have the ability to export their data to such a file.

TABLE 1.4

Hypothetical Data for a Slimming Club

1023	red	189	165
1049	yellow	145	124
1219	red	210	192
1246	yellow	194	177
1078	red	127	118
1221	yellow	220	.
1095	blue	135	127
1157	green	155	141
1331	blue	187	172
1067	green	135	122
1251	blue	181	166
1333	green	141	129
1192	yellow	152	139
1352	green	156	137
1262	blue	196	180
1087	red	148	135
1124	green	156	142
1197	red	138	125
1133	blue	180	167
1036	green	135	123
1057	yellow	146	132
1328	red	155	142
1243	blue	134	122
1177	red	141	130
1259	green	189	172
1017	blue	138	127
1099	yellow	148	132
1329	yellow	188	174

1.4.3 Infile Statement

The `infile` statement specifies the file where the raw data are stored. The full path name of the file is given. If the file is in the current directory (i.e., the one specified at the bottom right of the SAS window), the file name could have been specified simply as `'SlimmingClub.dat'`. The name of the raw data file must be in quotes. In many cases, the `infile` statement will only need to specify the file name, as in this example.

In some circumstances, additional options on the `infile` statement will be needed. One such instance is where the values in the raw data file are not separated by spaces. Common alternatives are files where the data values are separated by tabs or commas. The `expandtabs` option changes tab characters into a number of spaces. The `delimiter` option can be used to specify a separator. For example, `delimiter=','` could be used for files where the data values are separated by commas. More than one delimiter can be specified. Tab- and comma-separated data are discussed in more detail later.

Another situation where additional options may be needed is to specify what happens when the program requests more data values than a line in the raw data file contains. This can happen for a number of reasons, particularly where character data are being read. Often the solution is to use the `pad` option, which adds spaces to the end of each data line as it is read.

There is one situation where an `infile` statement is not needed: when the data are contained within the SAS program itself. This is referred to as 'instream' data. If data are instream, an `infile` statement is only needed when additional options are required. When data are instream, SAS automatically expands tabs according to the tab size setting for the editor (see Figure 1.2), so the `expandtabs` option is not needed. In practice, raw data are more commonly contained in an external file.

1.4.4 Input Statement

The `input` statement in the example specifies that four variables are to be read in from the raw data file: `idno`, `team`, `startweight`, and `weightnow`. The dollar sign after `team` indicates that it is a character variable. SAS only has two types of variables: numeric and character.

The function of the `input` statement is to name the variables, specify their type as numeric or character, and indicate where in the raw data the corresponding data values are. If the data values are separated by spaces, as they are here, a simple form of the `input` statement is possible in which the variable names are merely listed in order and character variables are indicated by a dollar sign after their name. This is the so-called 'list' form of input. SAS has three main modes of input[*]:

- List—for data separated by spaces
- Column—for data arranged in columns
- Formatted—for data in nonstandard formats

There is often a choice of which mode of input to use and it is a question of which mode is more convenient for the data at hand.

1.4.4.1 List Input

List input is the simplest and is usually preferred for that reason. However, the requirement that the data values be separated by spaces has some important implications. The first is that missing values cannot be represented by spaces in the raw data; a period (.) should be used instead. In the example, the value of `weightnow` is missing for member number 1221.

---

[*] There is a fourth form, named input, but data suitable for this form of input occur so rarely that its description can safely be omitted.

The second is that character values cannot contain spaces. With list input, it is also important to bear in mind that the default length for character variables is eight.

When using list input *always* examine the SAS log. Check that the correct number of variables and observations have been read in. The message 'SAS went to a new line when INPUT statement reached past the end of a line' often indicates a problem in reading the data. If so, the pad option on the infile statement may be the answer.

With small data sets, it is advisable to print them out with proc print or open the data set via the explorer window and check that the raw data have been read in correctly. It is worth paying particular attention to checking the first and last observations.

1.4.4.2 Column Input

If list input is problematic and the data are arranged in columns, column input may be simpler. Table 1.5 shows the slimming club data with members'

TABLE 1.5

Hypothetical Slimming Data with
Members' Names

David Shaw	red	189	165
Amelia Serrano	yellow	145	124
Alan Nance	red	210	192
Ravi Sinha	yellow	194	177
Ashley McKnight	red	127	118
Jim Brown	yellow	220	
Susan Stewart	blue	135	127
Rose Collins	green	155	141
Jason Schock	blue	187	172
Kanoko Nagasaka	green	135	122
Richard Rose	blue	181	166
Li-Hwa Lee	green	141	129
Charlene Armstrong	yellow	152	139
Bette Long	green	156	137
Yao Chen	blue	196	180
Kim Blackburn	red	148	135
Adrienne Fink	green	156	142
Lynne Overby	red	138	125
John VanMeter	blue	180	167
Becky Redding	green	135	123
Margie Vanhoy	yellow	146	132
Hisashi Ito	red	155	142
Deanna Hicks	blue	134	122
Holly Choate	red	141	130
Raoul Sanchez	green	189	172
Jennifer Brooks	blue	138	127
Asha Garg	yellow	148	132
Larry Goss	yellow	188	174

names instead of their membership numbers. To read in the data in the column form of input statement would be the following:

```
input name $ 1-18 team $ 20-25 startweight 27-29 weightnow
31-33;
```

As can be seen, the difference between the two forms of input statement is simply that the columns containing the data values for each variable are specified after the variable name, or after the dollar in the case of a character variable. The start and finish columns are separated by a hyphen, but for single column variables it is only necessary to give the one column number. Note also that Jim Brown's current weight is missing, but the blank columns are treated as a missing value, so the period is not needed as it would be with list input.

1.4.4.3 Formatted Input

With formatted input, each variable is followed by its input format, referred to as its *informat*. Alternatively, a list of variables in parentheses is followed by a format list, also in parentheses. Formatted input is the most flexible, partly because a wide range of informats is available. To read the preceding data using formatted input, the following input statement could be used:

```
input name $19. team $7. startweight 4. weightnow 3.;
```

The informat for a character variable consists of a dollar sign, the number of columns occupied by the data values, and a period. The simplest form of informat for numeric data is simply the number of columns occupied by the data and a period. Note that the spaces separating the data values have been taken into account in the informat.

Formatted input must be used if the data are not in a standard numeric format. Such data are rare in practice. The most common use of special SAS informats is likely to be the date informats. When a date is read using a date informat, the resultant value is the number of days from January 1, 1960, to that date. The following data step illustrates the use of the ddmmyyw. informat. The width w may be from 6 to 32 columns. There is also the mmddyyw. informat for dates in American format. (There are also corresponding output formats, referred to simply as 'formats', to output dates in calendar form.)

```
data days;
input day ddmmyy8.;
cards;
020160
01/02/60
31 12 59
```

```
231019
231020
23101919
;
run;
proc print data=days;
run;
proc print data=days;
  format day ddmmyy10.;
run;
```

As the example illustrates, if the year is only given by its last two digits, values of 20 or above are assumed to be in the twentieth century (i.e., 1920, etc.). As the last date shows, the same format can be used for dates where the year is given as four digits, and this is clearly the safest option. If separators were used, the width of the informat would need to be increased (e.g., to ddmmyy10).

This data step is also an example of instream data. The data are contained between a `cards` statement (`datalines` is a synonym for `cards`) and a line with a single semicolon on it. The data must always be at the end of the data step.

Another instance where formatted input may be needed is when numeric data contain an implied decimal point. In this case, the informat has a second number after the period to indicate the number of digits to the right of the decimal point. For example, an informat of 5.2 would read five columns of numeric data and, in effect, move the decimal point two places to the left. Where the data contain an explicit decimal point, this takes precedence over the informat:

```
data decimals;
  input realnum 5.2;
cards;
1234
 4567
123.4
   6789
;
proc print;
run;
```

Leading or trailing spaces *within the field width,* as in lines 1 and 2, will not prevent the number from being read correctly. In the case of the last line, the final digit is outside the field width (i.e., in column 6), so it is not read as part of the number.

Formatted input can be much more concise than column input, particularly when consecutive data values have the same format. If the first 20 columns of the data line contain the single digit responses to 20 questions, the data could be read as follows:

```
input (q1 - q20) (20*1.);
```

In this case, using a numbered variable list makes the statement even more concise. The informats in the format list can be repeated by prefixing them with n*, where n is the number of times the format is to be repeated—20 in this case. If the format list has fewer informats than there are variables in the variable list, the whole format list is reused. Thus, the preceding input statement could be rewritten as

```
input (q1 - q20) (1.);
```

This feature is useful where the data contain repeating groups. If the answers to the 20 questions occupied one and two columns alternately, they could be read with

```
input (q1 - q20) (1. 2.);
```

The different forms of input may be mixed on the same input statement for maximum flexibility.

1.4.4.4 Multiple Lines per Observation

Where the data for an observation occupy several lines, the slash character (/), used as part of the input statement, indicates where to start reading data from the next line. Alternatively, a separate input statement could be written for each line of data, since SAS automatically goes on to the next line of data at the completion of each input statement.

1.4.4.5 Multiple Observations per Line

In some circumstances, it is useful to be able to prevent SAS from automatically going on to the next line; this is done by adding an @ character to the end of the input statement. The usual reason for doing this is that there are data for more than one observation on the same line. These features of data input will be illustrated in later chapters.

1.4.4.6 Delimited Data

There are two commonly occurring forms of raw data that are worth commenting on specifically: tab-separated data and comma-separated data. Whilst list input is most commonly used for data separated by spaces, it can also be used to read data with other separators, referred to as 'delimiters'. One question which arises when delimiters other than spaces are used is how to treat two consecutive delimiters. With spaces as delimiters, list input by default treats consecutive spaces as a single delimiter. This is why spaces cannot be used for missing values. With comma-separated data, it is more likely that two consecutive commas are intended to indicate that the value that would have been between them is missing. Tabs are more commonly treated like spaces but could be intended to be read either way. To change the default so that two consecutive delimiters are treated as having a missing value between them, use the `dsd` (delimiter-sensitive data) option on the `infile` statement.

Tab-separated data. The simplest way to read tab-delimited data is to use list input with the `expandtabs` option on the `infile` statement. This substitutes a number of spaces for the tab character. If consecutive tabs indicate missing values, the `delimiter=` and `dsd` options are needed, as follows:

```
Infile 'filename' delimiter='09'x dsd;*
```

Comma-separated data. Comma-delimited data files may also be referred to as comma separate value (CSV) files, with a file extension of .csv; many PC programs can produce files in this format. For most of these, the `dsd` option on the `infile` statement will suffice, as it assumes that the delimiter is a comma. Some comma-delimited files will have data values enclosed in quotes to avoid problems where data values include commas. The `dsd` option deals with this, too, by ignoring commas within quotes and removing the quotes from the data values. The `missover` option is also recommended for CSV files to prevent SAS going to a new line where the last value on a data line is missing (see example in Chapter 14). CSV files may also contain the names of the variables as the first line of the file. To skip this line when reading the data, use the `firstobs=2` option. Thus, the recommended form of infile statement is

```
infile 'filename' dsd missover;
```

or

```
infile 'filename' dsd missover firstobs=2;
```

where the variable names are on the first line.

1.4.5 Reading Data—Proc Import

For tab- and comma-delimited data, particularly where the first line contains the variable names, proc import is a useful alternative to reading in the data with a data step. For example, to read a tab-delimited file with the variable names in the first line, use

```
proc import datafile='c:\amsus\data\SlimmingClub.tab'
out=SlimmingClub dbms=tab replace;
  getnames=yes;
run;
```

For comma-separated value files, substitute `dbms=csv`.

---

* The value 09 is the hexadecimal code for the tab character in the ASCII character set.

In order to determine whether variables are numeric or character, proc import looks at the first 20 rows to see whether they contain non-numeric characters. This usually gives the correct result, but does need to be checked.

An alternative way of using proc import is via the import wizard. From the `file` menu, select `import data....`

SAS has a comprehensive set of modules enabling data held in proprietary databases to be read directly into SAS. This needs the appropriate SAS/ACCESS module to be licensed and is beyond the scope of this book. In the PC context, however, it is worth mentioning that the SAS/ACCESS module for PC file formats will enable proc import to read data from Access, Excel, Dbase, and Lotus files. The first screen of the import wizard will show which data sources have been licensed.

1.4.6 Reading and Writing Excel Files

Microsoft Excel is probably the most commonly occurring proprietary data format. If the SAS/ACCESS module for PC file formats is licensed, data in this format can be read or written using `proc import` and `proc export`, respectively:

```
proc import datafile='c:\amsus\data\usair.xls' out=usairmiss
dbms=excel replace;
   sheet=usairmiss;
run;
```

This example reads the worksheet named 'usairmiss' from the usair workbook and creates the SAS data set usairmiss. If there were only one worksheet in the Excel file, the sheet statement would not be needed.

To read a range of cells from a worksheet, the range statement is used:

```
proc import datafile='c:\amsus\data\usair.xls' out=usairsub
dbms=excel replace;
   getnames=no;
   range="usairfull$a8:f42";
run;
```

The range comprises the name of the worksheet followed by a $, the upper left cell number, a colon and the lower right cell number. In this example, we also specify getnames=no as it is unlikely that the first row of the range does include the variable names.

To create an Excel file from a SAS data set, `proc export` is used in an analogous fashion:

```
proc export data=usairmiss file='c:\amsus\data\myExcel.xls'
dbms=excel replace;
run;
```

1.4.7 Temporary and Permanent SAS Data Sets—SAS Libraries

So far, all the examples have shown temporary SAS data sets. They are temporary in the sense that they will be deleted when SAS is exited. To store SAS data sets permanently on disk and to access such data sets, the `libname` statement is used and the SAS data set referred to slightly differently:

```
libname db 'c:\amsus\data';
data db.SlimmingClub;
 set SlimmingClub;
run;
```

The `libname` statement specifies that the *libref* db refers to the directory `'c:\amsus\data'`. Thereafter, a SAS data set name prefixed with `'db.'` refers to a data set stored in that directory. When used on a data statement, the effect is to create a SAS data set in that directory. This data step reads data from the temporary SAS data set `SlimmingClub` and stores it in a permanent data set of the same name.

Since the `libname` statement is a global statement, the link between the libref db and the directory `'c:\amsus\data'` remains throughout the SAS session, or until it is reset. If SAS has been exited and restarted, the `libname` statement will need to be submitted again.

In Table 1.2 we saw that the temporary data set `bodyfat` was referred to in the log notes as `'WORK.BODYFAT'`. This is because work is the libref pointing to the directory where temporary SAS data sets are stored. SAS automatically sets up this directory when it starts and deletes the directory and its contents when SAS is closed.

To use the SAS explorer window to examine the contents of a temporary data set, or its variables, double click on `libraries` in the explorer window and then double click on `work`. To do the same for permanently stored data sets, after opening the libraries folder, double click on the libref (e.g., db in the previous example).

1.4.8 Reading Data from an Existing SAS Data Set

To read data from a SAS data set, rather than from a raw data file, the `set` statement is used in place of the `infile` and `input` statements. For example, to retrieve a previously stored data set and continue working with a temporary copy,

```
libname db 'c:\amsus\data';
data SlimmingClub;
set db.SlimmingClub;
run;
```

creates a new, temporary, SAS data set `SlimmingClub` (which will be referred to as WORK.SLIMMINGCLUB in the log) reading in the data from the stored version of `SlimmingClub`.

1.5 Modifying SAS Data

As well as creating a SAS data set, the data step may also be used to modify the data in a variety of ways.

1.5.1 Creating and Modifying Variables

The assignment statement can be used both to create new variables and to modify existing ones. The statement

```
weightloss=startweight-weightnow;
```

creates a new variable `weightloss` and sets its value to the starting weight minus the current weight. The following statement will convert the starting weight from pounds to kilograms:

```
startweight=startweight * 0.4536;
```

SAS has the normal set of arithmetic operators: + (add), − (subtract), / (divide), * (multiply), and ** (exponentiate), plus various arithmetic, mathematical, and statistical functions, some of which will be illustrated in later chapters.

1.5.1.1 Missing Values in Arithmetic Expressions

The result of an arithmetic operation performed on a missing value is itself a missing value. When this happens, a warning message is printed in the log. Missing values for numeric variables are represented by a period (.) and a numeric variable can be set to a missing value by an assignment statement such as

```
age = . ;
```

With any arithmetical operation, it is worth considering what the effect of missing values will be. Say that we want to calculate the mean of five variables, x1–x5. An assignment of the form xmean=(x1+x2+x3+x4+x5)/5; will result in a missing value if *any* of x1–x5 are missing. On the other hand, xmean=mean(x1,x2,x3,x4,x5); will only result in a missing value if *all* of them are missing.

To assign a value to a character variable, the text string must be enclosed in quotes—for example,

```
team='green';
```

A missing value may be assigned to a character variable as follows:

```
team='';
```

To modify the value of a variable for some observations and not others, or to make different modifications for different groups of observations, the assignment statement may be used within an `if then` statement:

```
reward=0;
if weightloss > 10 then reward=1;
```

If the condition `weightloss > 10` is true, then the assignment statement `reward=1` is executed; otherwise, the variable `reward` keeps its previously assigned value of 0. In cases like this, an `else` statement could be used in conjunction with the `if then` statement:

```
if weightloss > 10 then reward=1;
   else reward=0;
```

The condition in the `if  then` statement may be a simple comparison of two values. The form of comparison may be one of the following:

Operator		Meaning	Example
EQ	=	Equal to	`a = b`
NE	~=	Not equal to	`a ne b`
LT	<	Less than	`a < b`
GT	>	Greater than	`a gt b`
GE	>=	Greater than or equal to	`a >= b`
LE	<=	Less than or equal to	`a le b`

Comparisons can be combined into a more complex condition using and (&), or (|), and not (~):

```
if team='blue' and weightloss gt 10 then reward=1;
```

In more complex cases, it may be advisable to make the logic explicit by grouping conditions together with parentheses.

Some conditions involving a single variable can be simplified. For example, the following two statements are equivalent:

```
if age > 18 and age < 40 then agegroup = 1;
if 18 < age < 40 then agegroup = 1;
```

Conditions of the form

```
x = 1 or x = 3 or x = 5
```

may be abbreviated to

```
x in(1, 3, 5)
```

using the `in` operator. If the data contain missing values, it is important to allow for this when recoding.

In numeric comparisons, missing values are treated as smaller than any number. For instance,

```
if age >= 18 then adult=1;
   else adult=0;
```

would assign the value 0 to `adult` if `age` were missing, whereas it may be more appropriate to assign a missing value. The missing function could be used to do this by following the `else` statement with

```
if missing(age) then adult=.;
```

Care needs to be exercised when making comparisons involving character variables, since these are case sensitive and sensitive to leading blanks.

A group of statements may be executed conditionally by placing them between a do statement and an end statement:

```
If weightloss > 10 and weightnow < 140 then do;
target=1;
reward=1;
team ='blue';
end;
```

Every observation that satisfies the condition will have the values of `target`, `reward`, and `team` set as indicated. Otherwise, they will remain at their previous values.

Where the same operation is to be carried out on several variables, it is often convenient to use an `array` and an iterative do loop in combination. This is best illustrated with a simple example. Suppose we have 20 variables, q1 to q20, for which 'not applicable' has been coded –1 and we wish to set those to missing values, we might do it as follows:

```
array qall {20} q1-q20;
do i= 1 to 20;
  if qall{i}=-1 then qall{i}=.;
end;
```

The `array` statement defines an array by specifying the name of the array (`qall` here), the number of variables to be included in it in braces, and the list of variables to be included. All the variables in the array must be of the same type—that is, all numeric or all character.

The iterative do loop repeats the statements between the do and the end a fixed number of times, with an index variable changing at each repetition. When used to process each of the variables in an array, the do loop should start with the index variable equal to 1 and end when it equals the number of variables in the array.

The array is a shorthand way of referring to a group of variables. In effect, it provides aliases for them so that each variable can be referred to by using the name of the array and its position within the array in braces. For example, q12 could be referred to as qall{12} or, when the variable i has the value 12, as qall{i}. However, the array only lasts for the duration of the data step in which it is defined.

1.5.2 Deleting Variables

Variables may be removed from the data set being created by using the drop or keep statements. The drop statement names a list of variables that are to be excluded from the data set, and the keep statement does the converse; that is, it names a list of variables that are to be the only ones retained in the data set, with all others excluded. Thus, the statement drop x y z; in a data step results in a data set that does not contain the variables x, y, and z, whereas keep x y z; results in a data set that contains only those three variables.

1.5.3 Deleting Observations

It may be necessary to delete observations from the data set—for example, if they contain errors. Deleting erroneous observations is best done by using the if then statement with the delete statement:

```
if weightloss > startweight then delete;
```

In a case like this, it would also be useful to write out a message giving more information about the observation that contains the error:

```
if weightloss > startweight then do;
put 'Error in weight data' idno= startweight= weightloss=;
delete;
end;
```

The put statement writes text (in quotes) and the values of variables to the log.

1.5.4 Subsetting Data Sets

If analysis of a subset of the data is needed, it is often convenient to create a new data set containing only the relevant observations. This can be achieved with either the subsetting if statement or the where statement. The subsetting if statement consists simply of the keyword if followed by a logical condition. Only observations for which the condition is true are included in the data set being created:

```
data women;
   set bodyfat;
   if sex='F';
run;
```

The statement `where sex='F';` has the same form and could be used to the same effect. The difference between the subsetting `if` statement and the `where` statement will not concern most users, except that the `where` statement may also be used with `proc` steps as discussed below. More complex conditions may be specified on either statement in the same way as for an `if then` statement.

1.5.5 Concatenating and Merging Data Sets

Two or more data sets can be combined into one by specifying them on a single `set` statement:

```
data survey;
   set men women;
run;
```

This is also a simple way of adding new observations to an existing data set. First, read the data for the new cases into a SAS data set and then combine this with the existing data set as follows:

```
data survey;
  set survey newcases;
run;
```

1.5.6 Merging Data Sets—Adding Variables

Data for a study may arise from more than one source, or at different times, and need to be combined. For instance, demographic details from a questionnaire may need to be combined with the results of laboratory tests. To deal with this situation, the data are read into separate SAS data sets and then combined using a merge with a unique subject identifier as a key. Assuming that the data have been read into two data sets, `demographics` and `labtests`, and that both data sets contain the subject identifier `idnumber`, they can be combined as follows:

```
proc sort data=demographics;
   by idnumber;
proc sort data=labtests;
   by idnumber;
```

```
data combined;
 merge demographics (in=indem) labtest (in=inlab);
 by idnumber;
 if indem and inlab;
run;
```

First, both data sets must be sorted by the matching variable, `idnumber`. This variable should be of the same type, numeric or character, and same length in both data sets. The `merge` statement in the data step specifies the data sets to be merged. The option in parentheses after the name creates a temporary variable which indicates whether that data set provided an observation for the merged data set. The by statement specifies the matching variable. The subsetting `if` statement specifies that only observations that have both the demographic data and the lab results should be included in the combined data set. Without this, the combined data set may contain incomplete observations (i.e., those where there are demographic data but no lab results, or vice versa). An alternative might be to retain the incomplete observations but print messages in the log to identify them as follows:

```
If not indem then put idnumber 'no demographics';
If not inlab then put idnumber 'no lab results';
```

This method of match merging is not confined to situations where there is a one-to-one correspondence between the observations in the data sets; it can be used for one-to-many or many-to-one relationships as well. A common practical application is in the use of lookup tables. For example, the research data set might contain the respondent's post code (or zip code), and another file might contain information on the characteristics of the area. Match merging the two data sets by post code would attach area information to the individual observations. A subsetting `if` statement would be used so that only observations from the research data were retained.

1.5.7 Operation of the Data Step

In addition to learning the statements that may be used in a data step, it is useful to understand how the data step operates.

The statements that comprise the data step form a sequence according to the order in which they occur. The sequence begins with the data statement and finishes at the end of the data step and is executed repeatedly until the source of data runs out. Starting from the `data` statement, a typical data step will read in some data with an `input` or `set` statement and use that data to construct an observation. The observation will then be used to execute the statements that follow. The data in the observation may be modified or added to in the process. At the end of the data step the observation will be written to the data set being created. The sequence will begin again from the data statement, reading the data for the next observation, processing it, and writing it to the output data set. This continues until all the data have been read in and processed. The data step will then finish and the execution of the program will pass on to the next step.

In effect, then, the data step consists of a loop of instructions executed repeatedly until all the data are processed. The automatic SAS variable (_n_) records the iteration number but is not stored in the data set. Its use will be illustrated in later chapters.

The point at which SAS adds an observation to the data set can be controlled by the use of the `output` statement. When a data step includes one or more `output` statements, an observation is added to the data set each time an `output` statement is executed, but not at the end of the data step. In this way the data being read in can be used to construct several observations. This will be illustrated in later chapters.

1.6 Proc Step

Once data have been read into a SAS data set, SAS procedures can be used to analyse the data. Roughly speaking, each SAS procedure performs a specific type of analysis. The `proc` step is a block of statements that specify the data set to be analysed, the procedure to be used, and any further details of the analysis. The step begins with a `proc` statement and ends with a `run` statement or when the next `data` or `proc` step starts. We recommend including a `run` statement for every proc step.

1.6.1 Proc Statement

The `proc` statement names the procedure to be used and may also specify options for the analysis. The most important option is the `data=` option, which names the data set to be analysed. If the option is omitted, the procedure uses the most recently created data set. Although this is usually what is intended, it is safer to specify the data set explicitly. When ODS graphics (described below) is enabled, the procedure may produce graphical output and this can be controlled by the `plots=` option.

Many of the statements that follow particular `proc` statements are specific to individual procedures and will be described in later chapters as they arise. A few, though, are more general and apply to a number of procedures.

1.6.2 Var Statement

The `var` statement specifies the variables that are to be processed by the proc step. For example,

```
proc print data= SlimmingClub;
   var name team weightloss;
run;
```

restricts the printout to the three variables mentioned, whereas the default would be to print all variables.

1.6.3 Where Statement

The `where` statement selects the observations to be processed. The keyword `where` is followed by a logical condition and only those observations for which the condition is true are included in the analysis:

```
proc print data= SlimmingClub;
   where weightloss > 0;
run;
```

1.6.4 By Statement

The `by` statement is used to process the data in groups. The observations are grouped according to the values of the variable named on the by statement and a separate analysis is conducted for each group. In order to do this, the data set must first be sorted on the by variable:

```
proc sort data= SlimmingClub;
   by team;
proc means;
   var weightloss;
   by team;
run;
```

1.6.5 Class Statement

The `class` statement is used with many procedures to name variables that are to be used as classification variables, or factors. The variables named may be character or numeric variables and will typically contain a relatively small range of discrete values. There may be additional options on the `class` statement depending on the procedure.

1.7 Global Statements

Global statements may occur at any point in a SAS program and remain in effect until reset. The `title` statement is a global statement and provides a title that will appear on each page of printed output *and* each graph until reset. An example would be

```
title 'Analysis of Slimming club data';
```

The text of the title must be enclosed in quotes. Multiple lines of titles can be specified with the `title2` statement for the second line, `title3` for the third line, and so on up to ten. The `title` statement is synonymous with `title1`. Titles are reset by a statement of the following form:

```
title2;
```

This will reset line two of the titles and all lower lines (i.e., title3, etc.), and `title1;` would reset all titles.

Comment statements are global statements in the sense that they can occur anywhere. There are two forms of comment statement. The first form begins with an asterisk and ends with a semicolon—for example,

```
* this is a comment;
```

The second form begins with /* and ends with */:

```
/* this is also a
   comment
*/
```

Comments may appear on the same line as a SAS statement—for example,

```
bmi=weight/height**2; /* Body Mass Index */
```

The enhanced editor colour codes comments green, so it is easier to see if the */ has been omitted from the end or if the semicolon has been omitted in the first form of comment.

The first form of comment is useful for 'commenting out' individual statements, whereas the second is useful for commenting out one or more steps, since it can include semicolons.

1.7.1 Options

The `options` global statement is used to set SAS system options. Most of the system options can be safely left at their default values. Some of those controlling the procedure output that may be considered useful include

- nocenter   aligns the output at the left, rather than centring it on the page (useful when the output line size is wider than the screen)
- nodate   suppresses printing of the date and time on the output
- ps=n sets the output page size to n lines long
- ls=n sets the output line size to n characters

- pageno=*n* sets the page number for the next page of output (e.g., pageno=1 at the beginning of a program that is to be run repeatedly)

Several options can be set on a single options statement, for example,

```
options nodate nocenter pagegno=1;
```

1.8 SAS Graphics

There are a number of ways of producing high-quality graphical output. The three main approaches include

- Graphical options within a statistical procedure
- Statistical graphics procedures
- Traditional graphics procedures

We concentrate on the first two of these.

As of version 9.3, the statistical graphics procedures have been incorporated into the BASE part of SAS, whereas the traditional graphics still require the SAS/GRAPH module to be licensed. By 'traditional' graphics procedures we mean those that have names beginning with 'g', such as gplot, gchart, etc. The statistical graphics procedures have names beginning with 'sg', such as sgplot, sgpanel, sgscatter, and sgrender. The new procedures, particularly sgplot, can produce a wide range of attractive graphs relatively simply and will be all that most users need.

The graphical options that are available within statistical procedures will be dealt with in later chapters as they arise.

1.8.1 *xy* **Plots**—proc sgplot

An *xy* plot is one in which the data are represented in two dimensions defined by the values of two variables. The simplest such plot is a scatter plot and can be illustrated using the bodyfat data set described earlier:

```
proc sgplot data=bodyfat;
  scatter y=pctfat x=age;
run;
```

The syntax is straightforward: A scatter statement is used and the *x* and *y* variables specified explicitly. For different types of plots, a statement other than scatter is used. Table 1.6 shows some *xy* plots that could be generated by sgplot. Most of these will be illustrated in later chapters.

TABLE 1.6

xy Plots Using sgplot

Type of Plot	Plotting Statement
Scatter plot—data values are plotted	`scatter`
Line plot—data values are joined with lines	`series`
Step plot—data values joined with stepped lines	`step`
Needle plot—vertical line joins the value to the x axis	`needle`
Regression plot—a scatter plot with a regression line	`reg`
Locally weighted regression	`loess`
Penalised beta splines	`pbspline`

For line plots and step plots, the points will be plotted in the order in which they occur in the data set, so it is usually necessary to sort the data by the x axis variable first.

A common variant of the *xy* plot distinguishes separate groups in the data by using different plotting symbols and/or different lines. This is done by the `group=var` option:

```
proc sgplot data=bodyfat;
  scatter y=pctfat x=age / group=sex;
run;
```

It is often useful to combine the information from two or more plots by overlaying them. Sgplot does this automatically when more than one plotting statement is included. For example, a plot to compare the fits from linear and locally weighted regression could be produced as follows (locally weighted regression is explained in Chapter 10):

```
proc sgplot data=bodyfat;
  reg y=pctfat x=age;
  loess y=pctfat x=age / nomarkers;
run;
```

The `nomarkers` option is specified on the `loess` statement to prevent the data points being plotted twice as sgplot uses different plotting symbols for each.

The basic *xy* plot can be enhanced with confidence bands (`band`) or lines (`highlow` or `vector`) and reference lines (`refline`). When used in conjunction with some data processing, quite sophisticated plots can be produced.

1.8.2 Summary Plots

Plots of summary statistics are often useful when comparing groups. Sgplot can produce plots of means, frequencies, or sums as a bar plot, line plot, or dot plot. The plot statements are `vbar/hbar` and `vline/hline`, depending on whether vertical or horizontal orientation is desired, and dot. To illustrate, age in the bodyfat data set is first recoded into 10-year bands:

```
data bodyfat;
   set bodyfat;
   decade=int(age/10);
run;

proc sgplot data=bodyfat;
   vline decade / response=pctfat stat=mean limitstat=stddev;
run;
```

Another useful summary plot is the box plot described in Chapter 2, which can be produced with the vbox/hbox statement as follows:

```
proc sgplot data=bodyfat;
   vbox pctfat / category=sex;
run;
```

Proc sgplot is used extensively throughout the book and many more options are illustrated in subsequent chapters.

1.8.3 Panel Plots

Both Proc sgpanel and proc sgscatter produce multiple plots contained within a grid of related panels. Within sgpanel, the grid is defined by the values of variables in the data set with the result that each plot contains a subset of the data. With sgscatter, each plot contains the full set of data and the grid is an arrangement of pairs of variables, with or without common axes. There are examples of both types in later chapters (see the index).

Proc sgrender is for bespoke plots programmed in the graphics template language which underlies the statistical graphics procedures. A detailed description is beyond the scope of this book but a simple example that could be easily adapted is given in Chapter 6.

1.9 ODS—Output Delivery System

The output delivery system began as a means of generating SAS output in different formats. From this beginning as something of a cosmetic luxury, ODS is now an essential part of SAS. There are three reasons for this:

- It produces publication-quality procedure output.
- Output can be saved in SAS data sets.
- ODS graphics are available.

1.9.1 ODS Procedure Output

The first of these might appear cosmetic, but the time and effort saved by using ODS should not be underestimated. Whatever the final form in which the results of an analysis are to be published, ODS simplifies the process by saving the output directly in the appropriate format. Html is the default format in SAS 9.3 and, together with rtf (rich text format), is probably the most commonly used of the formats, although there are many others, including xml, latex, and pdf. Rtf is specifically designed for incorporating into word processors. Each of these output formats is referred to as an 'ODS destination'. The plain text format, which is displayed in the output window, is referred to as the `listing` destination.

The output of one or more procedures can be saved in a particular format by opening the corresponding ODS destination beforehand and closing it afterwards.* The rtf destination is opened by the `ods rtf;` statement and closed by the `ods rtf close;` statement, as in the following example:

```
ods rtf;
proc print data=bodyfat;
proc corr data=bodyfat;
run;
ods rtf close;
```

The output appears in the output window as usual, but the formatted version is also saved in a file named `sasrtf.rtf` in the current directory. As this file will be overwritten the next time the rtf destination is opened, it is usually better to save the output to an explicitly named file with the `file='filename'` option on the `ods rtf` statement.

1.9.1.1 ODS Styles

ODS output can be formatted according to a number of built-in styles. Each output destination has a default style optimised for that destination. The default style for html is called `htmlblue` and that for rtf is called `rtf`. The output in this book has been produced with the `theme` style, so the preceding `ods rtf` statement could be replaced with

```
ods rtf file='c:\amsus\rtfexample.rtf' style=theme;
```

The names of other built-in styles can be listed by submitting

```
proc template;
  list styles;
run;
```

---

* The listing and html destinations can be permanently selected via the preferences menu as shown in Figure 1.3.

Where the final output is to be in black and white, with greyscale fills or shading, the `journal` style is a good choice.

The rtf output may also appear in a results viewer window and this may need to be closed before more rtf output is generated. The results viewer is switched on or off via the `View results as they are gener-`ated option as shown in Figure 1.3. If the output rtf file has been opened with a word processor, it will need to be closed before more output is sent to it.

1.10 Saving Output in SAS Data Sets—`ods output`

Another useful feature of ODS is the ability to save procedure output as SAS data sets. Prior to ODS, SAS procedures could save output—parameter estimates, fitted values, residuals, etc.—in SAS data sets via the `output` statement or other procedure-specific options. As part of the development of ODS, each procedure's output was broken down into a number of tables and any one of these may be saved to a SAS data set by including a statement of the form

```
ods output table = dataset;
```

within the proc step that generates the output.

The names of the tables created by each procedure are given in the details section of the procedure's documentation. To find the variable names, use the SAS explorer window, `proc contents data=dataset;`, or even `proc print` if the data set is small.

1.10.1 ODS Graphics

ODS graphics are a relatively recent development of ODS whereby many of the statistical procedures produce a range of useful plots either automatically or by specifying some optional plots, usually with the `plot` option on the `proc` statement. As with the ODS tables, information on the ODS graphics that are available for each procedure is given in the details section of the procedure's documentation. ODS graphics are switched on and off with the `ods graphics on;` and `ods graphics off;` statements or via the `Use ODS Graphics` option in the preferences window (Figure 1.3). Although ODS graphics are produced even when the listing (normal output) is the only destination open, they will more typically be used with another ODS destination open, so a full example might be

```
ods html;
ods graphics on;
```

```
<one or more procedures that produce graphs>
ods graphics off;
ods html close;
```

We could also have used `ods rtf;`, but there is a difference. With rtf, the graphs are included in the rtf document along with the tables. With html, the graphs are each in a separate file, even though they appear in the same results viewer window. The directories that html output and the graphs are stored in can be specified by the `path=` and `gpath=` options on the `ods html` statement. The default image file type of the graphs varies according to the ODS destination but GIF, JPEG, and PNG are alternatives that can be set via the `outputfmt=` option on the `ods graphics` statement. In the example, we could use the following to store JPEG format graphs in the named directory:

```
ods html gpath='c:\amsus\figures';
ods graphics on / outputfmt =jpeg;
```

Since the ODS graphics are sent to the currently open ODS destinations, they are also formatted with the same style as the tabular output. Any graphs produced independently using the new 'statistical' graphics procedures will also use the same style.

NOTE: *producing ODS graphics leads to longer processing times.* Those with large data sets to analyse may need to be selective in their use. In version 9.3 of SAS, ODS graphics are enabled by default; see Figure 1.3 to view how to deselect this option.

It is important to bear in mind that the output produced by ODS for the rtf destination is tailored to the current page setup and this should, therefore, match that of the document for which the output is intended. Whilst this can easily be done from the page setup menu (`File, Page Setup`), it can also be done via the `options` statement as in the following example:

```
options papersize=a4 orientation=portrait
    bottommargin=1in topmargin=1in
    leftmargin=1in rightmargin=1in;
```

The default for `papersize` is `letter`. Margins can also be specified in centimetres—for example, `bottommargin=2.5cm`.

When output is to be incorporated in a word processor document, the following options and settings can be useful:

`options nodate nonumber;`	Switches off date and page numbers
`ods noproctitle;`	Omits the procedure name from the output
`ods rtf bodytitle;`	Titles are placed in document body rather than the header
`title;`	Sets null titles

1.11 Enhancing Output

1.11.1 Variable Labels

Whereas variable *names* are limited to 32 characters with no spaces, variable *labels* can contain spaces and can be much longer—up to 256 characters. If a variable has been given a label, then this can be used in the output. Whether or not labels are used in the output is controlled by the `option label;` and `option nolabel;` statements. The default is on.

The `label` statement is used to give variables a label and has the form of

```
label variable ='variable label';
```

For example,

```
label pctfat='Fat as a % of body mass';
```

If the `label` statement is used in a `data` step, the label is permanently associated with the variable, whereas if it is used in a `proc` step, the label is only used for the output from that procedure. To remove a variable's label, include a statement of the form `label sex=' ';` in the data or proc step.

1.11.2 Value Labels—SAS Formats

SAS formats are used to give variable values more meaningful labels. `Proc format` is used to create the format and the `format` statement is used to associate the format with a variable. For example,

```
proc format;
  value $sex 'M'='Male' 'F'='Female';
run;
proc sgplot data=bodyfat;
  scatter y=pctfat x=age /group=sex;
  format sex $sex.;
  label pctfat='Fat as % of body mass';
run;
```

The `value` statement within `proc format` has the general form of

```
value format-name value1='label1' value2='label2';
```

There may be as many `value='label'` pairs as required. Where the values are character values, as in the example, they must be in quotes and the format name must begin with a $. Character values are case sensitive, so `'m'='Male'` would not have worked in the preceding example as all the values of `sex` are uppercase.

Format names are like variable names but should not end in a number. Note that in the `format` statement, the format name ends in a period but that it does not in the `value` statement. If, instead of the variable `sex`, the `bodyfat` data set contained a numeric variable called `gender`, the `value` and `format` statements might be

```
value gender 1='Male' 2='Female';
...
format gender gender.;
```

More than one variable can be associated with the same format. If a number of variables were coded 0 and 1, meaning 'no' and 'yes', the `value` and `format` statements might be

```
value yn10f 0='No' 1='Yes';
...
format q1-q20 yn10f.;
```

1.12 SAS Macros

SAS macros are general purpose SAS programs—'general purpose' in the sense that they can be run repeatedly using different data sets, variables, or settings. Of course, any SAS program can be adapted to use another data set and other variables by editing it and changing the names of the data sets and variables throughout. The advantage of a macro is that the user supplies the new names once and SAS does all the necessary substitution. A macro may also be a long and complicated program where manual substitution of new data set and variable names would be tedious and error prone.

It is useful to know how to use macros, even if one has no inclination to write any. A simple example will help to illustrate how they work. First, we write a macro definition:

```
%macro xyplot(data=,x=,y=);
proc sgplot data=&data;
   scatter y=&y x=&x;
run;
%mend plotxy;
```

This is a macro to plot two variables. The definition begins with a `%macro` statement, which declares the name of the macro, `xyplot`, and then in parentheses the values it needs when it is used. These are referred to as the macro's parameters. The body of the macro follows and the `%mend` statement signals the end of the macro definition. The body of the macro consists of a proc sgplot step, but with `&data`, `&y`, and `&x` in place of the data set and variable names,

```
options mprint;
```

will print in the log the statements that the macro creates when it is run. Before running the macro, we must submit the macro definition—that is, select and submit the whole macro definition. If the macro definition is stored in a file, this can be done by including it with, for example, `%inc 'c:\amsus\macros\xyplot.sas';`

The macro is run as follows:

```
%xyplot (data=bodyfat,x=age,y=pctfat);
```

and the log shows how the values provided have been substituted into the body of the macro:

```
MPRINT(XYPLOT): proc sgplot data=bodyfat;
MPRINT(XYPLOT): scatter y=pctfat x=age;
MPRINT(XYPLOT): run;
```

Macro parameters have two different forms. The form already illustrated is the so-called keyword form. The alternative is positional form. If the macro had been defined as

```
%macro xyplot (data,x,y);
proc gplot data=&data;
  plot &y*&x;
run;
%mend plotxy;
```

then it would have to be run with

```
%xyplot(bodyfat,age,pctfat);
```

A few macros that we have written will be used in later chapters. There are also macros supplied by SAS, and others are available on the SAS website and elsewhere. Often users will have written macros to perform a type of analysis that is not yet available in SAS. The keyword form of parameters is the more common, partly because the parameters can be given default values. A macro will usually come with some documentation on how to use it: what the parameters are, which form they take, and what the default values are.

1.13 Some Tips for Preventing and Correcting Errors

When writing programs:

- Have one statement per line, where possible.
- End each step with a run statement.
- Indent each statement within a step (i.e., each statement between the data or proc statement and the run statement) by a couple of spaces. This is automated in the enhanced editor.
- Give the full path name for raw data files on the infile statement.

Before submitting a program:

- Check that each statement ends with a semicolon.
- Check that all opening and closing quotes match.

Use the enhanced editor colour coding to double check.

- Check any statement that does not begin with a keyword (blue or navy blue) or a variable name (black).
- Large blocks of purple may indicate a missing quotation mark.
- Large areas of green may indicate a missing */ from a comment.

'Collapse' the program to check its overall structure. Hold down the Ctrl and Alt keys and press the numeric keypad minus key. Only the data, proc statements and global statements should be visible. To expand the program, press the numeric keypad plus key while holding down Ctrl and Alt.

After running a program:

- Examine the SAS log for warning and error messages.
- Check for the message 'SAS went to a new line when INPUT statement reached past the end of a line' when using list input.
- Verify that the number of observations and variables read in is correct.
- When reading raw data, check the number of lines read and the maximum and minimum line lengths reported.
- Print out small data sets to ensure that they have been read correctly.

If there is an error message for a statement that appears to be correct, check whether the semicolon was omitted from the previous statement.

The message that a variable is 'uninitialised' or 'not found' usually means that it has been misspelled. If not, it might have been included in a `drop` statement or left out of a `keep` statement.

To correct a missing quote, submit: `'; run;` or `"; run;` and then correct the program and resubmit it.

2

Statistics and Measurement in Medicine

2.1 Introduction

> Statistics is a general intellectual method that applies wherever data, variation, and chance appear. It is a fundamental method because data, variation, and chance are omnipresent in modern life. It is an independent discipline with its own core ideas, rather than, for example, a branch of mathematics.... Statistics offers general, fundamental, and independent ways of thinking. (Moore 1998)

Quintessentially, statistics is about solving problems: Data (measurements or observations) relevant to these problems are collected, and statistical analyses are used to provide useful answers. But the path from data collection to analysis and interpretation is often not straightforward. Most real-life applications of statistical methodology have one or more nonstandard features, meaning in practice that there are few routine statistical questions, although there are questionable statistical routines. Many statistical pitfalls lie in wait for the unwary. Indeed, statistics is perhaps more open to misuse than most other subjects, particularly by the nonstatistician with access to powerful statistical software. The misleading average, the graph with 'fiddled axes', the inappropriate p-value, and the linear regression fitted to nonlinear data are just four examples of horror stories that are part of statistical folklore.

Medical statistics is simply the application of the science of statistics in medical studies and nowadays medical statistics is ubiquitous throughout medicine from the analysis of data from *clinical trials* (see Chapter 3) to the investigation of *high-dimensional data* (see Everitt 2011) arising from imaging research (see Glasbey and Horgan 1996) and the application of microarray technology in genetics (see Kafadar 2011). But how and when did medical statistics begin?

2.2 A Brief History of Medical Statistics

The first attempts at 'medical statistics' might perhaps be considered the early efforts to keep track of births and deaths through church records of weddings, christenings, and burials. But, more ambitious statistical procedures than simple counting would have been largely unwelcome to physicians until well into the seventeenth century simply because they might have raised the unthinkable spectre of questioning the invulnerability most of them still claimed. Medical practices at the time were largely based on uncritical reliance on past experience, *post hoc, ergo propter hoc* reasoning, and veneration of the 'truth' as proclaimed by authoritative figures such as Galen (130–200), a Greek physician whose influence dominated medicine for many centuries. Such attitudes largely stifled any interest in experimentation or proper scientific investigation or explanation of medical phenomena. Even the few clinicians who did strive to increase their knowledge by close observation or simple experiment often interpreted their findings in the light of the currently accepted dogma.

But by the late seventeenth and early eighteenth centuries, medicine had begun its slow progress from a sort of mystical certainty to a scientifically more acceptable uncertainty about many of its procedures. The taking of systematic observations and carrying out of experiments became more widespread. For example, John Graunt (1620–1674), the son of a London draper, published in 1662 his *Natural and Political Observations Made upon the Bills of Mortality* and derived the first ever life table. Graunt was what might today be termed a *vital statistician:* He examined the risk inherent in the process of birth, marriage, and death and used bills of mortality (weekly reports on the numbers and causes of death in an area) to compare one disease with another and one year with another by calculating mortality statistics. Graunt's work and ideas had considerable influence and bills of mortality were also introduced in Paris and other cities in Europe.

Early experimental work in medicine is illustrated by the oft quoted example of James Lind's (1716–1794) study undertaken on board the ship the *Salisbury* in 1747. Lind assessed several different possible treatments for scurvy by giving each to a different pair of sailors with the disease. He observed that the two men given oranges and lemons made the most dramatic recovery, although it was another 40 years before the Admiralty were convinced enough by Lind's finding to issue lemon juice to members of the British Navy.

The 1700s also saw the first appearance of a procedure that looks remarkably similar to a modern day significance test—specifically, a sign test. This arose from John Arbuthnot's (1667–1735) attempt to argue the case for divine providence in the stability of the ratio of number of men to women. Arbuthnot maintained that the guiding hand of a divine being was to be discerned in the nearly constant ratio of male to female christenings recorded annually in London over the years 1629–1710. The data presented by Arbuthnot showed that in each of the 82 years in this period, the annual number of male christenings had been consistently higher than the number of female christenings, but never very much higher. He then essentially tested a null hypothesis of 'chance' determination of sex at birth against an alternative of divine providence by calculating, under the assumption that the null hypothesis is true, a probability defined by reference to the observed data. Arbuthnot's representation of chance in this context was the toss of a fair two-sided die, in which case the distribution of births would be

$$\left(\frac{1}{2} + \frac{1}{2}\right)^{82}$$

Therefore, the observed excess of male christenings on each of 82 occasions had an extremely small probability, thus providing support for the divine providence hypothesis.

Arbuthnot offered an explanation for the greater supply of males as a wise economy of nature, as the males are more subject to accidents and diseases, having to seek their food and deal with danger. Therefore, to repair the loss, provident nature brings forth more males. The near equality of the sexes is designed so that every male may have a female of the same country and of suitable age.

Other mathematical developments in the eighteenth century that were of special relevance for medical statistics included Daniel Bernoulli's (1700–1782) development of the normal approximation to the binomial distribution. This was also used in studies of the stability of the sex ratio at birth.

The power of medical statistics in pursuing reform is illustrated by the work of Florence Nightingale (1820–1907). In her efforts to improve the squalid hospital conditions in Turkey during the Crimean War and in her subsequent campaigns to improve the health and living conditions of the British Army, the sanitary conditions and administration of hospitals, and the nursing profession, Florence Nightingale was not unlike many other Victorian reformers. But in one important respect she was very different, since she marshalled massive amounts of data and carefully arranged, tabulated, graphed, and presented this material to ministers, viceroys, and others, to convince them of the justice of her case. No other major national cause had previously been championed through the presentation of sound statistical data and those who opposed Florence Nightingale's reforms went down to defeat because her data were unanswerable; their publication led to an outcry.

Another telling example of how careful arrangement of data was used in the nineteenth century to save lives is provided by the work of the epidemiologist John Snow (1813–1858). After an outbreak of cholera in central London in September 1854, Snow used data collected by the General Register Office and plotted the location of deaths on a map of the area and also showed the location of the area's 11 water pumps. The resulting map is shown in Figure 2.1 (deaths are marked by dots and water pumps by crosses). Examining the scatter over the surface of the map, Snow observed that nearly all the cholera deaths were among those who lived near the Broad Street pump.

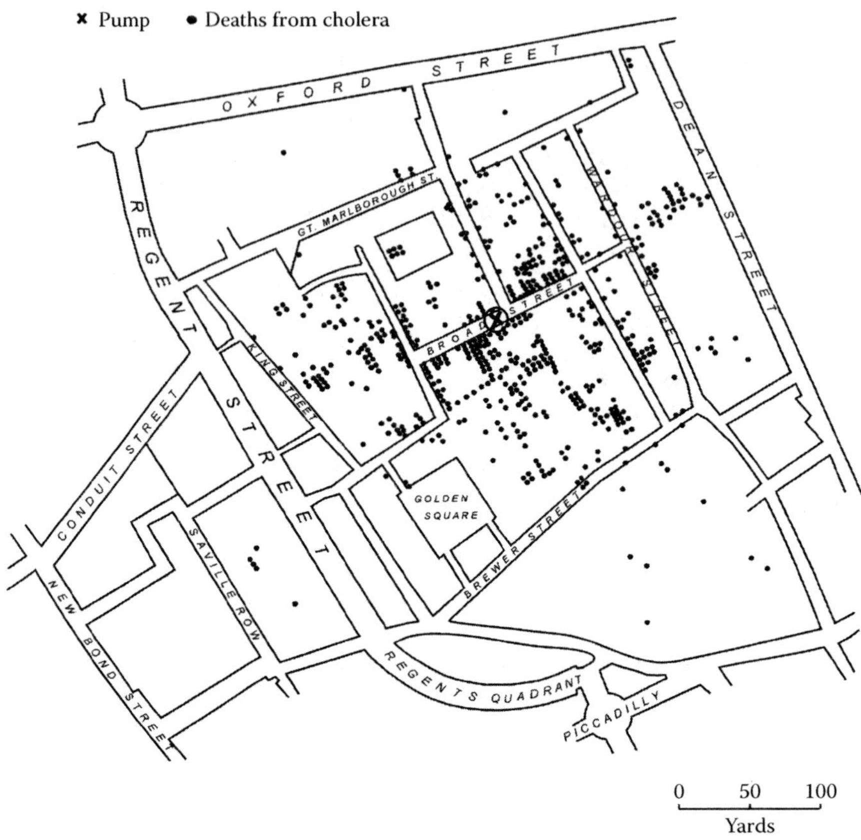

FIGURE 2.1
A map constructed by John Snow in 1854 showing that most of the deaths due to cholera clustered around the Broad Street water pump. (From Dunn, G. 2004. *Statistical Evaluation of Measurement Errors*. London: Arnold.)

But before claiming that he had discovered a possible causal connection, Snow made a more detailed investigation of the deaths that had occurred near some other pump. He visited the families of ten of the deceased and found that five of them, because they preferred its taste, regularly sent for water from the Broad Street pump. Three others were children who attended a school near the Broad Street pump. One other finding that initially confused Snow was that there were no deaths amongst workers in a brewery close to the Broad Street pump, a confusion that was quickly resolved when it became apparent that the workers drank only beer, never water! Snow's findings were sufficiently compelling to persuade the authorities to remove the handle of the Broad Street pump and, in days, the neighbourhood epidemic that had taken more than 500 lives had ended.

Later in the nineteenth century and in the early twentieth century, the work of people like Sir Francis Galton (1822–1911), Wilhelm Lexis (1837–1914) and, in particular, Karl Pearson (1857–1936) began to change the emphasis in statistics from the descriptive to the mathematical. The concept of correlation and its measurement by a correlation coefficient was introduced. Statistical inference began to develop and enter most areas of scientific investigation, including medical research. And, in 1909, Ronald Aylmer Fisher (later, Sir Ronald Fisher; 1890–1962) entered Cambridge to study mathematics, the first step to becoming the most influential statistician of the twentieth century. Fisher developed *maximum likelihood estimation,* worked on evolutionary theory, made massive contributions to genetics, and invented the *analysis of variance* (ANOVA; see Chapter 6).

But perhaps Fisher's most important contribution to medical statistics was his introduction of *randomisation* as a principle in the design of certain experiments. In Fisher's case the experiments were in agriculture and were concerned with which fertilisers led to the greatest crop yields. Fisher divided agricultural areas into plots and randomly assigned the plots to different experimental fertilisers. But the principle was soon adopted in medicine in studies to compare competing therapies for a particular condition, leading, of course, to the *randomised clinical trial* (RCT) described by Sir David Cox as 'the most important contribution of twentieth century statistics'. The first properly performed RCT is now generally acknowledged to be that carried out in 1948 by another giant of twentieth century medical statistics, Sir Austin Bradford Hill (1897–1991), who investigated the use of streptomycin in the treatment of pulmonary tuberculosis. Nowadays, over 8,000 RCTs are undertaken annually. Clinical trials are covered in detail in the next chapter.

At about the time that Bradford Hill was busy with the first randomised clinical trial, another development was taking place that by revolutionising man's ability to calculate was to have a dramatic effect on the science of statistics and the work of statisticians. The computer age was about to begin, although it would be some years before statisticians were entirely relieved of the burden of undertaking large amounts of laborious arithmetic on some precomputer calculator. But in the 1960s the first statistical software packages, which made the application of many complex statistical procedures easy and routine, began to appear.

The influence of increasing, inexpensive computing power on statistics continues to this day and, over the last 20 years, its almost universal availability has meant that research workers in statistics in general, and medical statistics in particular, no longer have to keep one eye on the computational difficulties when developing new methods of analysis. The result has been the introduction of many exciting and powerful new statistical methods, many of which are of great importance in medical statistics. Notable examples include

- Cox's regression (see Chapter 16)
- Logistic regression (see Chapter 9)

- Multiple imputation (see Chapter 18)
- Generalised estimating equations (see Chapter 14)

In addition, Bayesian methods (see Chapter 17), at one time little more than an intellectual curiosity without practical implications because of their associated computational requirements, can now be applied relatively routinely.

2.3 Measurement in Medicine

> Stone-dead has no fellow, and preeminent therefore stands the number of patients who die. No statistician, so far as I know, has in this respect accused the physician of an over-reliance upon the clinical impression. (Bradford Hill 1962)

The basic material, the data that are the foundation of all medical investigations, consists of the measurements and observations that are made on the patients or subjects of interest. Measurements are central to clinical practice and medical and health research and form the basis of diagnosis, prognosis, and evaluation of the results of medical interventions (deVet et al. 2011). Clearly, such measurements need to be objective, precise, and reproducible for reasons nicely summarised by the following extract from Fleiss (1999):

> The most elegant design of a clinical study will not overcome the damage caused by unreliable or imprecise measurement. The requirement that one's data be of high quality is at least as important a component of a proper study design as the requirement for randomization, double blinding, controlling where necessary for prognostic factors, and so on. Larger sample sizes than otherwise necessary, biased estimates, and even biased samples are some of the untoward consequences of unreliable measurements that can be demonstrated.

As Bradford Hill points out in the quotation which began this section, the death of a patient is the most objective outcome observation that might be made in a study. Fortunately, however, most medical investigations are concerned with diseases that are not lethal and where the assessment of the patient's condition or outcome depends on a measure or observation that is less drastic than simply dead or alive. The appropriate measurements and observations that are needed will depend on the particular area of investigation and could range from measurements of blood pressure, weight, and temperature to a rating of anxiety or depression or even simply a classification as to 'improved' or 'not improved' in respect of some course of treatment. The characteristics of the observations will, in part at least, help to determine the appropriate methods of statistical analysis.

Measurements differ according to the degree of precision they give; for example, saying that an individual's serum uric acid level is high is not as precise as saying that the individual has 8.5 mg/100 mm of serum uric acid. The comment that a woman is obese is less precise than saying that she is 1.6 m tall and weighs 95 kg. Certain patient characteristics will be more amenable to precise measurement than others; for example, given an accurate thermometer, a patient's temperature can be measured with great precision. Assessing the degree of pain of a patient suffering from migraine is a far more difficult task. It is time to say a little about scales of measurement.

2.3.1 Scales of Measurement

Four levels of measurement scales are generally distinguished.

2.3.1.1 Nominal or Categorical Measurements

Nominal measurements allow patients to be classified with respect to some characteristic. Examples of such measurements are marital status, sex, and blood group. The following are properties of a nominal scale:

- The categories are mutually exclusive (an individual can belong to only one category).
- The categories have no logical order—numbers may be assigned to categories but merely as convenient labels.

2.3.1.2 Ordinal Scale Measurements

The next level of measurement is the ordinal scale. This scale has one additional property over those of a nominal scale—a logical ordering of the categories. With such measurements, the numbers assigned to the categories indicate the amount of a characteristic possessed. A psychiatrist may, for example, grade patients on an anxiety scale as 'not anxious', 'mildly anxious', 'moderately anxious', or 'severely anxious' and use the numbers 0, 1, 2, and 3 to label the categories, with lower numbers indicating less anxiety.

The psychiatrist cannot infer, however, that the difference in anxiety between patients with scores of, say, 0 and 1 is the same as the difference between patients assigned scores of 2 and 3. The scores on an ordinal scale, however, do allow patients to be ranked with respect to the characteristic being assessed.

The following are the properties of an ordinal scale:

- The categories are mutually exclusive.
- The categories have some logical order.
- The categories are scaled according to the amount of a particular characteristic that they indicate.

2.3.1.3 Interval Scales

The third level of measurement is the interval scale. Such scales possess all the properties of an ordinal scale plus the additional property that equal differences between category levels, on any part of the scale, reflect equal differences in the characteristic being measured. An example of such a scale is temperature on the Celsius (C) or Fahrenheit (F) scale; the difference between temperatures of 80°F and 90°F represents the same difference in heat as that between temperatures of 30° and 40° on the Fahrenheit scale. An important point to make about interval scales is that the zero point is simply another point on the scale; it does not represent the starting point of the scale or the total absence of the characteristic being measured. The properties of an interval scale are as follows:

- The categories are mutually exclusive.
- The categories have a logical order.
- The categories are scaled according to the amount of the characteristic that they indicate.
- Equal differences in the characteristic are represented by equal differences in the numbers assigned to the categories.
- The zero point is completely arbitrary.

2.3.1.4 Ratio Scales

The final level of measurement is the ratio scale. This type of scale has one property in addition to those listed for interval scales—namely, the possession of a true zero point that represents the absence of the characteristic being measured. Consequently, statements can be made about both the differences on the scale and the ratio of points on the scale. An example is weight, where not only is the difference between 100 and 50 kg the same as that between 75 and 25 kg, but an object weighing 100 kg can also be said to be twice as heavy as one weighing 50 kg. This is not true of, say, temperature on the Celsius or Fahrenheit scales, where a reading of 100° on either scale does not represent twice the warmth of a temperature of 50°. If, however, two temperatures are measured on the Kelvin scale, which does have a true zero point (absolute zero or −273°C), then statements about the ratio of the two temperatures can be made.

The properties of a ratio scale are the following:

- The categories are mutually exclusive.
- The data categories have a logical order.
- The categories are scaled according to the amount of the characteristic that they possess.

- Equal differences in the characteristic being measured are represented by equal differences in the numbers assigned to the categories.

- The zero point represents an absence of the characteristic being measured.

In many statistical textbooks, discussion of different types of measurements is often followed by recommendations as to which statistical techniques are suitable for each type. For example, analyses on nominal data should be limited to summary statistics such as the number of cases, the mode, etc., and for ordinal data, means and standard deviations are said not to be suitable; Andersen (1990) gives a nice illustration of why this is the case. But Velleman and Wilkinson (1993) make the important point that restricting the choice of statistical methods in this way may be a dangerous practice for data analysis. In essence, the measurement taxonomy described is often too strict to apply to real-world data. This is not the place for a detailed discussion of measurement, but we think a fairly pragmatic approach to such problems is advisable. For example, we would not agonise too long over applying statistical techniques that strictly require interval scale data to variables such as measures of depression or anxiety, although they are essentially ordinal.

2.4 Assessing Bias and Reliability of Measurements

In all medical studies, it is important to ensure that the data collected are as accurate as possible and that measurement error is absent or very small. In assessing the accuracy of any particular measuring 'instrument' (where this term is used for any type of measurement situation from, say, using a thermometer to assessing the presence or absence of some particular property in a patient) it is usual to distinguish between the *reliability* of the data collected and their *validity*. Reliability is essentially the degree to which the measurement provided by the measuring instrument is free from measurement error, and validity is the extent to which a measurement provides a true assessment of the characteristic which it purports to measure. There are several comprehensive accounts that deal with the reliability and validity of measurements— for example, Fleiss (1999), Dunn (2004), and de Vet et al. (2011).

The question of measurement validity is complex and we will not deal with it here; readers can find a detailed discussion of validity in the three references given in the previous paragraph. But we will now say a little about reliability where the issues usually involve whether different observers making the same measurement agree (*inter-rater reliability*) or whether two measurements of a patient characteristic that does not change with time made at different times by the same observer agree (*intra-rater reliability*). In the following subsections we give a relatively brief account of determining the reliability of different types of measurements primarily via some numerical examples. We begin in the next subsection with an example of assessing the reliability and bias of a simple categorical 'measurement' with just two categories (i.e., a *binary variable*) and then, in Subsection 2.4.2, we consider an example that involves quantitative measurements.

2.4.1 Assessing Reliability and Bias for Binary and Other Categorical Observations

Landis and Koch (1977) and Fleiss (1999) suggest that, when studying the variability of observer ratings, two components of possible lack of accuracy must be distinguished. The first is *interobserver bias*, which will be reflected in differences in the marginal distributions of the observation for each of the observers. The second is *observer disagreement*, which is indicated by how observers classify individual subjects into the same category on the measurement scale. We will illustrate how both interobserver bias and observer disagreement can be investigated using the data shown in Table 2.1 which arise from histological assessments of 118 biopsy slides made by seven

TABLE 2.1

Histology Assessment Made by Seven
Pathologists on the Presence or Absence
of Cancer of the Cervix

A	B	C	D	E	F	G	Frequency
1	1	1	1	1	1	1	16
1	1	1	1	1	0	1	10
1	1	1	0	1	1	1	5
1	1	0	1	1	1	1	3
1	1	1	0	1	0	1	13
1	1	0	1	1	0	1	2
1	1	0	0	1	1	1	1
1	1	0	1	0	0	1	1
1	1	0	0	1	0	1	7
1	0	1	0	1	0	1	1
1	1	0	0	1	0	0	2
1	1	0	0	0	0	1	1
0	1	0	0	1	0	1	5
1	1	0	0	0	0	0	2
0	1	0	0	1	0	0	4
0	1	0	0	0	0	1	1
1	0	0	0	0	0	0	2
0	1	0	0	0	0	0	6
0	0	0	0	1	0	0	2
0	0	0	0	0	0	0	34

independent pathologists of the presence (1) or absence (0) of cancer of the cervix (the data are given in Dunn 2004).

The proportions of the 118 slides perceived to be displaying carcinoma by each of the seven pathologists can be found using the following SAS code:

```
data pathologists;
infile 'c:\AMSUS\data\pathologists.dat';
 input A B C D E F G;
run;
proc means data=pathologists;
 var a--g;
run;
```

The 118 ratings made by the seven pathologists are in the file `patholo-gists.dat` represented by seven variables, labelled A to G and coded zero or one. These are read in using list input. As a positive rating is coded 1, the proportions rated positive by each of the pathologists can be calculated using `proc means`. The default output from `proc means` is as shown, but a wide range of other descriptive statistics is also available.

The calculated proportions are the following:

Variable	N	Mean	Std Dev	Minimum	Maximum
A	118	0.5593220	0.4985856	0	1.0000000
B	118	0.6694915	0.4724022	0	1.0000000
C	118	0.3813559	0.4877910	0	1.0000000
D	118	0.2711864	0.4464679	0	1.0000000
E	118	0.6016949	0.4916366	0	1.0000000
F	118	0.2118644	0.4103718	0	1.0000000
G	118	0.5593220	0.4985856	0	1.0000000

Pathologists A, B, E, and G appear to have reasonably similar marginal proportions (average 0.597) and pathologists C, D, and F also have reasonably similar proportions, although their average proportion, 0.288, is considerably different from that of the other group. We can formally test the marginal homogeneity of the seven pathologists with Cochran's Q-test, calculated as follows:

$$Q = \frac{r(r-1)\sum_{j=1}^{r}(y_{.j} - y_{..}/r)^2}{ry_{..} - \sum_{i=1}^{n} y_{i.}^2} \tag{2.1}$$

where
$n = 118$ is the number of slides
$r = 7$ is the number of pathologists
y_{ij} equals 1 if the ith slide is rated by the jth pathologist as showing the presence of carcinoma and 0 otherwise

$y_{i.}$ is the total number of pathologists who judge the ith slide as showing the presence of carcinoma

$y_{.j}$ is the total number of slides the jth pathologist judges to show the presence of carcinoma

$y_{..}$ is the total number of slides judged to show the presence of carcinoma.

If the null hypothesis of marginal homogeneity is true (i.e., all seven pathologists have an equal probability of judging that a slide in the population of such slides shows the presence of carcinoma and there is, consequently, no interobserver bias), then for large samples, Q will be approximately distributed as a chi-square with $r - 1$ degrees of freedom.

Cochran's Q is one of the statistics options available in `proc freq` for square symmetric tables via the `agree` option. In most cases this will be for a two-way table. To obtain the value of Q for all seven pathologists together, we specify the seven-way table formed by crossing all seven of the variables. As we are only interested in the value of Q and not the contents of this table itself, we use the `noprint` option to suppress printing of the table:

```
proc freq data=pathologists;
 tables a*b*c*d*e*f*g /noprint agree;
run;
```

The resulting Cochran's Q-test value is

Cochran's Q, for A by B by C by D by E by F by G	
Statistic (Q)	181.5947
DF	6
Pr > Q	<.0001

The test statistic is highly significant, so the hypothesis of marginal homogeneity for the seven pathologists is rejected. Having established that there are highly significant differences between the seven pathologists in their probabilities of identifying carcinoma from the biopsy slides, we can move on to look at differences between pairs of pathologists. (An alternative would be to examine differences in a priori contrasts between groups of pathologists, but here there is no justification for such an approach.) Table 2.2 sets out a standard notation for the general 2×2 contingency table for the comparison of a binary variable made by each of two raters.

In the case of just two raters ($r = 2$ in Equation 2.1), Cochran's Q-test is equivalent to the well-known McNemar test for the comparison of two correlated proportions (McNemar 1947); using the notation in Table 2.2, the relevant test statistic can be written as

$$X^2 = \frac{(n_{01} - n_{10})^2}{n_{01} + n_{10}} \tag{2.2}$$

TABLE 2.2

Two-Way Contingency Table for Assessment of Bias and Agreement between Two Binary Measurements Giving Observed Counts and Corresponding Proportions

		Rater 2	Category		
		0	1	Total	
Rater 1	0	$n_{00}(p_{00})$	$n_{01}(p_{01})$	$n_{0.}$	$p_{0.} = n_{0.}/n$
Category	1	$n_{10}(p_{10})$	$n^{11}(p_{11})$	$n_{1.}$	$p_{1.} = n_{1.}/n$
	Total	$n_{.0}$	$n_{.1}$	n	
		$p_{.0} = n_{.0}/n$	$p_{.1} = n_{.1}/n$		

Under the null hypothesis of marginal homogeneity, X^2 will have an asymptotic chi-squared distribution with a single degree of freedom. We can find the X^2 values and the associated p-values for each of the possible 21 paired comparisons amongst the seven pathologists in our example using the McNemar test (available as an ODS table, called `McNemarsTest`) when the `agree` option is specified on the `tables` statement. The ODS output statement is used to save the table in the SAS data set mcn. To save having to type all 21 pairs of variables out explicitly, variable lists are used in the `table` statement. Thus, `a*(b--g)` is equivalent to `a*b a*c a*d a*e a*f a*g`. The `noprint` option is used to suppress printing of the 21 separate tables.

```
ods output McNemarsTest=mcn;
proc freq data=pathologists;
   tables a*(b--g)
          b*(c--g)
        c*(d--g)
        d*(e--g)
        e*(f--g)
        f*g
   / agree noprint;
run;

proc transpose data=mcn out=mcn2;
 var nvalue1;
 id name1;
idlabel label1;
by table;
run;
proc sort data=mcn2; by p_mcnem; run;
proc print label;
 format p_mcnem pvalue6.4;
run;
```

The mcn data set contains three observations for each of the tables: one each for the test statistic, its degrees of freedom (DF), and *p*-value, along with variables indicating which is which (`name1` and `label1`) and the table to which they relate. We can use `proc transpose` to restructure the data set so that the three values are part of a single observation. `Proc transpose` swaps around the rows and columns of a data set so that the variables become observations and vice versa. It can also do this separately for groups of observations using a by group.

Here we want the three values in separate observations for each table to become three variables in a single observation. The variable that contains these values, `nValue1`, is specified on the `var` statement. (The variable called `cValue1` is a character representation of the same value.) The `id` and `idlabel` statements specify variables in the input data set that are used to provide names and labels for the transposed values. The default names would be `col1`, `col2`, and `col3`. The `out` option on the `proc` statement names the transposed data set.

The resulting data set is then sorted in ascending order of p-value and printed. By convention, p-values that would otherwise appear as 0.0000 are printed as <.0001 instead; this is achieved by using the `pvalue` format, which is one of the many formats built into SAS. The numbers specify the field with and number of decimal places (i.e., a field width of 6 with four decimal places). The `label` option on the `proc print` statement uses the variable labels as column headers instead of the variable names. The output is shown in Table 2.3.

As we have carried out 21 tests, we should adjust the nominal significance level of, say, 0.05 in some way to take account of the multiple tests. The simplest way to do this is to use the *Bonferroni adjustment* (see Fleiss 1999), which is to divide the nominal significance level by the number of comparisons being made; in this case, this leads to a revised significance level of 0.05/21 = 0.0024 with a corresponding critical value for a single degree of freedom chi-squared of about 9.5. Examining the critical values and significance levels in Table 2.3, we see that many of the comparisons between pairs of pathologists remain significant even when using the Bonferroni adjusted significance level. And the results in Table 2.3 strongly suggest that the pathologists make up two distinct groups: [A, B, E, and G] and [C, D, and F], as suggested previously by their different average proportion values. Perhaps the pathologists in each group have had different levels of training or experience?

In the original study involving the seven pathologists, they each classified the 118 biopsy slides into one of the following five categories based on the most involved lesion:

- Category 1: negative
- Category 2: a typical squamous hyperplasia
- Category 3: carcinoma in situ
- Category 4: squamous carcinoma with early stromal invasion
- Category 5: invasive carcinoma

TABLE 2.3

Results of McNemar's Test on All 21 Pairs of Pathologists

Obs	Table	NAME OF FORMER VARIABLE	Statistic (S)	DF	Pr > S
1	Table B * F	nValue1	54.000000	1.000000	<.0001
2	Table B * D	nValue1	47.000000	1.000000	<.0001
3	Table E * F	nValue1	46.000000	1.000000	<.0001
4	Table A * F	nValue1	41.000000	1.000000	<.0001
5	Table F * G	nValue1	41.000000	1.000000	<.0001
6	Table D * E	nValue1	37.097561	1.000000	<.0001
7	Table A * D	nValue1	34.000000	1.000000	<.0001
8	Table D * G	nValue1	34.000000	1.000000	<.0001
9	Table B * C	nValue1	32.111111	1.000000	<.0001
10	Table C * E	nValue1	26.000000	1.000000	<.0001
11	Table A * C	nValue1	21.000000	1.000000	<.0001
12	Table C * G	nValue1	21.000000	1.000000	<.0001
13	Table C * F	nValue1	14.285714	1.000000	0.0002
14	Table B * G	nValue1	11.266667	1.000000	0.0008
15	Table A * B	nValue1	8.894737	1.000000	0.0029
16	Table C * D	nValue1	6.760000	1.000000	0.0093
17	Table B * E	nValue1	4.571429	1.000000	0.0325
18	Table D * F	nValue1	2.578947	1.000000	0.1083
19	Table E * G	nValue1	2.272727	1.000000	0.1317
20	Table A * E	nValue1	1.470588	1.000000	0.2253
21	Table A * G	nValue1	0	1.000000	1.0000

(In the example analysed previously, the two categories were the result of combining categories 1 and 2 for the 'carcinoma absence' rating and categories 3, 4, and 5 for the 'carcinoma present' rating.)

Here we look at the results for just two of the pathologists, as given in Table 2.4. How do we assess the agreement between the two pathologists from this table? Intuitively, we might be tempted to use the simple proportion of agreement found as $(22 + 7 + 36 + 7 + 3)/118 = 0.064$. But this ignores the *chance agreement* that would result if the two pathologists simply rated according to their respective marginal proportions without regard to the nature of the slides. Aware of this problem, Cohen (1960) introduced a chance-corrected agreement index now known as Cohen's kappa (κ) and given by

$$\kappa = \frac{P_0 - P_c}{1 - P_c} \qquad (2.3)$$

where P_0 is the observed proportion of agreement and P_c is the chance agreement based on the observed marginal values of the two raters.

TABLE 2.4

Observed Frequencies of Biopsy Slides Classified by Two Pathologists according to the Most Involved Lesion of Uterine Cervix

	Category	1	2	3	4	5	Total
				Pathologist 2			
	1	22	2	2	0	0	26
Pathologist 1	2	5	7	14	0	0	26
	3	0	2	36	0	0	38
	4	0	1	14	7	0	22
	5	0	0	3	0	3	6
	Total	27	12	69	7	3	118

We see that κ is simply the ratio of the difference in observed and chance agreement to the maximum possible excess of observed over chance agreement; κ takes values in the interval [0,1]. The variance of κ is given in Everitt (1994) and can be used to test hypotheses about κ and to construct confidence intervals. The value of κ and its confidence intervals also form part of the output generated by the `agree` option on the `tables` statement.

First, the 5×5 table is read into a SAS data set. Two iterative do loops are used to form the rows and columns of this table. The count for each cell is read into the variable num and the trailing @ prevents the `input` statement from going to the next line. The `output` statement writes an observation for each of the 25 cells to the data set p12. This is one occasion when the message in the log, 'NOTE: SAS went to a new line when INPUT statement reached past the end of a line', is to be expected. A more detailed explanation of this process is given with the medical imaging example later in this chapter. The `weight` statement in `proc freq` specifies the number of observations for each cell:

```
data p12;
  do p1=1 to 5;
    do p2=1 to 5;
    input num @;
    output;
    end;
  end;
datalines;
22 2  2 0 0
 5 7 14 0 0
 0 2 36 0 0
 0 1 14 7 0
 0 0  3 0 3
;

proc freq data=p12;
  tables p1*p2 /agree;
  weight num;
run;
```

TABLE 2.5

Results for Kappa Statistic Calculated from Data in Table 2.4
(Statistics for Table of p1 by p2)

Statistic	Kappa Statistics			
	Value	ASE	95% Confidence Limits	
Simple kappa	0.4984	0.0566	0.3875	0.6094
Weighted kappa	0.6492	0.0487	0.5538	0.7446

TABLE 2.6

Landis and Koch Benchmarks for Evaluating
the Kappa Statistic

Kappa	Strength of Agreement
0.00	Poor
0.00–0.20	Slight
0.21–0.40	Fair
0.41–0.60	Moderate
0.61–0.80	Substantial
0.81–1.00	Almost perfect

The resulting output is shown in Table 2.5. The 95% confidence interval for kappa shows that there is strong evidence that it differs from zero, so the two pathologists' agreement is beyond the chance value. But is the level of agreement satisfactory? Judged against the arbitrary but practically useful benchmarks for evaluating observed values of kappa given in Landis and Koch (1977), which are given in Table 2.6, the agreement between the two pathologists is only between fair and moderate.

2.4.2 Assessing the Reliability of Quantitative Measurements

In this section, we will consider assessing the reliability of quantitative measurements. We will begin by constructing a simple model for such variables in which we let x represent the observed value for a particular patient; if the measurement were made a second time—say, some days later or by a different investigator or by a different measurement instrument—it would almost certainly differ to some degree from the first recording. If we now let t represent the 'true' value of the measurement for a patient—a value which the measurement process is seeking to record—then a model for x is

$$x = t + \varepsilon \tag{2.4}$$

where ε represents measurement error (i.e., the difference between the true value t and the observed value x).

We now assume that, in the population of patients under investigation, t has a distribution with mean μ and variance σ_t^2 and the error terms have a distribution with mean zero and variance σ_ε^2; in addition, we assume that the true score and the error are not correlated. A consequence of this model is that the variability in the observed values is a combination of true score variance and error variance (i.e., the variability in the observed values equals the sum of σ_t^2 and σ_ε^2). An index that reflects the relative magnitude of the two *components of variance* is the *intraclass correlation coefficient, R,* given by

$$R = \frac{\sigma_t^2}{\sigma_t^2 + \sigma_\varepsilon^2} \tag{2.5}$$

This can be rewritten as

$$R = \frac{1}{1 + \sigma_\varepsilon^2 / \sigma_t^2} \tag{2.6}$$

As $\sigma_\varepsilon^2/\sigma_t^2$ decreases (i.e., the error variance forms a decreasing part of the variability in the observations), R increases with its upper limit of one being achieved when the error variance is zero. In the reverse case, when σ_ε^2 forms an increasing proportion of the observed variance, R decreases to a lower limit of zero reached when all the variability in the measurements results from the error term in Equation (2.6). The intraclass correlation coefficient can be directly interpreted as the proportion of variance of a measurement due to between-subject variability in the true scores.

The interclass correlation coefficient is most often used as a measure of reliability in situations when each of a number of investigators (or measuring instruments) independently records the value of some characteristic of interest on a number of patients or subjects. For this, we need a slightly more complicated model to represent the observations with a new term (o) to allow for differences between observers/investigators being added to the basic model in Equation (2.4) to give

$$x = t + o + \varepsilon \tag{2.7}$$

The term o represents a randomly selected observer's effect on a measurement and is assumed to have a distribution with zero mean and variance, σ_o^2. The three terms x, t, and o are assumed to be independent of one another with the result that the variance of an observation is

$$\sigma^2 = \sigma_t^2 + \sigma_o^2 + \sigma_\varepsilon^2 \tag{2.8}$$

The corresponding intraclass correlation is

$$R = \frac{\sigma_t^2}{\sigma_t^2 + \sigma_o^2 + \sigma_\varepsilon^2} \tag{2.9}$$

In Equation 2.9, R is given in terms of population variances; thus, the question arises: 'How do we estimate R?' This involves carrying out a two-way

TABLE 2.7

Analysis of Variance Table for Reliability Data

Source of Variation	DF	Mean Square	Expected Mean Square
Patients	$n-1$	PMS	$\sigma_\varepsilon^2 + r\sigma_t^2$
Raters	$r-1$	RMS	$\sigma_\varepsilon^2 + n\sigma_o^2$
Error	$(n-1)(r-1)$	EMS	σ_ε^2

analysis of variance of the observers' measurements on a number of patients. (We shall have a more detailed look at analysis of variance in Chapter 6.) The analysis of variance table and the expected values of the relevant mean squares are given in Table 2.7.

From the expected mean squares, we can derive the following unbiased estimators for the three components of variance in the model:

$$\hat{\sigma}_t^2 = \frac{\text{PMS} - \text{EMS}}{r} \tag{2.10}$$

$$\hat{\sigma}_o^2 = \frac{\text{RMS} - \text{EMS}}{n} \tag{2.11}$$

$$\hat{\sigma}_\varepsilon^2 = \text{EMS} \tag{2.12}$$

The estimator of the intraclass correlation coefficient is found from

$$\hat{R} = \frac{\hat{\sigma}_t^2}{\hat{\sigma}_t^2 + \hat{\sigma}_o^2 + \hat{\sigma}_\varepsilon^2} \tag{2.13}$$

We will now look at an example of estimating the intraclass correlation using the data shown in Table 2.8. These data arise from computer-aided tomographic scans (CAT scans) of the heads of 25 psychiatric patients (see Turner, Toone, and Brett-Jones 1986). The primary aim of such scans is to determine the size of the brain ventricle relative to that of the patient's skull to given ventricle–brain ratio (VBR), which is usually calculated as VBR = 100 ventricle size/brain size. For a given scan of 'slice', the VBR is determined from measurements of the perimeter of a patient's ventricle together with the perimeter of the inner surface of the skull.

Such measurements can be made in two ways using either a hand-held planimeter or a projection of the x-ray image. We will label this measurement PLAN. The second way of making the required measurements is from an automated pixel count based on the image displayed on a television screen, and this we will label PIX. Table 2.8 shows the logged VBRs from single scans of the 25 patients; the first three columns in the table show the results obtained from repeated measurements using the planimeter and the last three rows to repeated measurement by the pixel count approach.

TABLE 2.8

CAT Scan Data (Logged VBRs)

Plan1	Plan2	Plan3	Pix1	Pix2	Pix3
2.05	2.13	2.10	1.79	1.77	1.81
1.72	1.28	1.83	1.53	1.55	1.54
1.93	1.79	1.65	1.57	1.57	1.56
2.16	1.96	2.01	1.65	1.70	1.60
2.27	1.95	1.78	2.05	2.12	2.10
2.53	2.17	2.40	2.03	1.98	2.16
1.79	1.67	1.80	1.63	1.65	1.67
1.87	1.48	1.90	1.51	1.49	1.50
1.57	1.57	1.60	1.69	1.79	1.62
1.39	1.39	1.43	1.50	1.55	1.53
1.89	1.84	1.75	1.74	1.72	1.81
2.39	2.26	2.18	1.95	1.89	1.93
1.67	1.72	1.71	1.74	1.77	1.78
1.57	1.39	1.45	1.67	1.69	1.69
2.30	2.25	2.18	1.91	1.74	1.81
2.03	1.93	2.08	2.03	1.99	2.00
1.19	1.70	1.61	0.88	0.96	1.00
1.13	0.41	0.75	1.25	1.28	1.27
1.63	1.22	1.71	1.79	1.77	1.81
1.93	2.03	1.95	1.84	1.89	1.78
1.89	1.50	1.82	1.22	1.22	1.24
1.63	2.03	1.71	1.90	1.99	1.91
1.70	1.96	2.01	2.11	2.15	2.07
2.82	2.84	2.87	2.19	2.03	2.01
0.53	0.99	1.01	1.10	1.19	1.21

Source: Turner, S. W., Toone, B. K., Brett-Jones, J. R. 1986. *Psychological Medicine*, 16:219–225.

We begin by reading the data in from the text file `cat_scan.dat` using list input. The first line of the file contains the variable names, so the `firstobs` option is used to begin reading the data values at line 2. The automatic SAS variable `_n_` is used to generate an id variable to identify the individual observations, if needed. `Proc means` is then used to list summary statistics:

```
data cat_scan;
infile 'c:\AMSUS\data\cat_scan.dat' firstobs=2;
 input plan1-plan3 pix1-pix3;
 patient=_n_;
run;
proc means data=cat_scan;
 var plan1-plan3 pix1-pix3;
run;
```

The resulting output is shown in the following table. The means and standard deviations of the three PIX measurements are lower than those of the three PLAN recordings:

Variable	N	Mean	Std Dev	Minimum	Maximum
plan1	25	1.8232000	0.4777440	0.5300000	2.8200000
plan2	25	1.7384000	0.4853923	0.4100000	2.8400000
plan3	25	1.8116000	0.4179581	0.7500000	2.8700000
pix1	25	1.6908000	0.3245243	0.8800000	2.1900000
pix2	25	1.6980000	0.2996109	0.9600000	2.1500000
pix3	25	1.6964000	0.2965479	1.0000000	2.1600000

The Pearson correlation coefficients for each pair of the six measures can be generated with `proc corr`. The `nosimple` option suppresses the listing of descriptive statistics for the variables, as these have already been given by `proc means`:

```
proc corr data=cat_scan nosimple;
 var plan1-plan3 pix1-pix3;
run;
```

The resulting correlations, etc. are given in Table 2.9. We see that correlations between the PIX and PLAN measurements are somewhat lower than those for the repeated PIX and PLAN measurements.

TABLE 2.9

Pearson Correlations for the Data in Table 2.8[a]

	plan1	plan2	plan3	pix1	pix2	pix3
Pearson Correlation Coefficients, N = 25						
Prob > |r| Under H0: Rho = 0						
plan1	1.00000	0.81205	0.89031	0.74323	0.64867	0.69970
		<.0001	<.0001	<.0001	0.0005	<.0001
plan2	0.81205	1.00000	0.89891	0.69510	0.63683	0.65682
	<.0001		<.0001	0.0001	0.0006	0.0004
plan3	0.89031	0.89891	1.00000	0.69169	0.59762	0.64382
	<.0001	<.0001		0.0001	0.0016	0.0005
pix1	0.74323	0.69510	0.69169	1.00000	0.97917	0.97964
	<.0001	0.0001	0.0001		<.0001	<.0001
pix2	0.64867	0.63683	0.59762	0.97917	1.00000	0.97226
	0.0005	0.0006	0.0016	<.0001		<.0001
pix3	0.69970	0.65682	0.64382	0.97964	0.97226	1.00000
	<.0001	0.0004	0.0005	<.0001	<.0001	

[a] Six variables: plan1, plan2, plan3, pix1, pix2, and pix3.

We can now move on to the estimation of the intraclass correlation coefficients for the two types of measurement, PIX and PLAN. To carry out the necessary separate analyses of variance for the PLAN and PIX measurements, we first need to restructure the data so that each rating is a separate observation with new variables indicating the type of measurement and the rater. To do this, we include all six measurements in an `array` and process them with an iterative do loop. The output statement is placed within the do loop to write an observation out on each pass through the loop:

```
data cat_long;
 set cat_scan;
 array pl {*} plan1-plan3 pix1-pix3;
 do i=1 to 6;
  rater=i;
  type='plan';
  vbr=pl{i};
  if i>3 then do;
        rater=i-3;
        type='pix';
        end;
  output;
 end;
 keep patient rater type vbr;
run;


proc sort data=cat_long; by type; run;
proc anova data=cat_long;
   class rater patient;
   model vbr=rater patient;
by type;
run;
```

The data set is then sorted by the type of measurement so that the two ANOVAs can be produced with the same `proc anova` step with the `by` statement. The relevant output is contained in two `proc anova` subtables and is shown in Table 2.10(a) and (b).

Taking first the results for the planimeter recordings, we obtain the following estimates of the variance components: $\hat{\sigma}_i^2 = 0.182817$, $\hat{\sigma}_o^2 = 0.0009128$, $\hat{\sigma}_\varepsilon^2 = 0.03003$ leading to an estimated intraclass correlation coefficient of 0.855. For the pixel method, the corresponding estimates are $\hat{\sigma}_i^2 = 0.09195$, $\hat{\sigma}_o^2 < 0$, $\hat{\sigma}_\varepsilon^2 = 0.00239$ with an estimated intraclass correlation coefficient of 0.975. (Here the error mean square is greater than that due to raters so that $\hat{\sigma}_o^2 < 0$ and thus, in the calculation of the intraclass correlation, is set to zero.) The results suggest that the pixel method is considerably more reliable than the older planimetry-based approach.

TABLE 2.10

Analysis of Variance Table for the Pix and Plan Measurements

(a) *Dependent variable: vbr* (type = pix)

Source	DF	Sum of Squares	Mean Square	F Value	Pr > F
Model	26	6.67878933	0.25687651	107.70	<.0001
Error	48	0.11448533	0.00238511		
Corrected total	74	6.79327467			

Source	DF	ANOVA SS	Mean Square	F Value	Pr > F
Rater	2	0.00071467	0.00035733	0.15	0.8613
Patient	24	6.67807467	0.27825311	116.66	<.0001

(b) *Dependent variable: vbr* (type = plan)

Source	DF	Sum of Squares	Mean Square	F Value	Pr > F
Model	26	13.98914667	0.53804410	17.92	<.0001
Error	48	1.44136800	0.03002850		
Corrected total	74	15.43051467			

Source	DF	ANOVA SS	Mean Square	F Value	Pr > F
Rater	2	0.10569867	0.05284933	1.76	0.1830
Patient	24	13.88344800	0.57847700	19.26	<.0001

2.5 Diagnostic Tests

Some of the most important observations and measurements that clinicians make (at least from the patient's point of view) are those used in diagnosis. Although diagnosis is an essential part of clinical practice, the field of diagnostic medicine is complex and it is often difficult to formulate straightforward scientific questions that can be addressed with simple study designs. In this section we will ignore the complex nature of diagnosis and give a relatively simple account of the evaluation of the tests used in terms of their accuracy and therefore their usefulness to the clinician.

A diagnostic test is said to have high accuracy if it achieves a high overall proportion of correct diagnoses. There are actually two aspects of accuracy— namely, the proportion of patients that the diagnostic test correctly identifies as having the disease of interest (the *sensitivity* of the test) and the proportion of patients that the test correctly identifies as not having the disease (the *specificity* of the test). The calculation of both assumes that we have a 'gold standard' diagnosis against which to evaluate the performance of our diagnostic test. For

TABLE 2.11

Relation between Results of Liver Scan and an Autopsy Diagnosis in 344 Patients

Liver scan prediction	Autopsy Assessment of Pathology		
	Abnormal (+)	Normal (−)	Total
Abnormal (+)	231 (True positive)	32 (False positive)	263
Normal (−)	27 (False negative)	54 (True negative)	81
Total	258	86	344

Source: Altman, D. G. 1991. *Practical Statistics for Medical Research.* London: CRC/Chapman & Hall.

example, after patients for whom we have the results of the diagnostic test die, they are examined by a pathologist and given a 'true' diagnosis. In the account that follows, we shall assume that we are assessing how well our diagnostic test predicts this true diagnosis and conveniently ignore the complications that may arise if the diagnosis against which the test is evaluated is itself fallible.

The simplest way to start describing how to evaluate the performance of a diagnostic test is where the test classifies the patients into two groups: 'disease' and 'no disease'. It will be useful to have a particular example in mind and the one we will use is shown in Table 2.11. This table shows the comparison between the results of what a liver scan predicts about the pathology of a patient's liver (abnormal or normal) and that found on the later autopsy of the patient.

We could simply calculate the agreement between the two classifications using the methods described earlier in the chapter, but here the problem is rather different because of the asymmetry of the relationship between the two classifications. Our interest lies in assessing how well or otherwise the liver scan diagnosis predicts the true autopsy classification. Let us first return to the sensitivity and specificity of a diagnostic test as defined previously. In this case the sensitivity is explicitly

Sensitivity = probability (liver scan positive|autopsy result positive)

The sensitivity reflects how well the liver scan can identify patients who truly have a liver abnormality. The estimate of sensitivity for the liver data in Table 2.11 is 231/258 = 0.8953.

Moving on to specificity, we have

Specificity = probability (liver scan negative|autopsy result negative)

The specificity reflects the ability of the liver scan to identify patients who in truth have no liver abnormality. The estimate of specificity for the liver data in Table 2.11 is 54/86 = 0.6279.

We now need to consider whether the estimated sensitivity and specificity give us all the information we need to judge the performance of the diagnostic test. A little thought shows that they do not; for example, the main concern of a patient who gets a positive liver scan will be his or her chance of actually having abnormal liver pathology. Understandably, perhaps, most patients who get a positive result will quickly conclude that they have problems with their liver or at least that there is a very high probability that this is the case. But statisticians (and some clinicians) know that the probability of a positive liver scan given that the patient has a liver abnormality is *not* the same as the probability that the patient has abnormal liver pathology given a positive liver scan. To evaluate the diagnostic test properly, we need to estimate the following two further probabilities:

Positive predictive value (PPV) = probability that a patient with a positive liver scan truly has a liver abnormality

Negative predictive value (NPV) = probability that a patient with a negative liver scan does not have liver abnormality

The PPV and the NPV give a direct assessment of the usefulness of the test in practice. But to calculate their values, we need to know the *prevalence* of liver abnormality in the population from which our patients are taken (i.e., the proportion of subjects in the population having the abnormality). It is then relatively easy to apply Bayes's theorem to show that

$$PPV = \frac{\text{sensitivity} \times \text{prevalence}}{\text{sensitivity} \times \text{prevalence} + (1 - \text{specificity}) \times (1 - \text{prevalence})}$$

and

$$NPV = \frac{\text{specificty} \times (1 - \text{prevalence})}{(1 - \text{sensitivity}) \times \text{prevalence} + \text{specificity} \times (1 - \text{prevalence})}$$

When the calculations for the liver data are performed assuming a prevalence of 0.5, a patient with a positive test result has a 71% chance of having a liver abnormality. However, if the prevalence were 0.1, this would be 21%. This demonstrates how the conclusion from the application of a diagnostic test that is most relevant to the patient depends heavily on the prevalence of the condition in the population.

Now let us consider the situation where the diagnostic test result is continuous or quasicontinuous. Figure 2.2 shows an idealised graph of the distributions (assumed normal for convenience) of the test result for patients with and without a disease of interest. The two distributions overlap and the test (like all diagnostic tests) cannot distinguish normal from diseased with 100% accuracy. In practice, we choose a cut point (a possible cut point is indicated in the figure by the vertical line) above which we consider the test to suggest the presence of the disease and below which we consider its value to suggest that the patient is disease free. The position of the cut point will determine the number of true positives (TPs), the number of true negatives (TNs),

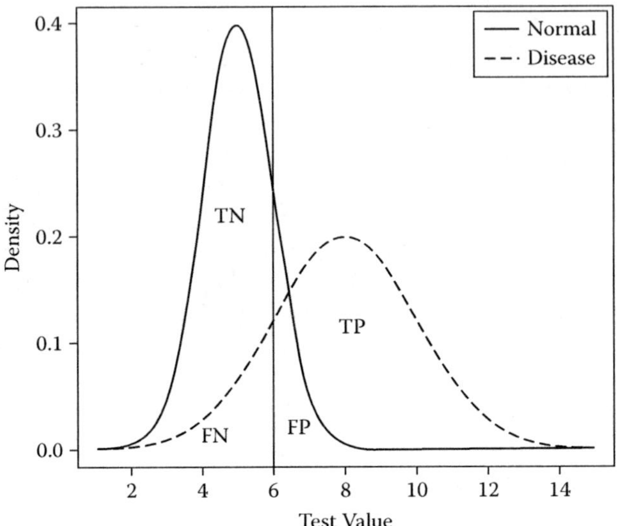

FIGURE 2.2
Distributions of the values of a continuous diagnostic test for diseased and disease-free patients.

TABLE 2.12

Data Arising from a Medical Imaging Study

True Disease Status	Rating					
	(1)	(2)	(3)	(4)	(5)	Total
Healthy	28	14	5	2	1	50
Diseased	2	4	10	14	20	50
Total	30	18	15	16	21	100

the number of false positives (FPs), and the number of false negatives (FNs). How do we evaluate the performance of such a test?

An example of data from the application of a 'continuous' valued diagnostic test is shown in Table 2.12. The data (taken from Faraggi and Reiser 2011) arise from a medical imaging study in which a clinician is asked to look at 100 images—50 from healthy subjects and 50 from people with a particular disease—and to rate each image on a scale from 1 to 5 with (1) definitely normal, (2) probably normal, (3) questionable, (4) probably abnormal, and (5) definitely abnormal. (Here the test is actually on an ordinal scale rather than a truly continuous scale but we shall ignore this relatively minor point in what follows.)

We begin by reading the cell counts into a SAS data set using two iterative do loops, one nested within the other. The first of the two data lines contains the cell counts for the healthy cases and the first iteration of the outer do loop sets disease = 0. Then each iteration of the inner do loop reads one of the five cell counts for the ratings 1 to 5 and writes an observation to the data. The trailing @ on the `input` statement holds the data line so that further values can be read from it. Without the trailing @, only the first value from each line would be read since, by default, the `input` statement would go to the next line.

The `output` statement forces an observation to be written to the data set being created. Having read and written the five values for healthy cases, the inner do loop ends. The outer do loop then sets disease = 1 and the inner do loop starts again with rating = 1 and the next five values are read. The trailing @ is still holding the first line, but as there are no more data values to be read from it, SAS automatically goes on to the next line and the log will contain the note 'SAS went to a new line when INPUT statement reached past the end of a line':

```
data imaging;
do disease= 0 to 1;
 do rating=1 to 5;
 input count @;
 output;
 end;
end;
datalines;
28      14      5       2       1
2       4       10      14      20
;
```

A useful graph to display these data is the *stacked bar chart*, which can be produced with the `vbar` statement within `proc sgplot`:

```
proc sgplot data=imaging;
 vbar rating /group=disease freq=count;
run;
```

The `rating` variable is used to form the categories for which separate bars are to be produced. The `group=disease` option names disease as the variable that will be used to subdivide the bars into sections and the `freq=count` option specifies that each observation corresponds to a number of cases. The result is given in Figure 2.3.

Now we will compute the sensitivity and specificity of the test for each possible threshold from (1) to (5). The principal use of `proc logistic` for logistic regression is described in Chapter 9, but it is also useful for this type of method comparison. Here the model statement is predicting the definitive diagnosis, as made at autopsy, from the results of the liver scan. The value of the autopsy variable corresponding to a positive diagnosis is indicated by `event='1'` in parentheses. By default, proc logistic predicts the lower value. Note that the value '1' must be in quotes even though autopsy is a numeric variable. Alternatives are `event=first` or `event=last`. The `outroc` option on the `model` statement saves the results we are interested in to a SAS data

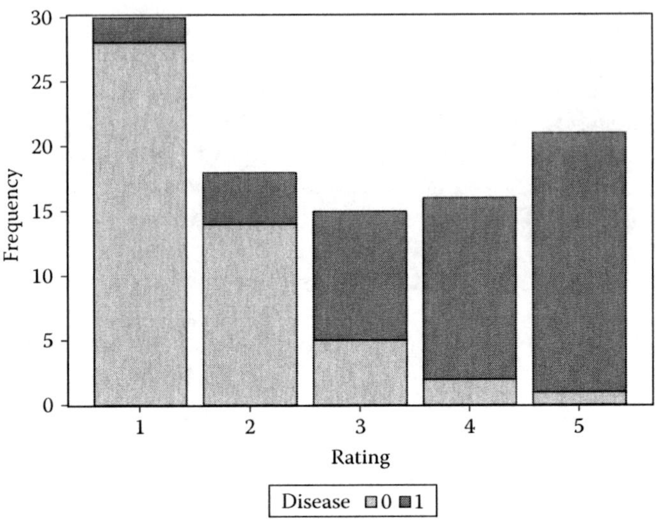

FIGURE 2.3
Stacked bar chart for medical imaging data.

set, rocres. As the data are in the tabular format, the freq statement is used
to indicate how many observations there are in each cell.

A short data step calculates the PPV and NPV assuming a population
prevalence of 0.5, and the results are printed out. The label option is used
on the proc print statement so that the variable labels are used for the column headings in the output and a format is used to print the PPV and NPV
values with two decimal places:

```
proc logistic data=imaging;
  model disease(event='1')=rating /outroc=rocs;
  freq count;
run;
data rocs;
  set rocs;
  sensitivity=_sensit_;
  specificity=1-_1mspec_;
  prevalence=0.5;
  PPV=(sensitivity*prevalence)/((sensitivity*prevalence) +
(1-specificity)*(1-prevalence));
  NPV=(specificity*(1-prevalence)) / ((1-sensitivity)*
prevalence+specificity*(1-prevalence));
  drop _sensit_;
run;

proc print data=rocs label;
format PPV NPV 4.2;
run;
```

TABLE 2.13

Sensitivities, Specificities, PPVs, and NPVs for the Data in Table 2.12

Obs	Probability Level	No. of Correctly Predicted Events	No. of Correctly Predicted Nonevents	No. of Nonevents Predicted as Events	No. of Events Predicted as Nonevents
1	0.96910	20	49	1	30
2	0.87371	34	47	3	16
3	0.60414	44	42	8	6
4	0.25187	48	28	22	2
5	0.06913	50	0	50	0

Obs	1-Specificity	sensitivity	specificity	prevalence	PPV	NPV
1	0.02	0.40	0.98	0.5	0.95	0.62
2	0.06	0.68	0.94	0.5	0.92	0.75
3	0.16	0.88	0.84	0.5	0.85	0.88
4	0.44	0.96	0.56	0.5	0.69	0.93
5	1.00	1.00	0.00	0.5	0.50	

Each line of the output in Table 2.13 shows the results of choosing one of the predicted probabilities from the model as the cut point to classify observations. The first line corresponds to a rating of 5, the second to a rating of 4, and so on.

Altman (1991) makes it clear that the choice of a cut-off is not a statistical decision as it involves a consideration of the relative 'costs' (not necessarily only financial costs) associated with false positive and false negative test results.

A useful way to display the sensitivities and specificities in Table 2.13 is by means of a *receiver operating characteristic* (ROC) curve. This is simply a plot of specificity versus 1−sensitivity and is one of the ODS graphics that can be produced by `proc logistic`. When ODS graphics is on, the ROC curve plot will be generated if one of the ROC options is used (such as the `outroc=` option on the `model` statement). Thus,

```
ods graphics on;
proc logistic data=imaging;
  model disease(event='1')=rating /outroc=rocs;
  freq count;
run;
```

will produce the plot shown in Figure 2.4. The `plots=` option on the `proc` statement could also have been used.

A diagnostic test performs well in correctly discriminating between healthy and diseased subjects if both sensitivity and specificity are high for a reasonable range of threshold values. In terms of the ROC plot, this means that the closer the curve comes to the left-hand border and then the

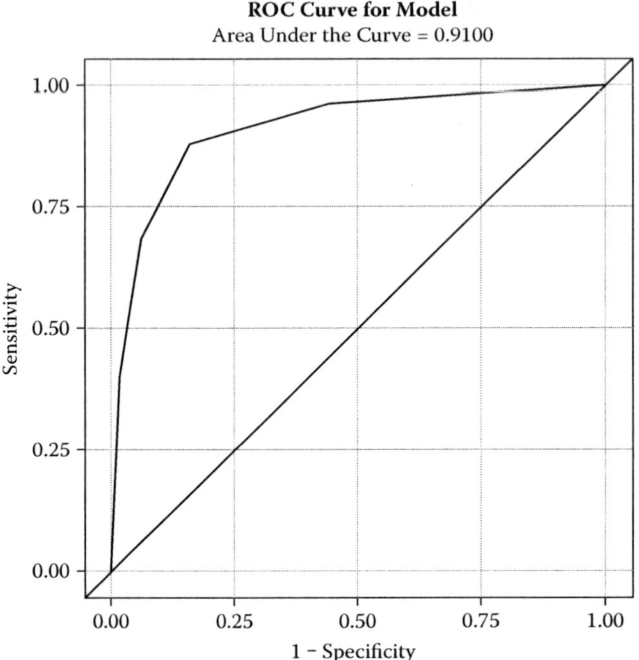

FIGURE 2.4
ROC curve for medical imaging data.

top border, the better the test is. The closer the ROC curve of a diagnostic test is to the diagonal (45°) line, the worse the test performance is.

The area under an ROC curve of a test (AUC) is an index of how well the test discriminates between healthy and diseased subjects (or images in our example). This area is an estimate of the probability that for one subject randomly selected from the healthy group and one subject randomly selected from the diseased group, the value of the diagnostic test is lower for the healthy subject (assuming that larger values of the test are more indicative of disease). A larger area implies a more accurate test, with an area of one representing a perfect test and an area of a half representing a worthless test, which is no better than allocating patients to the healthy and diseased group by the toss of an unbiased coin. For this example, the AUC is given in Figure 2.5 and its value is 0.91; such a high value indicates the high discriminatory ability of the test.

The effectiveness of alternative diagnostic tests for identifying the same disease can be assessed by comparing the areas under the respective ROC curves. The file `imaging.dat` contains the ratings already examined plus a second set from a (hypothetical) second rater. To produce a comparative ROC curve plot, we include both ratings on the `model` statement and one each on two `roc` statements with optional labels in quotes. By default, an ROC curve is generated for the overall model including both ratings. The `nofit` option

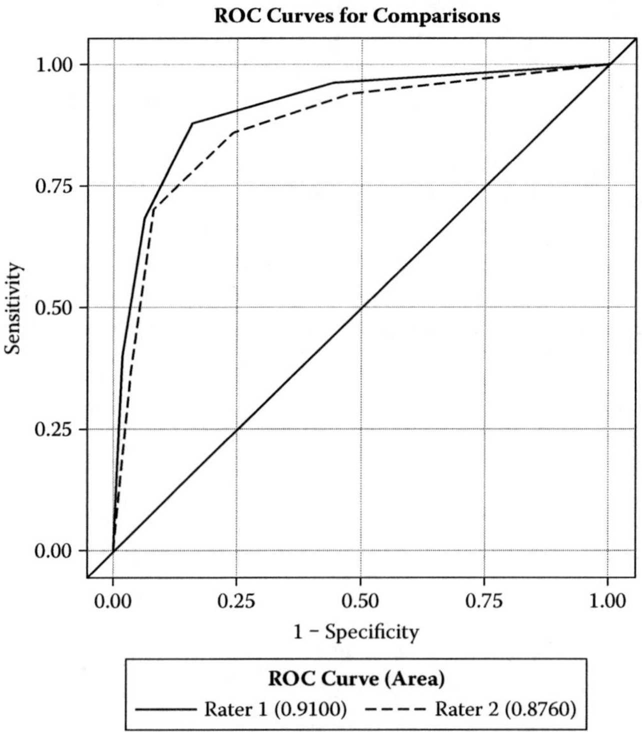

FIGURE 2.5
Comparative ROC curve for medical imaging data.

on the `model` statement suppresses this. A test for the difference between the ROC curves can be invoked with the `roccontrast` statement. The comparative ROC curve is shown in Figure 2.5. The second rater performs slightly less well, although this difference is not large:

```
data imaging2;
infile 'c:\AMSUS\data\imaging.dat';
 input disease rating1 rating2;
run;

ods graphics on;
proc logistic data=imaging2;
 model disease(event-last)- rating1 rating2 /nofit;
 roc 'rater 1' rating1;
 roc 'rater 2' rating2;
 roccontrast;
run;
ods graphics off;
```

The statistics of ROC curves is now a large area of research; interested readers are referred to Krzanowski and Hand (2009) for details.

2.6 Summary

Statistical methods have been used in medicine for some 200 to 300 years; in the twenty-first century—an era of evidence-based medicine and healthcare—statistics plays a crucial and central role. In this chapter we have looked at how statistical methods can be used to assess the reliability of measurements made in medical studies and in diagnoses. This is an important first stage in many investigations in medicine because, unless the measurements are objective, precise, and reproducible, irrespective of how elegant and acceptably designed is the rest of the study, the results will be almost worthless.

3

Clinical Trials

3.1 Introduction

Research investigations in medicine can be broadly divided into the experimental and the observational. The two classes are differentiated essentially by the amount of control the investigator has over what happens to the subjects/patients involved in the study. In an observational study, the investigator collects information but does not influence events. A number of people who smoke and a collection of nonsmokers, for example, may have their systolic blood pressures recorded and an estimate of the population difference in the mean systolic blood pressure for populations of smokers and nonsmokers calculated along with the relevant *confidence interval* (see later in this chapter). The investigator does *not*, however, have the option of allocating some individuals to be smokers and others to be nonsmokers (at least, not any option likely to pass an ethical committee). Observational studies are the foundation of epidemiology, the study of the possible causes or aetiology of disease. Such studies have three main aims:

- To describe the distribution and size of disease problems in human populations
- To identify possible aetiological factors in the pathogenesis of disease
- To provide data essential for the management, education, and planning of services for the prevention, control, and treatment of disease

Epidemiological studies will be the subject of the next chapter.

But in an experimental study, the investigator can deliberately influence events and then assess the effect of the intervention. The most common type of experimental study in medicine is, of course, the clinical trial—a topic we take up in the next section.

3.2 Clinical Trials

This chapter is concerned with a fundamental question for medicine: How do we tell if a treatment works, is ineffective, or even harmful? If a doctor claims that a certain type of psychotherapy will cure patients of their depression or a drug company maintains that a new product relieves the symptoms of asthma, how should these assertions be assessed? What sort of evidence do we need to decide that the claims made for the efficacy of clinical treatments are, indeed, valid? One thing is certain: We should not rely on the views of 'experts' unless they produce sound empirical evidence to support their views, nor should we credit the anecdotal evidence of people who have undergone the treatment and, in some cases, have been 'miraculously' cured. One of the principal changes in medical practice and culture during the last 100 years has been the increasing realisation that it is not enough for a doctor to say that his or her treatment works, nor it is enough for a patient to say likewise. These forms of anecdotal evidence, even if expanded into a series of anecdotes (dignified by the title of *case series*), are inadequate for the task.

Thus, if anecdote and number of people successfully treated alone is no real guide, how can we decide if a specific treatment works or not? We need to *experiment*, a fact recognised over 50 years ago by Pickering in his 1949 presidential address to the Section of Experimental Medicine and Therapeutics of the Royal Society of Medicine:

> Therapeutics is the branch of medicine that, by its very nature, should be experimental. For if we take a patient affected with a malady, and we alter his conditions of life, either by dieting him, or putting him to bed, or by administering to him a drug, or by performing on him an operation, we are performing an experiment. And if we are scientifically minded we should record the results. Before concluding that the change for better or for worse in the patient is due to the specific treatment employed, we must ascertain whether the result can be repeated a significant number of times in similar patients, whether the result was merely due to the natural history of the disease, or in other words to the lapse of time, or whether it was due to some other factor which was necessarily associated with the therapeutic measure in question. And if, as a result of these procedures, we learn that the therapeutic measure employed produces a significant, though not very pronounced improvement, we would experiment with the method, altering dosage or other detail to see if it can be improved. This would seem the procedure to be expected of men with six years of scientific training behind them. But it has not been followed. Had it been done we should have gained a fairly precise knowledge of the place of individual methods of therapy in disease, and our efficiency as doctors would have been enormously enhanced. (Pickering 1949)

The experimental procedure needed in the evaluation of competing treatments is the clinical trial, which is a medical experiment designed to evaluate which (if any) of two or more treatments is the more effective. It is based on one of the oldest principles of scientific investigation—namely, that new information is obtained from a comparison of alternate states. The three main components of a clinical trial are

- A group of patients given the treatment under investigation (the *treatment group*) is compared with another group of patients given either an older or standard treatment, if one exists, or an 'inert treatment' generally known as a placebo (the *control group*). (Some trials may, of course, involve several treatment groups and a control group, but it eases this general discussion to concentrate on the simple two-group situation.)
- There is a method of assigning patients to the treatment and control groups.
- There is a means of assessing effectiveness (i.e., a measure of *outcome*). This may range from a simple rating of 'improved/not improved' to a numerical measure of some characteristic of a patient such as his or her weight. Many clinical trials will involve several measures of outcome. All need to be precise, objective, and reproducible, as discussed in Chapter 2.

One of the most important aspects of a clinical trial is the question of how patients should be allocated to the treatment group and control group. Silverman (1986) states:

> How is the impossible decision made to choose between the accepted standard treatment and the proposed improved approach when a fellow human being must be assigned to one of the two (or more) treatments under test? Despite the most extensive preclinical studies, the first human allocation of a powerful treatment is largely a blind gamble and it is perhaps not surprising that so much has been written on the most appropriate fashion to allocate treatments in a trial.

The objective in allocation is that the treatment group and control group should be alike in all respects except the treatment received. As a result the clinical trial is more likely to provide an unbiased comparison of the difference between the two treatments. Let's begin by considering some flawed allocation procedures that are unlikely to achieve the desired degree of similarity of the two groups:

- Perhaps the clinician should decide which patient goes into which group? Possibly, but then the results of the trial would be viewed with a considerable amount of scepticism. For example, the clinician might allocate the patients with the worst prognosis to what was, in his or her opinion, a 'promising' new therapy and the better ones to the older treatment, no doubt with the best possible intention in respect of her patients. Or older patients might receive the traditional therapy and youngsters the new one, and so on. All of these procedures would tend to invalidate the results from the trial.

- Should the patients themselves decide what treatment to receive? Again, this would be highly undesirable. They are likely to believe that the new therapy is about to solve all of their problems. Why else would it be featuring in the trial? What patient would knowingly select a placebo?

- Perhaps the first patients to volunteer to take part in the trial should all be given the novel treatment, for example, and the later ones used as controls? Again, early volunteers might be more seriously ill, desperate to find a new remedy that works.

- What about putting alternate patients into each group? The objection to this is that the clinician will know who is receiving what treatment and may be tempted to 'tinker' with the scheme to ensure that his patients who are most ill receive the new treatment.

Therefore, how should we form treatment and control groups? The answer is deceptively simple: use *randomisation*. The group to which a participant in the trial is allocated is decided by chance. It *could* be arranged by flipping a coin each time a new eligible patient arrives and allocating the patient to the new treatment if the result is a head or to the control group if a tail appears. In practice, of course, a more sophisticated randomisation procedure will be used, as we shall see later in this chapter. The essential feature for now, however, is the randomisation rather than the mechanism used to achieve it.

Why is randomisation the allocation method of choice? There are a variety of reasons:

- It provides an impartial method of allocating patients to treatments free from possible personal biases. In other words, randomisation deals with the selection bias problem identified in the introduction of this chapter. It ensures that like is being compared with like and that hidden biases favouring one arm of the trial or the other have not crept in.

- Randomisation deals directly with confounders by ensuring that they are distributed randomly (and hence without bias) between those who do and those who do not receive the treatment. And here lies the real beauty of randomisation: It deals not only with the confounders that you had thought of and possibly even recorded, but also with those that you had not (Sibbald and Roland 1998). For example, you might be aware that response to a particular intervention is better in females than males. Gender would then be a confounder since, if you had one arm of the trial that had more females than males, then that treatment would falsely appear to be superior. You *could* deal with the situation by requiring that the two arms have equal numbers of males and females and thus eliminate the effect of the confounder, although if the trial were large enough you could reasonably rely on randomisation alone to take care of the problem. But much is mysterious in medicine, and we can say with confidence that there is much we do not known about why some people respond better to any given treatment than others. Here is the elegance of randomisation: It will take care of these 'mystery' confounders so that you no longer need to worry about them, either now or in the future—not least when you submit your papers!

- Randomisation provides a firm basis for the application of the statistical methodology likely to be needed when evaluating the results from a trial. Technically, it provides a probabilistic basis for inference from the observed results when considered in reference to all possible results.

What happens if you don't randomise? The answer is simple. You are more likely to come up with the wrong answer. In a series of studies, it has been established beyond all doubt that when you don't randomise, all sorts of biases creep in (Chalmers et al. 1983; Kleijnen 1997; Sacks et al. 1987; Schulz et al. 1995). These biases systematically overstate the effectiveness of the new treatment. Study after study that compares the results of evaluations of new treatments that do not include randomisation find that these designs are far more likely to report that the new treatment works. Now it could be that, for some perverse reason, doctors tend to perform randomised controlled trials on weaker, less effective treatments, reserving the inferior research designs for the more powerful treatments. However, one can show the same even within randomised controlled trials—the better the design of the trial is and the greater the protection from bias is, the less is the chance of showing that the new treatment works.

By ensuring a lack of selection bias and distributing both known and unknown confounders impartially among the treatment and control groups, random allocation goes a long way to making the interpretation of an observed treatment effect unambiguous; its cause is very likely to be in the different treatments received by the patients in the two groups—a long way, but not the whole way, because there remain questions of blinding and allocation concealment. But here we intend to concentrate on the randomisation aspect of clinical trials; for details of the other necessary aspects of treatment allocation, see, for example, Everitt and Wessely (2008).

3.2.1 Types of Randomisation

Randomisation is an elegant way of allocating participants to different treatments in a clinical trial that avoids selection bias, provides a sound basis for the estimation of the treatment effect, and deals directly with the problem of bias from potential confounders by distributing them randomly between the different treatments. It would seem, in principle at least, that randomisation would be simplicity itself, involving little more than the toss of a fair coin. In practice, however, things are a little more complicated. Simply tossing a coin and allocating a participant in the trial to, say, treatment A if the coin is a head and to treatment B if the coin comes down tails has a disadvantage that may make it unattractive in practice—namely, that there is the considerable potential for an imbalance in the number of participants allocated to each treatment, particularly when the trial is relatively small.

Randomisation by simply tossing a coin (or *complete randomisation*, as it is generally known) is no guarantee of equally sized groups. If, say, 60 patients are to be allocated randomly between two treatments, it is very unlikely that complete randomisation will result in 30 in each group; when randomising 50 patients to two treatments using this approach, there is about a 5% probability of ending up with an imbalance between the groups of 14 patients or worse (Rosenberger and Lachin 2002).

Let's see what happens when we use SAS to apply the 'coin toss' allocation method a number of times to allocate, say, 100 participants to two treatment groups. We can mimic coin tossing using one of SAS's random number functions. To create 10 repetitions of 100 'tosses', we use two iterative do loops, one nested within the other. For each value of set in the outer loop, the inner loop will create 100 tosses. The rand function is capable of producing random numbers with a variety of different distributions. The Bernoulli distribution gives a result of zero or one with the probability of a one specified by the second argument. The output statement writes an observation each time the inner loop iterates. The call streaminit statement gives a number that forms the start of the random number sequence, known as the seed. Although setting the seed explicitly like this is optional, it is useful as it enables the same random number sequence to be generated when the program is rerun. The SAS code is

```
data cointoss;
call streaminit(12345);
do set=1 to 10;
do toss=1 to 100;
  result=rand('bernoulli',.5);
  output;
  end;
end;
run;


proc freq data=cointoss;
  tables set*result /norow nocol nopercent;
run;
```

TABLE 3.1

Numbers of Subjects Allocated to Each of Two
Treatment Groups by a 'Coin-Tossing' Process
in Which Subject Has an Equal Probability of
Being Allocated to Each Group

Table of Set by Result			
Set	**Result**		
Frequency	**0**	**1**	**Total**
1	59	41	100
2	55	45	100
3	48	52	100
4	42	58	100
5	54	46	100
6	55	45	100
7	53	47	100
8	46	54	100
9	53	47	100
10	53	47	100
Total	518	482	1000

The results are given in Table 3.1. We see that, in the first repetition, the imbalance between the two groups is 18, which for many investigators would be unacceptable. Why does an imbalance in the size of treatment groups matter (or does it)? The reasons usually given are that the precision of an estimate of treatment effect will decrease and the *power* of the study (see later in this chapter) will be less than for an equal division of participants between treatment groups for the same overall total number of subjects. But these are, in fact, not very convincing reasons for seeking equally sized groups as precision and power will decrease only minimally for moderate imbalances (see Pocock 1983 and Rosenberger and Lachin 2002).

But despite the seeming lack of any dire statistical consequences resulting from an imbalance produced by complete randomisation, investigators designing clinical trials will often still hanker after equally sized groups. The reason is that very uneven treatment group sizes can cause problems in the administration or even financing of a trial, particularly if the treatment under investigation is a psychological one or a complex health intervention that may be subjected to limited resources. Consequently, a number of *restricted* randomisation methods have been developed that ensure similar numbers in each treatment group throughout the trial. The most commonly used of these procedures is *blocked randomisation*. (It should perhaps be mentioned here that, under certain conditions, unequal group sizes may be a sensible design requirement. Arranging to allocate a larger number of patients to a new treatment than to the standard treatment, for example, may be warranted by the need for fuller information about the general characteristics of the new treatment.)

3.2.1.1 Blocked Randomisation

This method, also known as *permuted block randomisation*, guarantees that at no time during randomisation will the imbalance be large and that, at certain points, the number of subjects in each group will be equal. The essential feature of this approach is that *blocks* of a particular number of patients are considered and a different random ordering of treatments assigned in each block; the process is repeated for consecutive blocks of patients until all have been randomised.

For example, with two treatments (A and B), the investigator may want to ensure that, after every sixth randomised subject, the number of subjects in each treatment group is equal. Then a block of size six would be used and the process would randomise the order in which three As and three Bs are assigned for every consecutive group of six subjects entering the trial. There are 20 possible sequences of three As and three Bs, and one of these is chosen at random and the six subjects are assigned accordingly. The process is repeated as many times as possible. When six patients are enrolled, the numerical balance between treatment A and treatment B is equal and the equality is maintained with the enrolment of the 12th patient, 18th patient, and so on.

Friedman, Furberg, and De Mets (1985) suggest an alternative method of blocked randomisation in which random numbers between 0 and 1 are generated for each of the assignments within a block, and the assignment order is then determined by the ranking of these numbers. For example, with a block of size six in the two-treatment situation, we might have the following:

Assignment	Random Number
A	0.112
A	0.675
A	0.321
B	0.018
B	0.991
B	0.423

This leads to the assignment order BAABAB.

In trials that are not double blind, one potential problem with blocked randomisation is that at the end of each block, alert clinicians can begin to guess the next allocation by noting the pattern of past assignments. Should the clinician become aware that the two groups are equal in size, for example, after every four participants, then it is not difficult to start influencing the allocation (Schultz and Grimes 2002). The smaller the block size is, the greater is the risk of the randomisation becoming predictable. For this reason, repeated blocks of size two should *not* be used. One common solution is to insist that clinicians do not know the block size or even to vary the block sizes themselves randomly, which makes it very difficult to determine the next assignment in a series.

The great advantage of blocking is that balance between the number of subjects is guaranteed during the course of the randomisation. The number in each group will never differ by more than $b/2$ where b is the size of the block. This can be important for two reasons. First, if enrolment in a trial takes place slowly over a period of months or even years, the type of patient recruited for the study may change during the entry period (temporal changes in severity of illness, for example, are not uncommon), so blocking will produce more comparable groups. A second advantage of blocking is that if the trial should be terminated before enrolment is completed because of the results of some form of *interim analysis* (see Everitt and Wessely 2008), balance will exist in terms of number of subjects randomised to each group.

Strictly speaking, the statistical analysis of a trial in which blocked randomisation is used needs to take into account the blocking procedure. In practice, however, there is some consensus that the complexities introduced are not worth the minimal extra gain in power (Wittes 2001).

The method suggested by Friedman et al. (1985) can be programmed with only minor alterations to the earlier coin toss example. The necessary SAS code is

```
data blkdes;
  call streaminit(12345);
  do block=1 to 50;
    do unit=1 to 6;
    rndx=rand('uniform');
    if unit<4 then assignment='A';
              else assignment='B';
    output;
    end;
  end;
run;
proc sort data=blkdes;
by block rndx;
run;
proc print data=blkdes(obs=12);
run;
```

The outer do loop generates 50 blocks and the inner one six units per block. The first three of these are assigned to treatment A and the second three to treatment B. A uniform random number is generated and the data set is then sorted by block and within each block by the random number. The first 12 observations are printed and shown in Table 3.2.

TABLE 3.2

Results of Friedman's Method for Blocked Randomisation

Obs	block	unit	rndx	assignment
1	1	6	0.28057	B
2	1	1	0.58330	A
3	1	3	0.58789	A
4	1	5	0.82469	B
5	1	4	0.85747	B
6	1	2	0.99363	A
7	2	2	0.38192	A
8	2	3	0.44896	A
9	2	5	0.51838	B
10	2	1	0.64740	A
11	2	6	0.84267	B
12	2	4	0.87578	B

An alternative approach is to use `proc plan`, which is specifically for generating experimental designs. Now the code is

```
proc plan seed=12345;
   factors block=50 ordered unit=6 random;
   output out=blkdes2 unit cvals=('A' 'A' 'A' 'B' 'B' 'B')
   random;
run;
```

The random number seed is specified on the `proc` statement. Then the `factors` statement gives the details of the design. Here, we want 50 blocks, ordered—that is, generated in order. Within each block there are to be six units in random order. The `output` statement writes the design to a SAS data set, `blkdes2`. The `unit` factor is to be given the character values 'A' and 'B' and in random order. An alternative to the `cvals=` option would be `nvals=(1 1 1 2 2 2)`. Whichever is used, there need to be the same number of values as there are levels of the factor. Again, the first 12 observations are printed in Table 3.3.

3.2.1.2 Stratified Randomisation

As mentioned before, one of the objectives in randomising patients to treatment groups is to achieve between-group comparability on certain relevant patient characteristics usually known as *prognostic factors*. Measured prior to randomisation, these are factors that it is thought will likely correlate with subsequent patient response or outcome. For example, if it is known that educated patients are more likely to respond to a particular psychotherapy than the less educated, then one would want levels of education to be reasonably

TABLE 3.3

Results from Using `proc plan`
for Blocked Randomisation

Obs	block	unit
1	1	A
2	1	B
3	1	B
4	1	A
5	1	A
6	1	B
7	2	A
8	2	A
9	2	B
10	2	A
11	2	B
12	2	B

comparable between the groups; otherwise, that might be an alternative explanation for why one group improved and the other did not.

Simple randomisation tends to produce groups that are, on average, similar in their entry characteristics, both known and unknown. The larger a trial is, the less chance there will be of any serious noncomparability of treatment groups; however, for a small study (and in many areas of medicine—for example, psychiatry—sample size is not always what it should be), there is no guarantee that all baseline characteristics will be similar in the two groups. If prognostic factors are not evenly distributed between treatment groups, it may give the investigator cause for concern. If so, the solution may be to use stratified randomisation, which is a procedure that helps to achieve comparability between the study groups for a chosen set of prognostic factors. According to Pocock (1983), the method is rather like an insurance policy in that its primary aim is to guard against the unlikely event of the treatment groups ending up with some major difference in patient characteristics. The method is frequently performed in multicentre trials because, despite every effort by the investigators, differences between centres are the rule rather than the exception.

The first issue to be considered when contemplating stratified randomisation is which prognostic factors should be considered. Experience of earlier trials may be useful here. When several prognostic factors are to be considered, a stratum for randomisation is formed by selecting one subgroup from each of them (continuous variables such as age are divided into groups of some convenient range). Since the total number of strata is therefore the product of the number of subgroups in each factor, the number of strata increases rapidly as factors are added and the levels within factors are

TABLE 3.4

Stratified Randomisation Example

Strata	Age	Sex	Group Assignment
1	40–49	Male	ABBA BABA…
2	40–49	Female	
3	50–59	Male	
4	50–59	Female	
5	60–69	Male	
6	60–69	Female	

Note: Male patients between 40 and 49 years old would be assigned to treatment groups A and B in the sequences ABBA BABA…. Similarly, random sequences would appear in the other strata.

refined. Consequently, only the most important variables should be chosen and the number kept to a minimum.

Within each stratum, the randomisation process itself could be simple randomisation, but in practice most clinical trials will use some blocked randomisation approach. As an example, suppose that an investigator wishes to stratify on age and sex, and to use a block size of four. First, age is divided into a number of categories—say, 40–49, 50–59, and 60–69. The design thus has 3 × 2 strata, and the randomisation might be as shown in Table 3.4.

Although the main argument for stratified randomisation is that of making the treatment groups comparable with respect to specific prognostic factors, it may also lead to increased power, if the stratification is taken into account in the analysis, by reducing variability in group comparisons. Such reduction allows a study of a given size to detect smaller group differences in outcome measures or to detect a specified difference with fewer subjects.

The disadvantage of stratification is its complexity. As the technical requirements of the chosen randomisation process increase, so do the chances of error. The costs of the trial also increase, and there is always the chance that some strata will have insufficient numbers, thus reducing power. The general advice if stratified randomisation is to be used is to keep it simple. For example, only stratify on variables that are easy to measure, such as gender or age (assuming that these are considered predictive of outcome).

Stratified randomisation is of most relevance in small trials, but even here it may not be profitable if there is uncertainty over the importance or reliability of prognostic factors or if the trial has a limited organisation that might not cope well with complex randomisation procedures. In many cases, it may be more useful to employ a stratified analysis (subgroup analysis) or *analysis of covariance* to adjust for prognostic factors when assessing treatment differences (see Chapter 6).

Designs for stratified randomisation can be produced in the same way as for blocked designs, but incorporating the strata as an extra level. If we had six age–sex strata, as in the preceding example, and wanted them to be blocked in blocks of four, we could use `proc plan` as follows:

```
proc plan seed=12345;
   factors stratum=6 ordered block=10 ordered unit=4 random;
   output out=stdesign unit cvals=('A' 'A' 'B' 'B') random;
run;
```

This would be assuming that the maximum in any given stratum would be 40. The number of blocks could be increased if this were not sufficient.

In any of the preceding designs, it might also be desirable to generate an id number that will be allocated at the time of randomisation. Sequential numbers could be generated using the SAS automatic variable _n_ , as follows:

```
data stdesign;
   set stdesign;
   id=_n_;
run;
```

3.2.1.3 Minimisation Method

A further approach to achieving balance between treatment groups on selected prognostic factors is to use an adaptive randomisation procedure in which the chance of allocating a new patient to a particular treatment is adjusted according to any existing imbalances in the baseline characteristics of the groups. For example, if sex is a prognostic factor and one treatment group has more women than men, the allocation scheme is such that the next few male patients are more likely to be randomised into the group that currently has fewer men. This method is often referred to as minimisation because imbalances in the distribution of prognostic factors are minimised.

In general, the method is applied in situations involving several prognostic factors and patient allocation is then based on the aim of balancing the marginal treatment totals for each level of each factor. As an example of the application of minimisation, imagine a clinical trial comparing a new treatment of depression (A) with the standard treatment (B). Table 3.5 shows 60 patients already allocated to the two treatments categorised by four prognostic factors. Suppose the next patient to be allocated is less than 40 years old, has a current episode of depression that has lasted longer than 6 months, is female, and is currently taking other antidepressant drugs. Then, for each treatment, the numbers of patients in the corresponding four rows of Table 3.5 are added to give the following:

Sum for A = 16 + 18 + 20 + 15 = 69

Sum for B = 15 + 16 + 22 + 14 = 67

TABLE 3.5

Treatment Assignments by Four Prognostic Factors for 60 Patients in a Trial for a New Treatment of Depression

Factor	Variable Name	Level	Code	A	B
Age	agegrp	Less than 40	1	16	15
		Greater than 40	2	14	15
Length of current episode	Lepi	Less than 6 months	1	12	14
		Greater than 6 months	2	18	16
Sex	sex	Male	1	10	8
		Female	2	20	22
Currently taking other antidepressants?	onmed	Yes	1	15	14
		No	2	15	16

Minimisation requires the new patient to be allocated to the treatment with the smallest marginal total, in this case treatment A. If the sums for A and B are equal, then simple randomisation is used to allocate the patient.

The aim of minimisation is to balance the distribution of specific characteristics within the treatment groups, but to do so efficiently. Although minimisation is a largely nonrandom method of treatment allocation, Scott et al. (2002) find evidence that it is highly effective and recommend its wider adoption in the conduct of clinical trials.

Minimisation randomisation using SAS can be applied as follows. Data on the prognostic factors and treatment assignments for the 60 patients as shown in Table 3.3 are in the SAS data set `minimize`. We first calculate the marginal totals used for the allocation:

```
libname db "c:\amdus2\data";
ods output OneWayFreqs(persist)=marginals;
proc freq data=db.minimize; tables treat; where agegrp=1; run;
proc freq data=db.minimize; tables treat; where Lepi=2;   run;
proc freq data=db.minimize; tables treat; where sex=2;    run;
proc freq data=db.minimize; tables treat; where onmed=1;  run;
ods output close;
```

The `libname` statement links the directory where the data set is stored to the *libref* db, which can then be used to identify the data set. The `ods output` statement specifies that the `OneWayFreqs` ODS table is to be saved in the data set `marginals`. The `persist` option in parentheses keeps the data set open to accumulate the frequencies from multiple proc steps until explicitly closed by the `ods output close` statement. Without this option, only the output from the first `proc freq` step would be saved. Four `proc freq` steps are then used to calculate the numbers already allocated to the two treatments for those with the same values of the four prognostic factors as the new patient. In each case, the `where` statement selects those with the appropriate value of a factor.

Having calculated the necessary marginal totals, we sum them and make the treatment allocation as follows:

```
proc means data=marginals sum;
   class treat;
   var frequency;
run;
```

The marginal totals for treatment A sum to 69 and those for B to 67, so the patient is allocated to treatment B. If the sums were the same, the allocation could be made with a coin toss or a short data step, such as

```
data _null_;
   rx=rand('bernoulli',.5);
   if rx=0 then put "allocation is to group A";
          else put "allocation is to group B";
run;
```

The newly allocated patient would then need to be added to the minimise data set ready for the next new patient, which could be done as follows:

```
data newpt;
  input id agegrp Lepi sex onmed treat $;
datalines;
61 1 2  2  1 B
;
data db.minimize;
  set db.minimize newpt;
run;
```

Blocking, stratified randomisation, and minimisation all have their part to play in allocating patients to treatments in some clinical trials. But as the sample size used in a trial increases to a respectable value (sample size estimation will be considered in Section 3.3), it is unlikely that the investigator will need to consider any other randomisation scheme than complete randomisation. Once the overall sample size has reached around 200, most authorities advise that stratification, etc. becomes unnecessary, and simple randomisation will be sufficient to minimise chance biases (Pocock 1983). Simple randomisation, properly performed, has the added powerful advantage of being impossible to predict. But whatever method of randomisation is used in a clinical trial, it needs to be reported in detail in any scientific paper that is generated by the study.

Sadly, however, there is evidence that this does not happen. A study by Ogundipe, Boardman, and Masterson (1999), for example, examined the adequacy of the reporting of details of randomisation in clinical trials published in the *British Journal of Psychiatry* (*BJP*) and the *American Journal of Psychiatry* (*AJP*) and found that of 183 such submissions (73 in the *BJP* and 110 in the *AJP*), only nine papers in the *AJP* and six in the *BJP* described the technique used to create the randomisation sequence employed in the trial. Only one paper in the *AJP* and five in the *BJP* described both the generation of the random numbers and the mechanism of allocating patients to treatment. Clearly, the reporting of randomisation details is very often inadequate and editors of medical journals need to be alert to the problem to ensure that the randomised clinical trial status of such papers is specifically established by the authors of papers.

3.3 How Many Participants Do I Need in My Trial?

One of the most frequent questions faced by a statistician dealing with investigators planning a clinical trial is 'how many participants do I need to recruit to each treatment group?' Answering the question requires consideration of a number of factors—for example, the amount of time available for the trial, the likely ease or difficulty in recruiting the type of patient required, and the possible financial constraints that may be involved. But the statistician may, initially at least, largely ignore these important aspects of the problem and apply a statistical procedure for calculating sample size that involves the following:

- Specifying the appropriate statistical test to be used in the analysis of the chosen response

- Setting the size of the type I error (i.e., the significance level)

- Assessing the likely variance of the response variable

- Agreeing with the investigators on the power they would like to achieve (For those readers who have forgotten—or perhaps never knew—the power of a statistical test is its probability of rejecting the null hypothesis when it is false.)

- Obtaining from the investigators a size of treatment effect that is of clinical important (i.e., a treatment difference that the investigators would not like to miss being able to declare to be statistically significant)

Thus, the investigators need to specify the size of the treatment difference considered clinically relevant (i.e., important to detect) and with what degree of certainty (i.e., with what power) it should be detected. Given such information, the calculation of the corresponding sample size is often relatively straightforward, although the details will depend on the type of response variable and the type of test involved (see later discussion for an example). In general terms, the sample size will increase as the variability of the response variable increases and decrease as the chosen clinically relevant treatment effect increases. In addition, the sample size will need to be larger to achieve a greater power and/or a more stringent significance level.

As an example of the calculations involved in sample size determination, consider a trial involving the comparison of two treatments for anorexia nervosa. Anorexic women are to be assigned randomly to each treatment and the gain in weight in kilograms after 3 months is to be used as the outcome measure. From previous experience gained in similar trials, it is known that the standard deviation (σ) of weight gain is likely to be about 4 kg. The investigator feels that a difference in weight gain of 1 kg (Δ) would be of clinical importance and wishes to have a power of 90% when the appropriate two-sided test is used with significance level of 0.05 (α). The formula for calculating the number of women required in each treatment group (n) is

$$n = \frac{2\left(Z_{\alpha|2} + Z_{\beta}\right)^2 \sigma^2}{\Delta^2} \tag{3.1}$$

where β is $1 - \text{power}$, and

- $Z_{\alpha|2}$ is the value of the normal distribution that cuts off an upper tail probability of $\alpha|2$. Thus, for $\alpha = 0.05$, $Z_{\alpha|2} = 1.96$.
- Z_{β} is the value of the normal distribution that cuts off an upper tail probability of β. Thus, for a power of 0.90, $\beta = 0.10$ and $Z_{\beta} = 1.28$.

In SAS, we can use `proc power` to find the required sample sizes as follows:

```
proc power;
   twosamplemeans
     meandiff=1
     stddev=4
     power=.9
     npergroup=.;
run;
```

Proc power covers a range of common tests that a power calculation might be based on, including the one- and two-sample tests, one-way ANOVA (analysis of variance), multiple regression, logistic regression, and comparison of two survival curves. Each of these scenarios is invoked by a corresponding statement (e.g., `twosamplefreq`, `twosamplesurvival`, `onewayanova`, `logistic`, `multreg`, and so on). The general principle is that the quantity that is to be calculated is set to missing; most typically this is either the sample size or power, and the other aspects enumerated previously are specified or left at their default value. In the preceding example, npergroup is set to missing as that is the quantity that we wish to calculate. The power is set to 90%, the significance level is left at its default (5%), and the variance of the response is specified, as is the treatment effect. The resulting value for the number of subjects needed in each group is 338. Note that twosamplemeans is a single statement with multiple options, so there is a semicolon only at the end.

Equivalent information can be provided in a number of different ways. Each of the groups could have separate means, variances, or *N*s specified, rather than the mean difference, common variance, and equal group sizes. For example, in a study of a welfare-to-work program, the potential health improvement associated with a return to work was thought to be around 2 points on the SF-12 scale (a short health questionnaire), but an increase in variability was also expected so that the standard deviation might be 12 as opposed to 8 in the control group. In this case, the SAS code would be

```
proc power;
   twosamplemeans
      groupmeans=0  |  2
      groupstddevs=8  |  12
      test=diff_satt
      power=.8
      npergroup=.;
run;
```

The means for the two groups are separated by a vertical bar on the groupmeans option and likewise the standard deviations. For unequal variances, the *Satterthwaite test* (see Everitt 2011) is selected on the test option. The results suggest a sample size of 410 in each group.

An obvious danger with the sample size determination procedure mapped out on page 89 is that investigators (and, in some cases, even their statisticians) may occasionally be led to specify an effect size that is unrealistically extreme (what Senn 1997 has described with his usual candour as 'a cynically relevant difference') so that the calculated sample size looks feasible in terms of possible pressing temporal and financial constraints. Such a possibility maybe what led Senn (1997) to describe power calculations as 'a guess masquerading as mathematics' and Pocock (1996) to comment that they are 'a game that can produce any number you wish with manipulative juggling of the parameter values'. Statisticians advising on clinical trials need to be active in estimating the degree of difference that can be realistically expected for a clinical trial based on previous studies of a particular disease or, when such information is lacking, perhaps based on subjective opinions of investigators and physicians *not* involved in the proposed trial.

Getting the sample size right in a clinical trial is generally believed to be critical; indeed, according to Simon (1991),

> An effective clinical trial must ask an important question and provide a reliable answer. A major determinant of the reliability of the answer is the sample size of the trial. Trials of inadequate size may cause contradictory and erroneous results and thereby lead to an inappropriate treatment of patients. They also divert limited resources from useful applications and cheat the patients who participated in what they thought was important clinical research. Sample size planning is, therefore, a key component of clinical trial methodology.

Certainly, many clinical trial investigators would (and have) argued that trials with 'inadequate' sample size are, in a very real sense, unethical in that they require patients to accept the risks of treatment, however small, without any chance of benefit to them or future patients. Freiman, Chalmers, and Smith (1978), for example, reviewed 71 'negative' randomised clinical trials (i.e., trials in which the observed differences between the proposed and control treatments were not large enough to satisfy a specified 'significance' level (the risk of a type I error) and the results were declared to be 'not statistically significant'. Analysis of these clinical studies indicated that the investigators often worked with numbers of enrolled patients too small to offer a reasonable chance of avoiding the opposing mistake—a type II error (accepting the null hypothesis when it is false). Fifty of the trials had a greater than 10% risk of missing a substantial difference (true treatment difference of 50%) in treatment outcome. The reviewers warned that many treatments labelled as 'not different from control' had not received a critical test because the trials had insufficient power to do the job intended. Freiman and colleagues' examples clearly illustrate the truth in that memorable phrase of Altman and Bland (1995): 'absence of evidence is not evidence of absence'.

This concern about patient numbers in many clinical trials being too small is echoed by Pocock (1996), who sees the problem as 'general phenomena whose full implications for restricting therapeutic progress are not widely appreciated'. In the same article Pocock continues:

> The fact is that trials with truly modest treatment effects will achieve statistical significance only if random variation conveniently exaggerated these effects. The chances of publication and reader interest are much greater if the results of the trial are statistically significant. Hence, the current obsession with significance testing combined with the inadequate size of many trials means that publications on clinical trials for many treatments are likely to be biased towards an exaggeration of therapeutic effect, even if the trials are unbiased in all other respects.

The primary purpose in making a trial as large as possible is to maximise the chance of detecting a treatment effect, particularly if that effect is not very big, and to provide a precise estimate of the size of the treatment effect. A large trial may also allow a few sensible and predefined subgroup analyses to try to assess for whom the treatment works best (see later in this chapter). The case against trials with inadequate numbers of subjects appears strong, but as Senn (1997) points out, sometimes only a small trial is possible. And misinterpreting a nonsignificant effect as an indication that a treatment effect is not effective, rather than as a failure to *prove* that it is effective, suggests trying to improve medical education rather than totally abandoning small trials. In addition, with the growing use of *systematic reviews* and *meta-analysis* (topics to be discussed in Chapter 5), the results from small trials may prove valuable in contributing to an overview of the evidence of treatment effectiveness, a view neatly summarised by Senn in the phrase 'some evidence is better than none'. Perhaps with clinical trials, as with other things, size is not *always* everything.

3.4 Analysis of Data from Clinical Trials

A clinical trial generates data that must be analysed. Such analysis will involve the use of statistics—not always the most popular topic amongst clinicians and applied medical researchers, although few, we hope, would go as far as Le Fanu (1999) in believing that 'statistics are numbers to which complex mathematical formulae can be applied to produce conclusions of dubious veracity and from which all wit and human life is ingenuously excluded'. In this section, we will examine a number of general statistical issues that we feel are of particular relevance in analysing data from clinical trials. In essence, analysis and design are two sides of the same coin, and if a poor design can make a clinical trial almost useless, the benefits of a good design can be undermined with a poorly planned (or executed) analysis.

3.4.1 *p*-Values and Confidence Intervals

The *p*-value is probably the most ubiquitous statistical index found in the applied sciences literature and is particularly widely used in biomedical research. The *p*-value is defined as the probability of obtaining the observed data (or data that represent a more extreme departure from the null hypothesis) if the null hypothesis is true; it was first proposed as part of a quasiformal method of inference by Fisher in his influential 1925 book, *Statistical Methods for Research Workers*. For Fisher, the *p*-value represented an attempt to provide a measure of evidence against the null hypothesis; however, he intended it to be used informally, with the smaller the *p*-value the greater the evidence against the null hypothesis, rather than providing a division of the results into 'significant' and 'nonsignificant'.

Unfortunately, it seems that despite the many caveats in the literature (see, for example, Gardner and Altman 1986 and Oakes 1986), the accept/reject philosophy of hypothesis testing remains seductive to many clinicians, who seem determined to continue to express joy on achieving a p-value of 0.049 and despair on finding one of 'only' 0.051 (0.05 being the almost universally accepted threshold for labelling results, significant or nonsignificant). Many clinicians seem to internalise the difference between a p-value of 0.05 and one of 0.06 as 'right' versus 'wrong', 'creditable' versus 'embarrassing', 'success' versus 'failure', and, perhaps, the renewal of grants versus termination. Such practice was definitely *not* what Fisher had in mind as is evidenced by the following quotation from the 1925 edition of *Statistical Methods for Research Workers:*

> A man who 'rejects' a hypothesis provisionally, as a matter of habitual practice, when the significance is 1% or higher, will certainly be mistaken in not more than 1% of such decision…However, the calculation is absurdly academic, for in fact no scientific worker has a fixed level of significance at which from year to year, and in all circumstances, he rejects hypotheses; he rather gives his mind to each particular case in the light of his evidence and his ideas.

The most common alternative to presenting results from a clinical trial in terms of p-values, in relation to a statistical null hypothesis, is to estimate the magnitude of the difference of a measured outcome between treatment groups, along with some interval that includes the population value of the difference with some specified probability. Such an approach is intuitively sensible since most clinical objectives translate into a need to estimate a particular quantity—for example, a treatment effect—along with some idea of the precision of the estimate. The resulting interval is known, of course, as a *confidence interval.*

Confidence intervals can be found relatively simply for many quantities of interest (see Gardner and Altman 1986), and although the underlying logic of interval estimation is essentially similar to that of significance testing, they do not carry with them the pseudoscientific hypothesis testing language of such tests. Instead, they give a plausible range of values for the unknown difference. As Oakes (1986) rightly comments, 'the significance test relates to what the population parameter is not; the confidence interval gives a plausible range for what the parameter *is*'.

According to Gardner and Altman (1986),

> Overemphasis on hypothesis testing—and the use of p-values to dichotomise significant or non-significant results—has distracted from more useful approaches to interpreting study results, such as estimation and confidence intervals…. The excessive use of hypothesis testing at the expense of other ways of assessing results has reached such a degree that levels of significance are often quoted alone in the main text and abstracts of papers, with no mention of actual concentration, proportions, etc., or

their differences. The implications of hypothesis testing—that there can always be a simple 'yes' or 'no' answer as the fundamental result from a medical study—[are] clearly false, and used in this way hypothesis testing is of limited value.

Gardner and Altman's comments are well illustrated by the following quotation taken from a report of a clinical trial comparing olanzapine and haloperidol for treating the symptoms of schizophrenia: 'Patients treated with olanzapine showed an average decrease of 10.9 points on the brief psychiatric rating scale; patients treated with haloperidol reported an average decrease of 7.9 points. This difference was statistically significant'. Note that neither a measure of the variation of the outcome measure nor an interval estimate of the treatment difference (i.e., a confidence interval) is given.

Perhaps partly as a result of Gardner and Altman's paper, the use and reporting of confidence intervals have become more widespread in the medical literature in the past decade. Indeed, many journals now demand such intervals rather than simply p-values. In many medical journals, however, there appears to be a continuing commitment to p-values; certainly, there is no discernable move away from their use. There should be.

3.4.2 Some Examples of Analysis of Data from Clinical Trials Using Familiar Statistical Methods

Clinical trials may often generate data that require sophisticated statistical analyses; for example, as mentioned previously, clinical trials are often longitudinal with values of the outcome measure (or outcome measures) being taken on several different occasions. The analysis of such longitudinal data needs relatively complicated statistical techniques and will be the subject of Chapters 12, 13, and 14. But in this subsection, we will look at some ways of analysing relatively simple data arising from clinical trials using straightforward inferential methods familiar from introductory statistical courses and/or books.

The first example is adapted from Altman (1991). Twenty-two patients undergoing cardiac bypass surgery were randomised to one of three ventilation groups:

In group I, patients received a 50% nitrous oxide and 50% oxygen mixture continuously for 24 hours.

In group II, patients received a 50% nitrous oxide and 50% oxygen mixture only during the operation.

In group III, patients received no nitrous oxide but received 35%–50% oxygen for 24 hours.

Table 3.6 shows red cell folate levels for the three groups after 24 hours' ventilation.

TABLE 3.6

Red Folate Levels[a] in Three Groups of
Cardiac Bypass Patients Given Different
Levels of Nitrous Oxide Ventilation

Group 1 (*n* = 8)	Group 2 (*n* = 9)	Group 3 (*n* = 5)
243	206	241
251	210	258
275	226	270
291	249	293
347	255	328
354	273	
380	285	
392	295	
	309	

Source: Amess, J. A. et al. 1978. *Lancet* ii: 339–342.
[a] Micrograms per litre.

We would like to assess if there is any evidence that red folate level differs
between the groups. As with the vast majority of data analysis exercises, the
initial step should be to graph the data in some way. Here we will look at *box
plots* of the data in each group. We begin with a data step to read the data in:

```
data folates;
  do group=1 to 3;
    input rfl 4. @;
    if rfl~=. then output;
  end;
datalines;
243 206 241
251 210 258
275 226 270
291 249 293
347 255 328
354 273
380 285
392 295
    309
;
```

An iterative do loop is used to read three values per line and assign them
to the appropriate group. Formatted input is used because the data lines contain blanks that need to be treated as missing values. The trailing @ on the
input statement holds the data line so that all three values can be read from
it. By default, the `input` statement would go to a new line each time it is

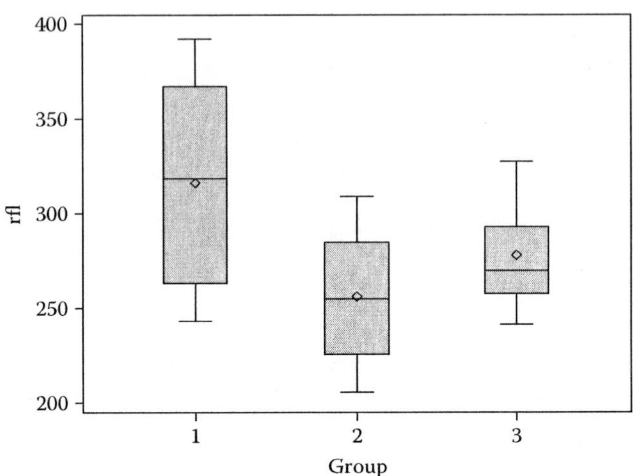

FIGURE 3.1
Box plots of data in Table 3.5.

used. The `output` statement writes an observation to the `folates` data set for each iteration of the `do` loop:

```
proc sgplot data=folates;
  vbox rfl / category=group;
run;
```

The `vbox` plot statement within `proc sgplot` will produce box plots. The response variable is `rfl` and the `category` option is used to produce separate plots for each group.

Examination of the box plots in Figure 3.1 suggests that the folate levels in group 1 are somewhat higher than those in groups 2 and 3. There is no evidence in the box plots of any potentially troublesome *outliers* and little evidence for *skewness* of the distribution of folate levels in any of the three groups which might have implications for the use of the statistical test that we shall use to assess folate levels in the three groups formally.

We shall compare red folate levels in each pair of groups by way of *Student's two independent samples t-test* (see Altman 1991). This is not the optimal analysis, which is a one-way *analysis of variance*, but we leave describing this approach until Chapter 6. We can apply the three *t*-tests for comparing each pair of groups using the following SAS code:

```
proc ttest data=folates;
  class group;
  var rfl;
where group in(1 2);
run;
```

```
proc ttest data=folates;
   class group;
   var rfl;
where group in(1 3);
run;

proc ttest data=folates;
   class group;
   var rfl;
where group in(2 3);
run;
```

For the `ttest` procedure, the `var` statement specifies the variable to be analysed and the `class` statement specifies the variable that divides the sample into two groups. In this case, the variable `group` has three values, but the `where` statement selects two at a time for comparison using the `in` operator. The results are shown in Table 3.7.

The two-sample *t*-test is based on three assumptions:

- The data are drawn from populations where red folate levels have a normal distribution.
- The normal distributions describing red folate levels in each group have the same variance.
- The samples in each group are independent of each other.

We can take the latter assumption as read because different subjects are used in each group. Informal support for the first two assumptions is given by the box plots and formal support for the second assumption is provided by the 'folded F'—the ratio of the larger of the two variances to the smaller, which is a test of the equality of variance of the two groups; for each pair of groups in these data, there is no evidence of a difference in variance. Consequently, we can use the 'pooled' *t*-test results rather than the 'Satterthwaite', which is used in situations when the group variances are considered to be unequal; the test is described in Everitt (2011).

Examining the results in Table 3.6, we find that the means of the three groups are

Group 1: 316.6

Group 2: 256.4

Group 3: 278.0

For each pair of groups, we find the 95% confidence intervals to be

Groups 1–2: [10.0,110.3]

Groups 1–3: [–25.5,102.7]

Groups 2–3: [–65.3,22.2]

TABLE 3.7

Independent Samples *t*-Tests for Red Folate Data

Variable: rfl						
group	N	Mean	Std Dev	Std Err	Minimum	Maximum
1	8	316.6	58.7171	20.7596	243.0	392.0
2	9	256.4	37.1218	12.3739	206.0	309.0
Diff (1−2)		60.1806	48.4136	23.5248		

group	Method	Mean	95% CL Mean		Std Dev	95% CL Std Dev	
1		316.6	267.5	365.7	58.7171	38.8222	119.5
2		256.4	227.9	285.0	37.1218	25.0742	71.1169
Diff (1−2)	Pooled	60.1806	10.0387	110.3	48.4136	35.7633	74.9292
Diff (1−2)	Satterthwaite	60.1806	7.3105	113.1			

Method	Variances	DF	t Value	Pr > |t|
Pooled	Equal	15	2.56	0.0218
Satterthwaite	Unequal	11.579	2.49	0.0291

Equality of Variances				
Method	Num DF	Den DF	F Value	Pr > F
Folded F	7	8	2.50	0.2223

Variable: rfl						
group	N	Mean	Std Dev	Std Err	Minimum	Maximum
1	8	316.6	58.7171	20.7596	243.0	392.0
3	5	278.0	33.7565	15.0964	241.0	328.0
Diff (1−2)		38.6250	51.0720	29.1155		

group	Method	Mean	95% CL Mean		Std Dev	95% CL Std Dev	
1		316.6	267.5	365.7	58.7171	38.8222	119.5
3		278.0	236.1	319.9	33.7565	20.2246	97.0011
Diff (1−2)	Pooled	38.6250	−25.4579	102.7	51.0720	36.1792	86.7141
Diff (1−2)	Satterthwaite	38.6250	−17.8799	95.1299			

Method	Variances	DF	t Value	Pr > |t|
Pooled	Equal	11	1.33	0.2115
Satterthwaite	Unequal	10.985	1.50	0.1606

TABLE 3.7 (*Continued*)

Independent Samples *t*-Tests for Red Folate Data

Equality of Variances				
Method	Num DF	Den DF	F Value	Pr > F
Folded F	7	4	3.03	0.3014

Variable: rfl						
Group	N	Mean	Std Dev	Std Err	Minimum	Maximum
2	9	256.4	37.1218	12.3739	206.0	309.0
3	5	278.0	33.7565	15.0964	241.0	328.0
Diff (1−2)		−21.5556	36.0350	20.0993		

Group	Method	Mean	95% CL Mean		Std Dev	95% CL Std Dev	
2		256.4	227.9	285.0	37.1218	25.0742	71.1169
3		278.0	236.1	319.9	33.7565	20.2246	97.0011
Diff (1−2)	Pooled	−21.5556	−65.3483	22.2371	36.0350	25.8402	59.4842
Diff (1−2)	Satterthwaite	−21.5556	−65.6223	22.5112			

Method	Variances	DF	t Value	Pr > |t|
Pooled	Equal	12	−1.07	0.3046
Satterthwaite	Unequal	9.1216	−1.10	0.2977

Equality of Variances				
Method	Num DF	Den DF	F Value	Pr > F
Folded F	8	4	1.21	0.9126

There is evidence that group 1 differs in average folate level from group 3, but no evidence for any other group difference.

As our second example, we will look at some data described in Williams et al. (1989) and also given in Altman (1991). The data are given in Table 3.8 and arise from a trial in which patients receiving chemotherapy as outpatients were randomised to receive either an active antiemetic treatment or placebo and asked to assess their nausea on a 100 mm linear analogue self-assessment scale on which higher values indicated more severe nausea.

The SAS code for both applying the two-independent samples *t*-test and producing some informative graphics of the data is as follows:

```
data nausea;
 do treatment='A', 'B';
 input nausea @;
```

```
   output;
  end;
 datalines;
 0         0
 0        10
 0        12
 .  .  .
30        82
52        86
76        95
 ;
```

The data step is similar to the previous example, but here list input can be used as the groups have equal numbers. This example also shows that iterative do loops can have character values, but they need to be in quotes and separated by commas. The graphics in Figure 3.2 are produced from the default ODS graphics for proc ttest:

TABLE 3.8

Self-Assessments of Nausea for Patients Receiving Chemotherapy Randomised to Active and Placebo Groups

Treatment Group	
Active (n = 20)	Placebo (n = 20)
0	0
0	10
0	12
0	15
0	15
2	30
7	35
8	38
10	42
13	45
15	50
18	50
20	60
20	64
21	68
22	71
25	74
30	82
52	86
76	95

Source: Williams, C. J., Davies, C., Ravel, M., Middleton, J., Luken, J., and Stone, B. 1989. *British Medical Journal*, 298:430–431.

```
ods graphics on;
proc ttest data=nausea;
   class treatment;
   var nausea;
run;
```

The results of the *t*-test are shown in Table 3.9, but, before looking at these, we need to look at the graphical material given in Figure 3.2. First in this figure are the histograms of the self-assessment scores in each treatment group enhanced by a fitted normal distribution and by a nonparametric estimate of the density function know as a *kernel estimator* (for details see, for example, Silverman 1986). In both groups, the plots give some evidence that the distributions are not normal; in the treatment group, there is considerable skewness and, in the placebo group, the appropriate distribution appears to be uniform rather than normal. The box plots given below the histograms also show the skewness of the observations in the active treatment group and the presence of an outlier in this group. The box plots are followed by normal probability plots of the data in each of the treatment groups. The deviation from linearity in the plot of the active treatment scores is apparent.

Looking now at the results from applying Student's two-independent samples *t*-test, we see that there is strong evidence of a difference in the mean

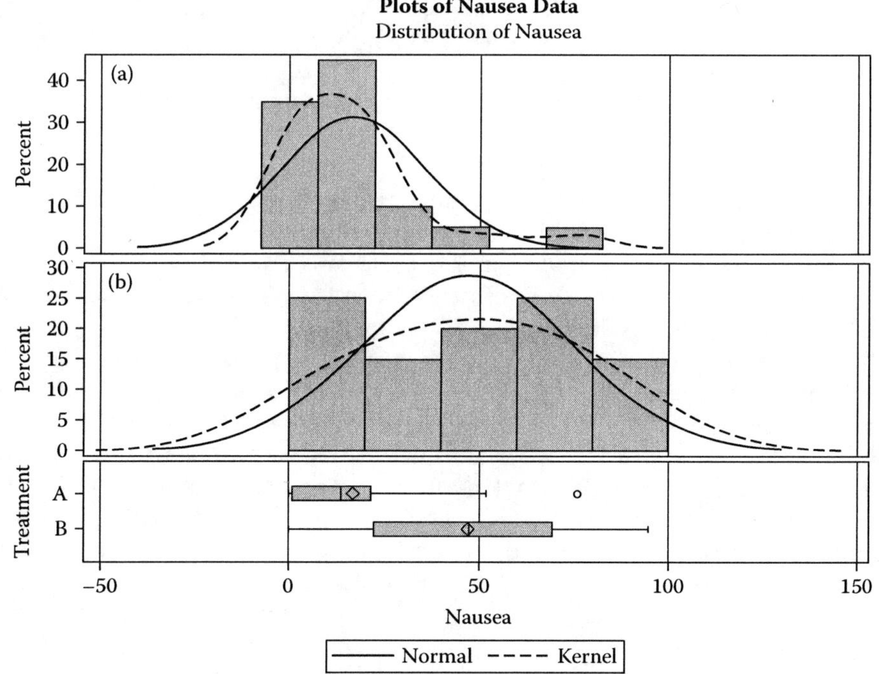

FIGURE 3.2
Proc ttest summary panel for nausea data.

TABLE 3.9

Results from Two-Independent Sample *t*-Tests on the Nausea Data

Variable: nausea						
Treatment	**N**	**Mean**	**Std Dev**	**Std Err**	**Minimum**	**Maximum**
A	20	16.9500	19.0829	4.2671	0	76.0000
B	20	47.1000	27.7828	6.2124	0	95.0000
Diff (1 − 2)		−30.1500	23.8332	7.5367		

Treatment	**Method**	**Mean**	**95% CL Mean**		**Std Dev**	**95% CL Std Dev**	
A		16.9500	8.0190	25.8810	19.0829	14.5123	27.8719
B		47.1000	34.0972	60.1028	27.7828	21.1286	40.5788
Diff (1 − 2)	Pooled	−30.1500	−45.4073	−14.8927	23.8332	19.4776	30.7157
Diff (1 − 2)	Satterthwaite	−30.1500	−45.4721	−14.8279			

Method	**Variances**	**DF**	**t Value**	**Pr > |t|**
Pooled	Equal	38	−4.00	0.0003
Satterthwaite	Unequal	33.664	−4.00	0.0003

Equality of Variances				
Method	**Num DF**	**Den DF**	**F Value**	**Pr > F**
Folded F	19	19	2.12	0.1101

self-assessment score for the active and placebo groups, with a 95% confidence interval for the mean difference being [−45.4,−14.9]. It is clear that the antiemetic given reduces nausea, and this claim is probably valid even given the departures from the assumption of normality of distributions of self-assessment scores indicated in Figure 3.2.

If we were concerned that the *t*-test is not appropriate for these data, we could apply the distribution-free equivalent of the two-independent samples *t*-test—namely, the *Wilcoxon Mann–Whitney rank sum test*, which is based on the joint ranking of the observations in the two groups (for details, see Altman 1991). Although it is not really necessary for this example as the evidence from what might be seen as a flawed *t*-test is so strong, we will demonstrate how to apply the distribution-free test. To do this, we use the `nparlway` procedure with the `wilcoxon` option:

```
proc nparlway data=nausea wilcoxon;
  class treatment;
  var nausea;
run;
```

TABLE 3.10

Results from Applying Wilcoxon Test to the Nausea Data in Table 3.8

Wilcoxon Scores (Rank Sums) for Variable nausea Classified by Variable Treatment					
treatment	N	Sum of Scores	Expected under H0	Std Dev under H0	Mean Score
A	20	288.50	410.0	36.893819	14.4250
B	20	531.50	410.0	36.893819	26.5750
Average scores were used for ties.					

Wilcoxon Two-Sample Test	
Statistic	288.5000
Normal approximation	
Z	−3.2797
One-sided Pr < Z	0.0005
Two-sided Pr > |Z|	0.0010
t Approximation	
One-sided Pr < Z	0.0011
Two-sided Pr > |Z|	0.0022
Z includes a continuity correction of 0.5.	

Kruskal–Wallis Test	
Chi-Square	10.8454
DF	1
Pr > Chi-Square	0.0010

The results shown in Table 3.10 confirm the results from the *t*-test described previously.

As a final example in this subsection, we will look at some data from a randomised controlled trial carried out on insulin-dependent diabetic patients with neuropathy (Hommel et al. 1986). The data in Table 3.11 show the systolic blood pressures of 16 patients before and after 1 week's treatment with captopril or placebo.

For the formal analysis, we shall begin by looking at the before and after values of blood pressure in the captopril group. Here, of course, we cannot use the independent samples *t*-test because the before and after values are taken on the same nine patients and thus are correlated rather than independent; we must use a *paired t-test* (see Altman 1996). This test assumes that the differences between the before and after blood pressures have a normal distribution; here there are very few (too few) observations on which to judge normality or otherwise, so we will simply proceed with using the paired *t*-test without trying to check assumptions.

TABLE 3.11

Blood Pressure Results from Trial Involving Dependent
Diabetic Patients with Neuropathy

	Captopril			Placebo	
	Baseline	After 1 week		Baseline	After 1 week
1	147	137	1	133	139
2	129	120	2	129	134
3	158	141	3	152	136
4	164	137	4	161	151
5	134	140	5	154	147
6	155	144	6	141	137
7	151	134	7	156	149
8	141	123			
9	153	142			

Source: Hommel, E., Parving, H., Mathiesen, E., Edsberg, B., Nielsen, M. D., and Giese, F. 1986. *British Medical Journal*, 293:467–470.

We begin with a data step that is similar to the one for the preceding `folates` data. The problem of different numbers of observations in each group is solved this time by adding missing values and using list input—but only outputting the observations with nonmissing ids. This data step also illustrates the use of an iterative do loop with character values.

```
data captopril;
   do treatment='Captopril', 'Placebo';
   input id basebp week1bp @;
   if id~=. then output;
   end;
datalines;
1 147 137 1 133 139
2 129 120 2 129 134
3 158 141 3 152 136
4 164 137 4 161 151
5 134 140 5 154 147
6 155 144 6 141 137
7 151 134 7 156 149
8 141 123 . .   .
9 153 142 . .   .
;
```

Now we can apply the paired t-test separately to the data in both groups, again using `proc ttest`. We could use two proc steps each with a `where` statement to select one of the groups, but instead we use a `by` statement. This requires that the data set first be sorted in order of `by` variable. The syntax for a paired t-test is largely self-explanatory, but note that the pair of variables needs to be joined with an asterisk. Several pairs of variables can be listed on the same statement.

```
proc sort data=captopril;
 by treatment;
run;
proc ttest data=captopril;
 paired basebp*week1bp;
 by treatment;
run;
```

The results are shown in Table 3.12. For the group treated with captopril, the paired *t*-test is highly significant, and the 95% confidence interval for the difference between baseline and week 1 means for blood pressure is [5.8,19.6]. In the placebo group, the paired *t*-test is not significant and the 95% CI for the difference, baseline to week 1, is [−2.6,12.0].

But before we use the results of the two separate paired *t*-tests to jump to the conclusion that captopril is more effective than placebo at reducing blood pressure, we should stop and think. If we do, we should quickly come to the conclusion that the two paired *t*-tests do *not* tell us all we wish to know about what is happening in this trial. The reason is that they do not provide

TABLE 3.12

Paired *t*-Test for Captopril Data

Difference: basebp − week1bp; treatment = Captopril					
N	**Mean**	**Std Dev**	**Std Err**	**Minimum**	**Maximum**
9	12.6667	8.9861	2.9954	−6.0000	27.0000

Mean	**95% CL Mean**		**Std Dev**	**95% CL Std Dev**	
12.6667	5.7593	19.5740	8.9861	6.0697	17.2153

DF	**t Value**	**Pr > |t|**
8	4.23	0.0029

Difference: basebp − week1bp; treatment = Placebo					
N	**Mean**	**Std Dev**	**Std Err**	**Minimum**	**Maximum**
7	4.7143	7.9102	2.9898	−6.0000	16.0000

Mean	**95% CL Mean**		**Std Dev**	**95% CL Std Dev**	
4.7143	−2.6014	12.0300	7.9102	5.0973	17.4188

DF	**t Value**	**Pr > |t|**
6	1.58	0.1659

an answer to whether the change in blood pressure over 1 week is the same in both treatment groups; the answers given by the separate tests—change of BP significant in one group and nonsignificant in the other—do *not* answer this question. To address the question of most interest about these data properly, we can apply a two-sample *t*-test to the differences in blood pressures in each group using the following SAS code:

```
data captopril;
  set captopril;
  bpdiff=basebp-week1bp;
run;

proc ttest data=captopril;
  class treatment;
  var bpdiff;
run;
```

The results are given in Table 3.13. The two-sample test is not significant at the 5% level and the 95% CI for the difference in the baseline to week 1 differences in blood pressure is [–1.3,17.20]. The trial produces no evidence that

TABLE 3.13

Results of Two Independent Sample *t*-Tests Applied to BP Differences, Baseline to Week, in the Two Treatment Groups in the Captopril Data

Variable: bpdiff						
treatment	N	Mean	Std Dev	Std Err	Minimum	Maximum
Captopril	9	12.6667	8.9861	2.9954	–6.0000	27.0000
Placebo	7	4.7143	7.9102	2.9898	–6.0000	16.0000
Diff (1 – 2)		7.9524	8.5416	4.3046		

treatment	Method	Mean	95% CL Mean		Std Dev	95% CL Std Dev	
Captopril		12.6667	5.7593	19.5740	8.9861	6.0697	17.2153
Placebo		4.7143	–2.6014	12.0300	7.9102	5.0973	17.4188
Diff (1 – 2)	Pooled	7.9524	–1.2800	17.1848	8.5416	6.2535	13.4710
Diff (1 – 2)	Satterthwaite	7.9524	–1.1420	17.0467			

Method	Variances	DF	t Value	Pr > |t|
Pooled	Equal	14	1.85	0.0859
Satterthwaite	Unequal	13.722	1.88	0.0816

Equality of Variances				
Method	Num DF	Den DF	F Value	Pr > F
Folded F	8	6	1.29	0.7773

the change in mean BP from baseline to 1 week differs for captopril and placebo. Of course, the number of patients in the trial is very small, so the tests performed are of rather low power.

Pocock et al. (2002) point out that clinical trial investigators often record a great deal of baseline data on each patient at randomisation. Such data can include, for example, details of previous disease events, current medication, age, sex, marital status, education, etc. In addition, it is very common to have one or more measurements of the main outcome variable(s) made before treatment begins, as in the example just discussed. How such baseline data can be incorporated into the analysis will be taken up in Chapter 6, where we shall also return to the captopril trial data.

3.5 Summary

No satisfactory alternative to the randomised controlled trial for evaluating competing therapies exists. 'All things being equal, randomised controlled trials are more able to attribute effects to causes' (Barton 2000) should be the motto etched on the hearts of all with treatments to compare.

But as Archie Cochrane once said, 'The randomised controlled trial is a very beautiful technique of wide applicability, but as with everything else there are snags' (Cochrane 1984). Clinical trials are certainly not perfect; for example, where they focus on narrow patient groups or exclude important segments of the population, there may be difficulties in generalising their results. Thus, although RCTs are often labelled as the 'gold standard' for research, Simon (2001) may be right that 'silver standard' might be more appropriate.

Nevertheless, clinical trials remain the essential methodology in the evaluation of the effectiveness of treatments and are a major contributor to improvements in health and well-being. This being so, the ethical issues associated with such studies (see Everitt and Wessely 2008) should not be allowed to cloud the judgement of potential participants in such trials. Clinicians and others need to work hard to convince an increasingly well-informed public that RCTs are necessary and valuable and that discarding this methodology will likely lead to confusion regarding the value of treatments and to the distinct possibility of worthless and even dangerous treatments becoming prevalent.

The discussion of clinical trials has of necessity been relatively brief, concentrating as it has on the use of SAS for such studies. For a full discussion of issues not covered here—for example, blinding, intention to treat, and sub-group analyses—see Everitt and Wessely (2008).

4

Epidemiology

4.1 Introduction

Epidemiology is the study of disease (in the widest sense and including both noncommunicable and infectious diseases) and its risk factors. Epidemiological studies are characterised by *observation* rather than *intervention*, which is the quintessential component of clinical trials. An early example of an epidemiological study is that of John Snow in 1854, who investigated deaths due to cholera that occurred in the same area of London (see Chapter 2.) More recently, epidemiologists have been involved with investigations into the proximity of nuclear power stations to the homes of people diagnosed with leukaemia, the question of the existence or otherwise of the so-called 'Gulf War Syndrome' amongst soldiers who fought in the Gulf War in 1990 and 1991, and the outbreak of severe acute respiratory syndrome (SARS) in 2002 and 2003.

Epidemiological studies are rarely as convincing as clinical trials in attributing a *causal mechanism*. In a well designed and well performed clinical trial, a significant treatment effect can, with some confidence, be said to be *caused* by the different treatments patients received. With an epidemiological study, attributing causality is far more problematic and would normally be claimed only after a range of studies carried out in a variety of settings had all found, say, the same relationship between some risk factor of interest and some particular disease. Investigators tempted to ascribe causality on the basis of a single, perhaps relatively small epidemiological study should think again.

The three main types of epidemiological study are described in the following section.

4.2 Types of Epidemiological Study

The three types of epidemiological study are

- Cross sectional (surveys)
- Case control
- Cohort

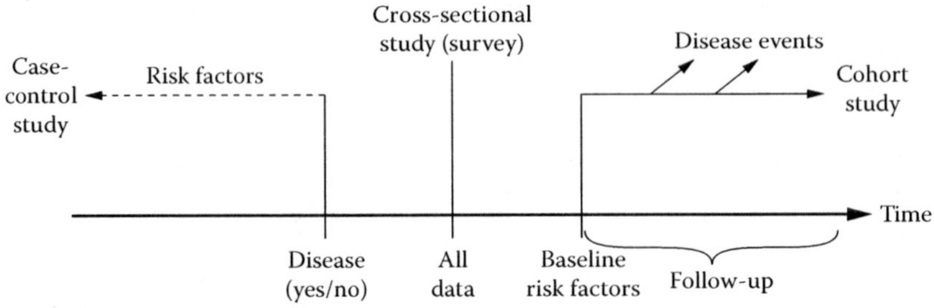

FIGURE 4.1
Schematic comparison of the three major study designs used in epidemiology. (Taken from Woodward, M. 2011. In *Encyclopaedic Companion to Medical Statistics*, 2nd ed., B. S. Everitt and C. Palmer, Eds., Chichester, England: Wiley. With permission.)

The diagram in Figure 4.1 shows a schematic comparison of these three types, each of which we will now describe in detail.

4.2.1 Surveys

Survey methods are based on the simple discovery that 'asking questions is a remarkably efficient way to obtain information from and about people' (Schuman and Kalton 1985, p. 635). Surveys involve an exchange of information between researcher and respondent; the researcher identifies topics of interest, and the respondent provides knowledge or opinion about these topics. Depending upon the length and content of the survey, as well as the facilities available, this exchange can be accomplished via written questionnaires, in-person interviews, or telephone conversations; in the twenty-first century, surveys via the Internet are increasingly common.

Surveys conducted by clinicians are usually designed to elicit information about the respondents' disease states and levels of risk factors for these diseases. But they may also ask about a person's lifestyle—even the most intimate parts of that lifestyle. One of the most famous surveys of the twentieth century, for example, was that conducted by Alfred Charles Kinsey, a student of human sexual behaviour in the 1940s and 1950s. The first Kinsey report, *Sexual Behaviour in the Human Male*, appeared in 1948 (see Kinsey, Wardell, and Martin 1948), and the second, *Sexual Behaviour in the Human Female*, in 1953 (see Kinsey et al. 1953). It is no exaggeration to say that both reports caused a sensation, and the first quickly became a bestseller.

An example of cross-sectional data from a survey is given in Table 4.1. The data come from Senie et al. (1981), who report the results of asking women about how frequently they carried out breast self-examination.

Surveys are often a flexible and powerful approach to gathering information of interest, but careful consideration needs to be given to several aspects of the survey if the information is to be accurate, particularly when

TABLE 4.1

Data on Breast Self-Examination

Age	Monthly	Occasionally/Never	Total
Younger than 45	91	141	232
45 or older	259	705	964
Total	350	846	1196

Source: Senie, R. T., Rosen, P. P., Lesser, M. L., and Kinne, D. W. 1981. *American Journal of Public Health*, 71:583–590. Please see back of this book for the complete table.

dealing with a sensitive topic. Having a representative sample, having a large enough sample, minimising nonresponse, and ensuring that the questions asked elicit accurate responses are just a few of the issues that the researcher thinking of carrying out a survey needs to consider. Readers are referred to Sudman and Bradburn (1982) and Tourangeau, Rips, and Rasinski (2000) for a detailed account of survey methodology.

Surveys give a 'snapshot' and have limited use in investigating causality; for example, in a survey of where a particular chronic disease is found to be less common among those who smoke, the obvious conclusion that smoking tends to protect people against the disease is not the only explanation of the finding. An alternative is that smokers, having developed the disease, give up the habit, thus leading to a predominance of the disease among those not smoking at the time of the survey. (This example and account are taken from Woodward 2011.)

4.2.2 Case-Control Studies

In case-control studies, a group of people with the disease of interest (the *cases*) is compared with a group of people without the disease (the *controls*) in respect of past exposure to a risk factor for the disease. The primary aim of a case-control study is to explore the aetiology of a disease by searching for difference in the prior exposure of the cases and controls to a range of suspect agents or factors. A classic case-control study is that described in Doll and Hill (1950), who recruited 649 male lung cancer cases and 649 male controls during an 18-month period in London. They were able to show a clear increase in risk with daily cigarette consumption.

An example of data collected from a case-control study is shown in Table 4.2. The data come from Adelusi (1977), who describes a case-control study for investigating whether age at first sexual intercourse (before and after the age of 15) is associated with the subsequent development of cervical cancer. The cases were married Nigerian women with a histological diagnosis of invasive cancer of the cervix. The control group consisted of healthy married women of child-bearing age. A questionnaire was administered to 47 cases and 173 controls; the subjects were asked about their sexual habits, in particular about their age at first intercourse.

TABLE 4.2

Data from a Case-Control Study of Sexual Habits Amongst Nigerian Women

Age at First Intercourse	Cases	Controls	Total
Younger than 15	36	78	114
Older than 15	11	95	106
Total	47	173	220

Source: Adelusi, B. 1977. *International Journal of Gynaecology and Obstetrics*, 15:5–11.

The prime advantages of the case-control study are that it is relatively simple to carry out and consequently is also relatively quick and cheap. The case-control study is also valuable when the disease of interest is rare. However, there are a number of disadvantages with this type of study. Sackett (1979) identified as many as 35 possible biases that can occur with case-control studies, including selection of cases and controls, recall bias, and inaccuracy of retrospective data.

To overcome some of the problems with selecting cases and controls, matched case-control studies are increasingly popular. One or more controls are chosen for each case and matched as closely as possible to the case for various factors that are not of intrinsic interest to the study; common matching factors are age and sex. One-to-one matching gives rise to a matched-pairs study. To increase the statistical power of the study, more than one control can be chosen for each case, although Woodward (2011) suggests that studying more than four controls per case is rarely worthwhile as the effort spent in collecting the data on the extra controls tends to outweigh the minimal increase in power.

An example of data from a matched case-control study is shown in Table 4.3. Here, the cases were 175 women of reproductive age (15–44) discharged alive from 43 hospitals in five cities after initial attacks of idiopathic thromboplebities, pulmonary embolism, or cerebral thrombosis or embolism. The controls were matched with their cases for hospital, residence, time of hospitalisation, race, age, marital status, and a number of other variables. The history of oral contraceptive use by the women was then determined. (Notice that it is counts of pairs that is important here, as we shall see when we come to the analysis of epidemiological data in Section 4.4.). For more details on case-control studies, see Schlesselman (1982) and Wacholder and Hartge (2005).

4.2.3 Cohort Studies

The cohort (or prospective) study is the design of choice for an epidemiological investigation. A study population is identified before the occurrence of disease and then followed in time until the first occurrence of the disease or the end of the study, whichever comes first. (In what follows, we shall ignore the complicating factor that at the end of the study some subjects will

TABLE 4.3

Data from a Matched Case-Control Study after Oral
Contraceptive Use in 175 Pairs of Married Women

Oral Contraceptive Use	Number of Pairs
Used by both members of the pair	10
Used by the case only	57
Used by the control only	13
Used by neither the case nor the control	95

not have contracted the disease but will do so later; their time to the event
of interest—that is, getting the disease—is *censored.* We shall deal with the
issue in Chapter 16.)

Typically, subjects are classified as exposed or not exposed to one or more
putative risk factors at the beginning of the study—for example, smoker
or nonsmoker—so that prevalence of disease amongst exposed and non-
exposed can be compared at the end of the study. After their case-control
study mentioned in the previous subsection suggested an association
between smoking and lung cancer, Doll and Hill undertook a large cohort
study beginning with a simple questionnaire about smoking habits being
sent to all doctors on a medical register and following up members of the
cohort until their deaths. The study is described in Doll and Hill (1954, 1956)
and the results provided compelling evidence that smoking was a cause of
lung cancer. There were some however who remained unconvinced; according to McMichael (2010) Fisher, used as he was to experimental studies of
randomly assigned agricultural plots, argued that epidemiological studies without randomisation were not 'scientific'. To underscore the point, he
hypothesised the existence of an underlying gene that caused both smoking behaviour and a disposition to lung cancer. He wrote abusive letters to
Doll and suggested publicly that he be stripped of his Fellow of the Royal
Society for having perpetrated poor science. (Fisher partly recanted in the
1960s.)

Some hypothetical data from a cohort study that mirrors that of Doll and
Hill are shown in Table 4.4. These data arise from a cohort of 1,000 people (400 smokers and 600 nonsmokers) followed up for 20 years; 50 subjects
developed lung cancer: 45 smokers and five nonsmokers.

The cohort study represents an improvement over the case-control
study in that it is less suspect to a number of biases (see Prentice 2005),
but there remain some difficulties, notably that they can take a very long
time and thus may be very expensive. And for studying rare events, it
would be necessary to follow a very large number of subjects to get an
adequate number contracting the disease to make a meaningful comparison possible.

For a detailed account of cohort studies, see Breslow and Day (1987).

TABLE 4.4

Data from a Cohort Study Investigating the Possible Link
between Smoking and Lung Cancer

Group	Lung Cancer	No Lung Cancer	Total
Smokers	45	355	400
Nonsmokers	5	595	600
Total	50	950	1000

4.3 Relative Risk and Odds Ratios

The data from many epidemiological studies can be arranged in a 2×2
table, three examples of which were given in the previous section. We can
imagine the population data arranged in a similar fashion as that shown in
Table 4.5, where the terms represent the probabilities of the various events
indexed by the rows and columns of the table. If the probabilities were
known, then probability of having the disease for those individuals having
the risk factor present would be $p_1/(p_1+p_3)$ and for those individuals not
having the risk factor present would be $p_2/(p_2+p_4)$. The ratio of these two
quantities,

$$\frac{p_1/(p_2+p_4)}{p_2/(p_1+p_3)} \tag{4.1}$$

is the population value of what is known as the *relative risk*. But, of course,
we do not know the probabilities in Table 4.5, so we have to turn to sample
data to estimate them.

The frequencies that result from sampling n values from the population
can also be written in a 2×2 table, as shown in Table 4.6. Let's now look
at the data in this table to see the different ways in which they arise for
a case-control and a cohort study. In the former, the investigation begins
with $a+c$ cases and a group of $b+d$ controls. Then a count of the numbers
exposed and not exposed to the risk factor is made and the 2×2 table
completed.

With a cohort study, the investigation begins with $a+b$ subjects who have
been exposed to the risk factor and $c+d$ who have not been exposed, and
these are followed for an appropriate time period (which, for convenience, is
assumed to be very long so that the problem of censored observations [see
Chapter 16] does not arise), thus enabling the table to be completed with the
numbers in each group contracting the disease.

In a cohort study, the relative risk and the two probabilities that make up
the relative risk can be estimated directly from the proportion of individuals

TABLE 4.5

Population Epidemiological Data

Risk Factor	Disease Present	Disease Absent	
Present	p_1	p_3	p_1+p_3
Absent	p_2	p_4	p_1+p_4
	p_1+p_2	p_3+p_4	1

TABLE 4.6

Sample Epidemiological Data

Risk Factor	Disease Present	Disease Absent	
Present	a	b	$a+b$
Absent	c	d	$c+d$
	$a+c$	$b+d$	

in the sample who develop the disease in the follow-up period in the risk-factor-present and risk-factor-absent groups. Thus, in a cohort study, the estimate for the probability of having the disease for those individuals having the risk factor is simply $a/(a+b)$ and, for those individuals not having the risk factor, it is $c/(c+d)$, leading to an estimate for the relative risk of $a(c+d)/c(a+b)$.

Now consider when the data in Table 4.6 arise from a case-control study. Here the proportion of cases in the study will not necessarily be comparable to the proportion of diseased persons in the population, with the consequence that the data cannot be used to estimate the relative risk directly, as is done in a cohort study. In this case, what can legitimately be estimated is the probability of the risk factor being present amongst people with the disease and similarly for the people without the disease. Therefore, for this type of study, we can estimate, for example, the conditional probability, Pr (having the risk factor |having the disease) but not the conditional probability of most interest, Pr (having the disease| having the risk factor), which can only be estimated directly from a cohort study. But when the disease is relatively rare so that the probability of having the disease is small, then in Equation (4.1) p_1 will be small compared to p_3 and p_2 will be small compared to p_4 and the relative risk becomes, approximately, $\dfrac{p_1/p_2}{p_3/p_4} = \dfrac{p_1 p_4}{p_2 p_3}$.

This is known as the *odds ratio* (OR): the ratio of the probabilities of having and not having the disease and having the risk factor present, divided by the ratio of the corresponding probabilities when not having the risk factor present. This approximation to the relative risk is often simply labelled relative risk and it can be estimated from both case-control and cohort studies as long as in the former the cases are a random, unbiased sample of all cases of the disease and the controls are a similar sample from all people without the disease. In both cases, the estimate of the population odds ratio (generally represented by ψ) is given by

$$\hat{\psi} = \frac{ad}{bc} \tag{4.2}$$

We shall return to consider more about the estimation of the relative risk and the odds ratio and about the analysis of epidemiological data in Section 4.5, but first we need to look at how to determine the sample sizes needed in observational studies.

4.4 Sample Size Estimation for Epidemiologic Studies

Consideration of sample size is as important for observational studies as it is for randomised clinical trials; the investigator needs to know whether his or her study will be large enough to answer the research question with sufficient statistical power. Therefore, in this section we will describe how to use SAS to estimate sample sizes—first for case-control studies and then for cohort studies.

4.4.1 Sample Size Estimation for Case-Control Studies

Using the nomenclature introduced in the previous section, the probability of having the risk factor present for the cases is $p_1/(p_1+p_2)$, which we shall denote as P_1; the probability of having the risk factor present for the controls is $p_3/(p_3+p_4)$, which we shall denote by P_0. For an unmatched case-control study with one control per case, the sample size, n, required in each group (we are assuming equally sized groups and two-sided tests) to achieve a power, $1-\beta$, when testing with significance level α, is given by

$$n = \frac{\left(z_{\alpha/2}\sqrt{(2\bar{P}\bar{Q})} + z_\beta\sqrt{(P_1(1-P_1)+P_0(1-P_0))}\right)^2}{(P_1-P_0)^2} \tag{4.3}$$

where

$$\bar{P} = (P_1 + P_0)/2 \text{ and } \bar{Q} = (1-\bar{P})$$

This formula is obtained from a normal approximation to the test statistic for comparing two proportions—that is, the familiar chi-squared statistic with a single degree of freedom (examples of using the test will be given in the next section).

For a study with k controls per case, the value of n is found from

$$n = \frac{\left(z_{\alpha/2}\sqrt{\left[(1+1/k)\bar{P}'\bar{Q}'\right]} + z_\beta \sqrt{(P_1 Q_1 + P_0 Q_0)}\right)^2}{(P_1 - P_0)^2} \tag{4.4}$$

where

$$\bar{P}' = (P_1 + kP_0)/(1+k), \quad \bar{Q}' = (1 - \bar{P}'), \quad Q_0 = 1 - P_0 \text{ and } Q_1 = 1 - P_1$$

In Equations (4.3) and (4.4),

- $Z_{\alpha|2}$ is the value of the normal distribution that cuts off an upper tail probability of $\alpha|2$. Thus, for $\alpha = 0.05$, $Z_{\alpha|2} = 1.96$.
- Z_β is the value of the normal distribution that cuts off an upper tail probability of β. Thus, for a power of 0.90, $\beta = 0.10$ and $Z_\beta = 1.28$.

In practice, the exposure rate among controls, P_0, is usually obtained from previous studies and estimated from the general population. The odds ratio, which, as we have seen in the previous section, in a case-control study, acts as an approximation to the relative risk, is then specified under the alternative hypothesis in the calculation of sample size. (The corresponding null hypothesis is that the odds ratio is one implying that the risk factor and disease state are not related; see the next section.) When using the odds ratio in sample size estimation, the exposure rate among cases can be found as follows:

$$P_1 = \frac{P_0 \text{OR}}{\left[1 + P_0(\text{OR} - 1)\right]} \tag{4.5}$$

We will illustrate the sample size calculations using an example suggested in Liu (2005) involving a case-control study of a potential association between congenital heart defects and oral contraceptives used before the time of conception. We have a prior estimate of the exposure rate amongst controls of 30% and will apply a two-sided test with $\alpha = 0.05$ and $\beta = 0.10$, so that the power will be 0.90 and we will take one control per case. We can now calculate the required sample size in order to detect an OR = 2 using the following SAS code:

```
proc power;
   twosamplefreq
      oddsratio = 2
      refproportion = 0.3
      power = 0.9
      npergroup = .
      ;
run;
```

This gives the required sample size in each group to be 188.

Now let us see what happens if we repeat the calculation using five cases per control. To do this, we specify that the total number is to be calculated with the `ntotal` option and use the `groupweights` option to specify the ratio of controls to cases:

```
proc power;
   twosamplefreq
      oddsratio = 2
      refproportion = 0.3
      power = 0.9
      groupweights=(5 1)
      ntotal = .
      ;
run;
```

This leads to the result that 111 cases and 555 controls are needed.

4.4.2 Sample Size Estimation for Cohort Studies

The sample size formula here is the same as that given in Equation (4.3) but with P_1 now being the proportion of subjects who develop the disease in the risk-factor-present group and P_0 the corresponding probability for the risk-free group. As an example, we will consider a cohort study investigating a possible link between smoking cigarettes and suffering from lung cancer. We wish to detect a relative risk of 1.5 when the probability of the disease being

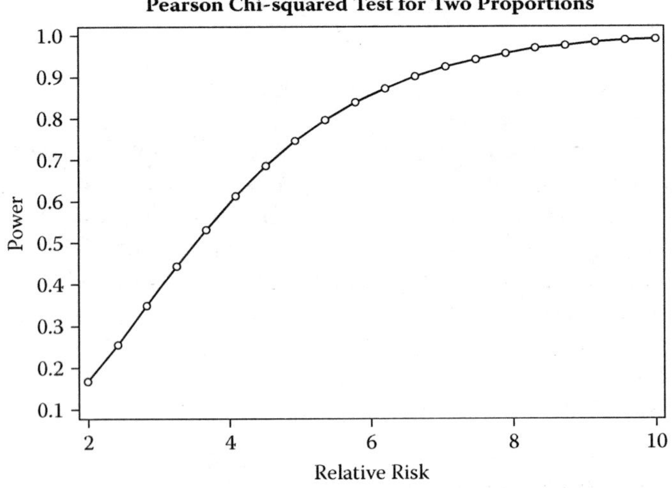

FIGURE 4.2
Power curve for fixed-size groups of 600 and 400.

present in the risk-factor-absent group is 0.005 and with $\alpha = 0.05$ and $\beta = 0.10$. The necessary sample size can be found from the following SAS code:

```
proc power;
   twosamplefreq
      relativerisk = 1.5
      refproportion = 0.005
      power = 0.9
      npergroup = .
      ;
run;
```

This gives the value 20,882! This demonstrates that, indeed, very large samples are needed to detect differences when the event of interest is rare.

Now let us look at how the power changes in this example as relative risk increases for fixed-size groups of 600 and 400. We can produce a *power curve* with the following SAS code:

```
proc power plotonly;
   twosamplefreq
      relativerisk = 2 to 10 by .5
      refproportion = 0.005
      power = .
      groupns =(600 400)
      ;
      plot x =effect;
run;
```

The resulting plot is shown in Figure 4.2.

4.5 Simple Analyses for Data from Observational Studies

Having considered the estimation of sample size, we can return to how we formally assess the 2×2 tables of data that arise from many epidemiological studies and how we can estimate and find confidence intervals for the two quantities of interest met in Section 4.3—namely, the relative risk and the odds ratio. More sophisticated analyses of such data will be the subject of later chapters, particularly Chapter 10 on *logistic regression*. We begin with the significance test that is used on 2×2 tables of counts from whatever type of study from which they arise.

4.5.1 Chi-Squared Test for Association

To test for association between the row and column classifications for 2×2 tables of frequencies, we apply the familiar chi-squared test given by

$$X^2 = \frac{n(ad - bc)^2}{(a+b)(c+d)(a+c)(b+d)} \tag{4.6}$$

Under the null hypothesis that the row and column variables are not related, the test statistic, X^2, has a chi-squared distribution with a single degree of freedom.

4.5.2 Finding a Confidence Interval for the Relative Risk and the Odds Ratio

The chi-squared test tells us whether there is any evidence between the row and column variables. However, in most cases, we would like to know a little more and this 'little more' is, in general, estimates and confidence intervals for the relative risks or, more commonly, for the odds ratio, reflecting that the odds ratio is more important when we come to more sophisticated of epidemiological data using logistic regression (see Chapter 10). But here we begin with the population relative risk, r, which we can estimate from the four frequencies in a 2×2 table as

$$\hat{r} = \frac{a/(a+b)}{c/(c+d)} \tag{4.7}$$

The estimate of the variance of $\log(\hat{r})$ is given by

$$\hat{\text{var}}(\log(r)) = \frac{1}{a} - \frac{1}{a+b} + \frac{1}{c} - \frac{1}{c+d} \tag{4.8}$$

This leads to a 95% confidence interval for the logarithm of the relative risk of

$$\log(\hat{r}) \pm 1.96\sqrt{\text{var}(\log(\hat{r}))} \tag{4.9}$$

The required confidence interval for the population relative risk can now be found by exponentiating the upper and lower limits in (4.9).

Moving on to the odds ratio, as we have already seen, this can be estimated as $\hat{\psi} = ad/bc$. A confidence interval for the odds ratio is again most easily found by initially considering its log value because the variance of $\log(\hat{\psi})$ can be estimated very simply from

$$\hat{\text{var}}(\ln \hat{\psi}) = \frac{1}{a} + \frac{1}{b} + \frac{1}{c} + \frac{1}{d} \tag{4.10}$$

This leads to the following 95% confidence interval for $\ln(\psi)$:

$$\ln(\hat{\psi}) \pm 1.96 \times \sqrt{\hat{\text{var}}[\ln(\hat{\psi})]} \tag{4.11}$$

The required confidence interval for ψ can now be found by exponentiating the upper and lower limits in (4.11).

4.5.3 Applying SAS to Analyse Examples of Epidemiological Data

In order to apply the chi-squared test to the data shown in Tables 4.1, 4.2, and 4.4 and to find estimates of odds ratios and relative risks, we first create a SAS data set from each of them as follows. We have used character variables to represent the rows and columns, but as these are case sensitive, care is needed to ensure consistency. For example 'monthly' and 'Monthly' would be different values for frequency:

```
data self_exam;
input agegroup $ frequency $ num;
datalines;
Under45  Monthly   91
Under45  Rarely    141
Over45   Monthly  259
Over45   Rarely   705
;

data ca_cervix;
  input debutage $ status $ num;
  datalines;
   Under15 case       36
   Under15 control   78
   Over15  case       11
   Over15  control   95
  ;

data ca_lung;
  input group $ lung_ca $ num;
  datalines;
   Smoker       Yes     45
   Smoker       No      355
   Nonsmoker    Yes     5
   Nonsmoker    No      595
  ;
```

Having created SAS data sets with the cell counts in, we can analyse them with proc freq:

```
proc freq data=self_exam order=data;
  tables agegroup*frequency /chisq;
  weight num;
run;

proc freq data=ca_cervix order=data;
  tables Debutage*status /chisq;
  weight num;
run;
```

```
proc freq data=ca_lung order=data;
 tables Group*lung_ca /chisq;
 weight num;
run;
```

`Proc freq` is used both to produce contingency tables and to analyse them. The `tables` statement defines the table to be produced and specifies the analysis of it. The variables that form the rows and columns are joined with an asterisk. These may be numeric or character variables. One-way frequency distributions are produced where variables are not joined by asterisks. Several tables may be specified on a single `tables` statement.

The options after the '/' specify the type of analysis. The `chisq` option requests chi-squared tests of independence and measures of association based on chi-squared. The `weight` statement specifies a variable that contains weights for each observation. The default weight is 1, so the `weight` statement is not usually needed when the data set consists of observations on individuals. In these examples, the data are in the form of a contingency table and the `weight` statement is used to specify the cell counts.

The `order=data` option on the `proc` statement specifies that the rows and columns are to be laid out in the order that they occur in the data. The default would be alphabetical order. This is for purely cosmetic purposes so that the tables in the output (see Table 4.7) match Tables 4.1, 4.2, and 4.4.

Looking first at the statistics for the breast self-examination data, we find that the chi-squared statistic is highly significant, implying that there is strong evidence for an association between age and breast self-examination. Older women are more likely to make a monthly examination of their breasts than are younger women. (The other tests mentioned in the table are variants of the chi-squared test, which we will not discuss here because they all give very similar results to the chi-squared test.)

Looking next at the statistics for the data on the sexual habits of Nigerian women, we find again a very significant chi-squared value. There is a greater proportion of the cases—here, women with cancer of the cervix—than the controls, having first sexual intercourse before the age of 15 years.

Lastly, the statistics for the smoking and lung cancer data give very strong evidence of an association between smoking and subsequent development of lung cancer.

The chi-squared statistic leads to a p-value for the null hypothesis that there is no association between the row and column classifications in the 2×2 table—that is, that the two variables forming the table are independent or, equivalently, the population odds ratio is one. But in most studies, a p-value is not really of very great interest; far more interesting is an estimate and confidence interval for the odds ratio (and on occasions the relative risk, although the odds ratio is more commonly reported).

TABLE 4.7

Analysis of Three Sets of Epidemiological Data

(a) Breast Self-Examination

Table of Agegroup by Frequency

agegroup	Frequency		
Frequency **Percent** **Row pct** **Col pct**	**Monthly**	**Rarely**	**Total**
Under 45	91	141	232
	7.61	11.79	19.40
	39.22	60.78	
	26.00	16.67	
Over 45	259	705	964
	21.66	58.95	80.60
	26.87	73.13	
	74.00	83.33	
Total	350	846	1196
	29.26	70.74	100.00

Statistics for Table of Agegroup by Frequency

Statistic	DF	Value	Prob
Chi-Squared	1	13.7936	0.0002
Likelihood Ratio Chi-Squared	1	13.2376	0.0003
Continuity Adj. Chi-Squared	1	13.2031	0.0003
Mantel–Haenszel Chi-Squared	1	13.7821	0.0002
Phi Coefficient		0.1074	
Contingency Coefficient		0.1068	
Cramér's V		0.1074	

Sample size = 1196

(b) Sexual Habits Amongst Nigerian Women

Statistics for Table of Debutage by Status

Statistic	DF	Value	Prob
Chi-Squared	1	14.6969	0.0001
Likelihood Ratio Chi-Squared	1	15.3913	<.0001
Continuity Adj. Chi-Squared	1	13.4620	0.0002
Mantel–Haenszel Chi-Squared	1	14.6301	0.0001
Phi Coefficient		–0.2585	
Contingency Coefficient		0.2502	
Cramér's V		–0.2585	

(Continued)

TABLE 4.7 (*Continued*)

Analysis of Three Sets of Epidemiological Data

(c) Smoking And Lung Cancer

Statistics for Table of Group by Lung_ca

Statistic	DF	Value	Prob
Chi-Squared	1	54.8246	<.0001
Likelihood Ratio Chi-Squared	1	57.8290	<.0001
Continuity Adj. Chi-Squared	1	52.6535	<.0001
Mantel–Haenszel Chi-Squared	1	54.7697	<.0001
Phi Coefficient		0.2341	
Contingency Coefficient		0.2280	
Cramér's V		0.2341	

The relative risk and odds ratio and their confidence intervals are requested via the `relrisk` option in the `tables` statement. Thus, for the data on self-examination, the tables statement would be `tables agegroup*frequency /relrisk;`. The rest of the proc step would remain as before. The `relrisk` option assumes that the groups to be compared form the rows of the table as they do in these examples. The relevant part of the output is shown in Table 4.8. For the data from the cross-sectional study concerned with breast self-examination, the 95% confidence interval for the odds ratio is [1.3,2.4]; the odds of an older women making monthly examinations of her breasts are between 1.3 and 2.4 times the odds for a younger woman doing so.

For the second data set on the sexual habits of Nigerian women, the corresponding confidence interval is [1.9,8.3]. The conclusion is that the odds of contracting cervical cancer in women who have first intercourse when they are relatively young are between about two and eight times the odds as those for women who have first intercourse when they are older than 15 years. (Note that as these data arise from a case-control study, the relative risk given is not an appropriate statistic to report.)

For the lung cancer and smoking data, which are the result of a cohort study, we can look at the relative risk; this is estimated as $\dfrac{45/400}{5/600} = 13.5$ with a 95% confidence interval of [5.4,33.7]. The evidence from the data is that the risk of somebody who smokes developing lung cancer is at least five times the risk for a nonsmoker and maybe nearly 34 times higher.

(It should always be remembered that although the odds ratio and relative risk are very important indices of the strength of an association between a risk factor and a disease, they say nothing about the probability that an individual will contract that disease. This may explain why, despite their high relative risks of being killed in an airplane crash, airplane pilots can still sleep easy in their beds. They know that the absolute risk of their being the victim of a crash remains extremely small.)

TABLE 4.8

Odds Ratios and Relative Risks for the Three Epidemiological Data Sets

(a) Breast Self-Examination

Statistics for Table of Agegroup by Frequency

Estimates of the Relative Risk (row1/row2)		
Type of Study	**Value**	**95% Confidence Limits**
Case-Control (Odds Ratio)	1.7568	1.3020 2.3703
Cohort (Col1 risk)	1.4599	1.2060 1.7673
Cohort (Col2 risk)	0.8310	0.7443 0.9279

(b) Sexual Habits of Nigerian Women

Statistics for Table of Debutage by Status

Estimates of the Relative Risk (row1/row2)		
Type of Study	**Value**	**95% Confidence Limits**
Case-Control (Odds Ratio)	3.9860	1.9043 8.3432
Cohort (Col1 risk)	3.0431	1.6349 5.6641
Cohort (Col2 risk)	0.7634	0.6633 0.8786

(c) Smoking and Lung Cancer

Statistics for Table of Group by Lung_ca

Estimates of the Relative Risk (row1/row2)		
Type of Study	**Value**	**95% Confidence Limits**
Case-Control (Odds Ratio)	15.0845	5.9324 38.3558
Cohort (Col1 risk)	13.5000	5.4057 33.7143
Cohort (Col2 risk)	0.8950	0.8636 0.9274

4.5.4 Fisher's Test

One of the requirements of the chi-squared test used in the preceding examples is that the expected values are not too small. Historically, this has been interpreted as requiring values greater than five for the test to be valid. Although there is some evidence that this recommendation is rather too conservative, very sparse contingency tables can be a problem for the usual chi-squared test. For a 2×2 table, the usual alternative suggested is *Fisher's exact test*. This test is based on the probability of any particular arrangement of the frequencies *a, b, c,* and *d* in a 2×2 contingency table, when the marginal totals are fixed and the two variables are independent; this probability, *P,* is given by

$$P = \frac{(a+b)!(a+c)!(c+d)!(b+d)!}{a!b!c!d!N!} \tag{4.12}$$

TABLE 4.9

Spectacle Wearing and Delinquency

Spectacle Wearer?	Juvenile Delinquents	Nondelinquents	Total
Yes	1	5	6
No	8	2	10
Total	9	7	16

This is known as the *hypergeometric distribution* (see Everitt and Skrondal 2010). Fisher's exact test employs this distribution to find the probability of the observed arrangement of frequencies and of every arrangement giving as much or more evidence of a departure from independence, when the marginal totals are fixed.

Fisher's test can be illustrated on the data shown in Table 4.9 that come from a study comparing the health of juvenile delinquent boys with a non-delinquent control group. They relate to the subset of the boys who failed a vision test and show the numbers who did and did not wear glasses. The question of interest is whether delinquents with poor eyesight are more or less likely to wear glasses than are nondelinquents with poor eyesight. (Note that Fisher's test is computed by default when the `chisq` option is used with a 2×2 table, but the result was edited out of the output from the three previous data sets.)

```
data delinquency;
   input specs$ delinquent$ n;
cards;
Y Y 1
Y N 5
N Y 8
N N 2
;

proc freq data=delinquency;
   tables specs*delinquent/chisq;
   weight n;
run;
```

The two-sided p-value obtained by applying Fisher's exact test can be found in the SAS output (which we do not give here) to be 0.035. There is some evidence of a difference in spectacle wearing between juvenile delinquents and non-juvenile delinquents with poor eyesight. A lower proportion of the delinquents wear spectacles. (For interest, the chi-squared test in this case gives a p-value of 0.051.)

As a small digression from the main theme of this chapter, we can look at the application of Fisher's test to tables larger than those 2×2 tables to which it has usually been applied when there is concern about small values in some cells of such tables. The last decade has seen a large amount of work

TABLE 4.10

Oral Lesions Data Set

Site of Lesion	Kerala	Gujarat	Andhra
Buccal mucosa	8	1	8
Commisure	0	1	0
Gingiva	0	1	0
Hard palate	0	1	0
Soft palate	0	1	0
Tongue	0	1	0
Floor of mouth	1	0	1
Alveolar ridge	1	0	1

on exact tests for contingency tables in which the counts are small (see, for example, Mehta and Patel 1986). To illustrate this use of Fisher's exact test, we shall use the data shown in Table 4.10; these data give the distribution of the oral lesion site found in house-to-house surveys in three geographic regions of rural India. Application of Fisher's test to the data requires the following SAS code:

```
data lesions;
   length region $8.;
   input site $ 1-16 n1 n2 n3;
   region='Keral'; n=n1;    output;
   region='Gujarat'; n=n2;  output;
   region='Anhara'; n=n3;   output;
   drop n1-n3;
cards;
Buccal Mucosa    8 1 8
Labial Mucosa    0 1 0
Commissure       0 1 0
Gingiva          0 1 0
Hard palate      0 1 0
Soft palate      0 1 0
Tongue           0 1 0
Floor of mouth   1 0 1
Alveolar ridge   1 0 1
;
run;

proc freq data=lesions order=data;
   tables site*region/exact;
   weight n;
run;
```

For tables larger than 2×2, exact tests are requested by using the exact option on the tables statement.

The resulting *p*-value of 0.01 taken from the SAS output indicates a strong association between site of lesion and geographic region. For comparison, the chi-squared statistic for these data takes the value 22.01, which with 14 degrees of freedom has an associated *p*-value of 0.14, suggesting no association. Here, the contingency table is so sparse that the usual chi-squared asymptotic distribution with 14 DF is unlikely to yield accurate *p*-values.

4.5.5 Matched Case-Control Data

When the data in a case-control study have been collected from matched pairs of cases and controls, the chi-squared test used previously is not valid; the appropriate test is now *McNemar's test* for correlated proportions, which we shall now describe.

The frequencies in a matched case-control data set can be written as shown in Table 4.11. Under the hypothesis that the two populations do not differ in their probability of having the risk factor of interest present, the test statistic X^2, which is based only on the *discordant pairs b* and *c*, is given by

$$X^2 = \frac{(b-c)^2}{b+c} \tag{4.13}$$

and has a chi-squared distribution with a single degree of freedom. For paired data, the odds ratio is again calculated from the discordant pair counts and is estimated as

$$\hat{\psi} = \frac{b}{c} \tag{4.14}$$

An approximate confidence interval for ψ can be constructed from knowing that the variance of $\ln(\psi)$ can be estimated from

$$\hat{var}(\ln(\hat{\psi})) = \frac{1}{b} + \frac{1}{c} \tag{4.15}$$

McNemar's test can be applied to the contraceptive pill data in Table 4.3 using the SAS code

TABLE 4.11

Frequencies in a Matched
Case-Control Data Set

		Controls	
		Present	**Absent**
Cases	Present	a	b
	Absent	c	d

```
data pill_use;
   input caseused $ controlused $ num;
cards;
Y Y 10
Y N 57
N Y 13
N N 95
;
run;

proc freq data=pill_use order=data;
  tables caseused*controlused/agree;
  weight num;
run;
```

The `agree` option is used for the McNemar test as well as measures of agreement.

Here, the value of the test statistic is 27.66 and the associated *p*-value is very small. There is a statistically significant association between thrombo-embolism and oral contraceptive use. The proportion of pairs in which only the case has used oral contraceptives is greater than the proportion in which only the control has used the pill. The estimated odds ratio is 4.38 with 95% CI of [2.40,8.01]. The odds of a case having used the contraceptive pill are between about 2.5 and 8 times the odds for a control.

4.5.6 Stratified 2×2 Tables

The interpretation of an estimated odds ratio is often made difficult because of the possibility that a confounding variable related either to the disease or to the risk factor has led to a spurious degree of association between the two. When a potential confounding variable is identified that is categorical, we can construct a series of 2×2 tables—one for each level of the confounder. The data *could* be collapsed over the categories of the confounder variable and then the chi-squared test in Equation (4.6) applied to the resulting 2×2 table, but the dangers of such a procedure are well known and it can generate spurious associations as well as mask true relationships (see Everitt 1992 for examples). How then do we test for association and how do we estimate the odds ratio and its associated confidence interval? The appropriate way to assess association is the *Mantel–Haenszel test*. For a series of k 2×2 contingency tables, the Mantel–Haenszel statistic for testing the hypothesis of no association is

$$X^2 = \frac{\left[\sum_{i=1}^{k} a_i - \sum_{i=1}^{k} \frac{(a_i + b_i)(a_i + c_i)}{N_i}\right]^2}{\sum_{i=1}^{k} \frac{(a_i + b_i)(c_i + d_i)(a_i + c_i)(b_i + d_i)}{N_i^2(N_i - 1)}} \tag{4.16}$$

TABLE 4.12

Number of Cases of Bronchitis by Level of Organic Particulates in
the Air and by Age

Age (years)	Organic Particulate Level	Bronchitis		Total
		Yes	No	
0–14	High	62	915	977
	Low	7	442	449
15–24	High	20	382	402
	Low	9	214	223
23–40	High	10	172	182
	Low	7	120	127
40+	High	12	237	339
	Low	6	183	189

where a_i, b_i, c_i, d_i represent the counts in the four cells of the ith table and N_i is the total number of observations in the ith table.

Under the null hypothesis, this statistic has a chi-squared distribution with a single degree of freedom. The test is only appropriate if the degree and direction of the association between the two variables are the same in each stratum. A possible test of this assumption is that due to Breslow and Day (see Agresti 1996).

We shall illustrate the use of this test on data collected to investigate the level of organic particulates in the air as a risk factor for bronchitis (shown in Table 4.12).

To apply the Mantel–Haenszel test to the data in Table 4.12, we use the following code:

```
data bronchitis;
  input agegrp level $ bronch $ num;
cards;
1 H Y 62
1 H N 915
1 L Y 7
1 L N 442
2 H Y 20
2 H N 382
2 L Y 9
2 L N 214
3 H Y 10
3 H N 172
3 L Y 7
3 L N 120
4 H Y 12
4 H N 327
4 L Y 6
```

```
4  L  N  183
;
proc freq data=bronchitis order=data;
  Tables agegrp*level*bronch / cmh noprint;
  weight num;
run;
```

The `tables` statement specifies a three-way tabulation with `agegrp` defining the strata. The `cmh` option requests the Cochran–Mantel–Haenszel statistics and the `noprint` option suppresses the tables.

The results are shown in Table 4.13. Looking first at the result of the Breslow–Day test for homogeneity of odds ratios, we see that it is significant: There is some evidence that the odds ratios in the four age groups are not the same. We can obtain the estimated odds ratios for each age group and their associated 95% confidence intervals using the `relrisk` option on the `tables` statement. We find that the 95% confidence intervals for the four age groups are

age 0–14:	[1.94,9.42]
age 15–24:	[0.56,2.78]
age 23–40:	[0.37,2.69]
age 40+:	[0.41,3.03]

We see that the odds ratio for the younger age group is quite different from those for the other three age groups. Therefore, we will now apply the Mantel–Haenszel test to the three older age groups, by rerunning the previous step but including the statement `where agegrp>1;`.

Now the Breslow–Day test is nonsignificant ($p = 0.943$) and now it makes sense to look at the result from the Mantel–Haenszel test: the test statistic is 0.22 with an associated p-value of 0.64.

TABLE 4.13

Mantel–Haenszel Results for the Data in Table 4.12

Cochran–Mantel–Haenszel Statistics Based on Table Scores				
Statistic	**Alternative Hypothesis**	**DF**	**Value**	**Prob**
1	Nonzero correlation	1	9.5778	0.0020
2	Row mean scores differ	1	9.5778	0.0020
3	General association	1	9.5778	0.0020

Breslow–Day Test for Homogeneity of the Odds Ratios	
Chi-Squared	8.2099
DF	3
Pr > ChiSq	0.0419

TABLE 4.14

Estimation of the Common Odds Ratio for the Three Older Age Groups
in Table 4.12

Estimates of the Common Relative Risk (row1/row2)				
Type of Study	**Method**	**Value**	**95% Confidence Limits**	
Case control	Mantel–Haenszel	1.1355	0.6693	1.9266
Odds ratio	Logit	1.1341	0.6678	1.9260
Cohort	Mantel–Haenszel	1.1291	0.6808	1.8728
Col1 risk	Logit	1.1272	0.6794	1.8704
Cohort	Mantel–Haenszel	0.9945	0.9725	1.0170
Col2 risk	Logit	0.9945	0.9729	1.0166

Having shown that the three older age groups can be assumed to have the
same odds ratio, how do we estimate this common value? One way is to take
separate estimates of $\ln(\psi)$ and weight them by the reciprocal of their variance. The estimates are then combined by taking a weighted mean. An alternative method—one that has a number of advantages (see Emerson 1994)—is
due to Mantel and Haenszel (1959). The common estimate for a series of
2×2 tables using the previously specified nomenclature is

$$\hat{\psi}_{pooled} = \frac{\sum_{i=1}^{k} a_i d_i / n_i}{\sum_{i=1}^{k} b_i c_i / n_i} \tag{4.17}$$

where k is the number of categories of the confounding variable. The variance of $\ln\left(\hat{\psi}_{pooled}\right)$ can be estimated as shown in Everitt (1994).

The relevant section of the SAS output from the previous run is shown in
Table 4.14. The estimate of the common odds ratio is 1.136 with a 95% confidence interval of [0.669,1.927].

4.6 Summary

Observational studies are necessary when active intervention is either impossible or unethical and thus there can be no question of using randomisation.
Consequently, ascribing causality is far more problematic in such a study
(although see the discussion of *propensity scores* in Chapter 10). Cohort studies are perhaps the 'gold standard' amongst observational studies, but they
can take a long time to complete and are expensive; case-control studies have
potentially more problems but can be carried out relatively speedily and

cheaply. For both types of studies, the sample odds ratio acts as an approximate estimate of relative risk. In this chapter we have described simple methods for the analysis of data from observational studies. But such studies can often have complexities not covered in this chapter and will then require more sophisticated methods of analysis, as we shall see in later chapters, particularly in Chapter 10.

5

Meta-Analysis

5.1 Introduction

Many individual clinical trials are not large enough to answer the questions we want to answer as reliably as we would want to answer them. (The same applies to epidemiological studies, but in this chapter we shall concentrate on clinical trials.) For example, trials are often too small for adequate conclusions to be drawn about potentially small advantages of particular therapies. Advocacy of large trials is a natural response to this situation, but it is not always possible to launch very large trials before therapies become widely accepted or rejected prematurely.

In the past, the problem has been addressed by the classical narrative review of a set of clinical trials with an accompanying informal synthesis of evidence from the different studies. And given that it is rare indeed that any single trial ever gives the definitive answer to a clinical question, it is via reviews of several trials that we finally arrive at a conclusion about the effectiveness or not of an intervention. Thus, we might reasonably expect that reviews, which after all are far more widely read by practicing clinicians, who rarely have the time or the expertise to evaluate and synthesise each individual trial, should be as rigorous as and perhaps more rigorous than the individual trials that they involve. Sadly, until relatively recently, this expectation was rarely met.

In a pivotal paper, Mulrow (1987) showed that looking only at four of the best medical journals, 86% of review articles depended upon qualitative synthesis of the literature, and only a handful contained any description of the methodology or rules by which papers were selected and conclusions reached. Since then, numerous studies have showed again and again the deficiencies of the single 'narrative review'. There is evidence that such narrative reviews can sometimes tell us more about the background and orientation of the writer(s) than about the subject under review (Joyce, Rabe-Hesketh, and Wessely 1998).

It appears, then, that narrative, qualitative review articles may be very misleading as a result of both the possibly biased selection of evidence and the emphasis placed upon it by the reviewer to support his or her opinion.

An alternative approach that has become increasingly popular in the last decade or so is the *systematic review,* which has essentially two components:

- *Qualitative:* the description of the available trials, in terms of their relevance and methodological strengths and weaknesses
- *Quantitative:* a means of mathematically combining results from different studies, even (possibly) when these studies have used different measures to assess the dependent variable

The quantitative component of a systematic review is usually known as a *meta-analysis,* defined in the *Cambridge Dictionary of Statistics in the Medical Sciences* as follows:

> A collection of techniques whereby the results of two or more independent studies are statistically combined to yield an overall answer to a question of interest. The rationale behind this approach is to provide a test with more power than is provided by the separate studies themselves.

It is now generally accepted that meta-analysis gives the systematic review an objectivity that is inevitably lacking in literature reviews and can also help the process to achieve greater precision and generalisability of findings than any single study. Chalmers and Lau (1993) make the point that both the classical review article and a meta-analysis can be biased, but that at least the writer of a meta-analytic paper is required by the rudimentary standards of the discipline to give the data on which any conclusions are based and to defend the development of these conclusions by giving evidence that all available data are included or the reasons for not including the data. Chalmers and Lau conclude that 'it seems obvious that a discipline that requires all available data be revealed and included in an analysis has an advantage over one that has traditionally not presented analyses of all the data on which conclusions are based'.

The meta-analysis approach, first used as far as we are aware by a psychologist (Glass 1976), has become increasingly popular in the last decade or so and it is probably fair to say that the majority of statisticians and clinicians are largely enthusiastic about the advantages of meta-analysis over the classical review. But the technique is not without its critics, particularly because of the difficulties of knowing which studies should be included and to which population final results actually apply. Those who remain sceptical do so because they feel that the conclusions from meta-analyses often go beyond what the technique and the data justify, a view nicely summarised in the following quotation from Oakes (1993):

> The term meta-analysis refers to the quantitative combination of data from independent trials. Where the result of such combination is

> a descriptive summary of the weight of the available evidence, the
> exercise is of undoubted value. Attempts to apply inferential methods,
> however, are subject to considerable methodological and logical difficul-
> ties. The selection and quality of trials included, population bias and the
> specification of the population to which inference may properly be made
> are problems to which no satisfactory solutions have been proposed.

Hans Eysenck, one of the earliest critics of meta-analysis, which he believed
to be combining apples and oranges, was, as ever, more pungently critical,
using the phrase 'mega silliness' to describe the procedure (Eysenck 1978).

Despite the concerns expressed by a small number of critics, the demand
for systematic reviews of health care interventions has developed rapidly
during the last decade, initiated by the widespread adoption of the principles of evidence-based medicine amongst both health care practitioners and
policy makers. Such reviews are now increasingly used as a basis for both
individual treatment decisions and the funding of health care and health
care research worldwide. This growth in systematic reviews is reflected in
the current state of the Cochrane Collaboration database, containing as it
does more than 1,200 complete systematic reviews, with a further 1,000 due
to be added soon.

Systematic reviews have a number of aims:

- To review systematically the available evidence from a particular
  research area
- To provide quantitative summaries of the results from each study
- To combine the results across studies if appropriate—such combination of results leading to greater statistical power in estimating
  treatment effects
- To assess the amount of variability between studies
- To estimate the degree of benefit associated with a particular study
  treatment
- To identify study characteristics associated with particularly effective treatments

Ideally, the trials selected by a systematic review and then subjected to a
meta-analysis should be clinically homogeneous. For example, they might all
study a similar type of patient for a similar duration with the same treatment
in the two arms of each trial. In practice, of course, the trials included are far
more likely to differ in some aspects, such as eligibility criterion, duration
of treatment, length of follow-up, and how ancillary care is used. On occasions, even treatment itself may not be identical in all the trials. According
to Thompson (1998), this implies that, in most circumstances, the objective of
a systematic review *cannot* be equated with that of a single large trial, even
if that trial has wide eligibility. Whilst a single trial focuses on the effect of

a specific treatment in specific situations, a meta-analysis aims for a more generalisable conclusion about the effect of a generic treatment policy in a wider range of areas.

When the trials included in a systematic review do differ in some of their components, therapeutic effects may very well be different, but these differences are likely to be in the *size* of the effects rather than their *direction*. It would, after all, be extraordinary if treatment effects were exactly the same when estimated from trials in different countries, in different populations, in different age groups, or under different treatment regimens. If the studies were big enough, it would be possible to measure these differences reliably, but in most cases this will *not* be possible. But meta-analysis allows the investigation of sources of possible heterogeneity in the results from different trials, as we shall see later, and discourages the common, simplistic, and often misleading interpretation that the results of individual clinical trials are in conflict because some are labelled 'positive' (i.e., statistically significant) and others 'negative' (i.e., statistically nonsignificant). A systematic approach to synthesising information can often estimate the degree of benefit from a particular therapy and whether the benefit depends upon specific characteristics of the studies.

5.2 Study Selection

The selection of the studies to be integrated in a systematic review will clearly have considerable bearing on the conclusions reached. Indeed, according to Pocock (1992), selection of studies is the *greatest* single concern in applying meta-analysis and he identifies three important components of the selection process: *breadth, quality,* and *representativeness*. Breadth relates to the decision as to whether to study a very specific narrow question (e.g., the same drug, disease, and setting for studies following a common protocol) or a more generic problem (e.g., a broad class of treatments for a range of conditions in a variety of settings). Pocock suggests that the broader the meta-analysis is, the more difficulty there is in interpreting the combined evidence as regards future policy. Consequently, the broader the meta-analysis is, the more it needs to be interpreted qualitatively rather than quantitatively.

The representativeness of the studies in a systematic review depends largely on having an acceptable *search strategy*. Once the researcher has established the goals of the systematic review, an ambitious literature search needs to be undertaken, the literature obtained, and then summarised. Possible sources of material include the published literature, unpublished literature, uncompleted research reports, work in progress, conference/symposia proceedings, dissertations, expert informants, granting agencies, trial registries, industry, and journal hand-searching.

The search will probably begin by using computerised bibliographic data-bases of published and unpublished research review articles, for example, MEDLINE. This is clearly a sensible strategy, although there are a number of papers illustrating the deficiencies of MEDLINE searches for randomised controlled trials, see, for example, Gotzsche and Lange (1991) and Hopewell et al. (2002). The latter report a comparison of hand-searching versus MEDLINE searching to identify reports of randomised controlled trials. A total of 714 reports of randomised trials (as defined by the Cochrane Collaboration) were found by using a combination of hand-searching and MEDLINE searching. Of these, 369 (52%) were identified only by hand-searching and 32 (4%) were identified only by MEDLINE searching. Of the reports identified only by hand-searching, 252 had no MEDLINE record, with 232 of these being meeting abstracts or published in supplements. The remaining 117 papers found only by hand-searching were included in the MEDLINE database, but were missed in the electronic search because they did not have either of the publication type terms 'randomised controlled trial' or 'controlled clinical trial'.

Not unreasonably, the authors conclude that 'a combination of MEDLINE and hand-searching is required to identify adequately reports of randomised trials'. Fortunately, help is at hand, since the databases of the two Cochrane groups that specialise in mental health contain the results of extensive hand-searching of a large range of journals, together with regularly updated 'state of the art' electronic searches of numerous databases, and can be readily searched. All trials identified are also located on the Cochrane Database of Clinical Trials.

Finally, the quality and reliability of a systematic review is dependent on the quality of the data in the included studies, although criticisms of meta-analyses for including original studies of questionable quality are typical examples of shooting the messenger who bears bad news. Aspects of quality of the original articles that are pertinent to the reliability of the meta-analysis include valid randomisation process (we are assuming that, in meta-analysis of clinical trials, *only* randomised trials will be selected); minimisation of potential biases introduced by dropouts; acceptable methods of analysis, particularly in regard to dropouts; level of blinding; and recording of adequate clinical details.

Several attempts have been made to make this aspect of meta-analysis more rigorous by using the results given by applying specially constructed *quality assessments scales* to assess the candidate trials for inclusion in the analysis. Moher et al. (1995), for example, present an annotated bibliography of 25 scales developed to assess quality, all of which the authors consider to have major weaknesses. Consequently, it is perhaps not too surprising that the use of such scales in meta-analysis has not been completely successful.

Juni et al. (1999), for example, used 25 different scales in a meta-analysis of 17 trials comparing low-molecular-weight heparin with standard heparin for prevention of postoperative thrombosis. They found that, for six scales, the trials rated as high quality corresponded to those showing no treatment effect, whereas those rated as low quality indicated a significant treatment difference. For another seven scales, the reverse was the case. For the remaining 12 scales, effect estimates were similar for those trials rated as high or low quality. In a regression analysis, summary quality scores were not significantly associated with treatment effects. The authors finally concluded that the use of the scales to identify trials of high quality was problematic; instead, they recommended that relevant methodological aspects of the trials should be assessed individually and their influence on effect size explored.

As an example of how the selection process in a meta-analysis operates in practice, we shall use the description provided by Kirsch and Sapirstein (1998) in their study of antidepressant medication. Studies assessing the efficacy of antidepressant medication were obtained through a number of previous reviews, supplemented by a computer search of PsycLit and MEDLINE databases from 1974 to 1995 using the search terms drug-therapy or pharmacotherapy or psychotherapy or placebo and depression or affective disorders. Approximately 1500 publications were identified by the literature search. Each of these was examined by one of the authors and those meeting the following criteria were included in the meta-analysis:

- Sample was restricted to patients with a primary diagnosis of depression. Studies were excluded if participants were selected because of other criteria (eating disorders, substance abuse, physical disabilities, or chronic medical conditions) as were studies in which the description of the patient population was vague (e.g., 'neurotic').

- Sufficient data were reported or obtainable to calculate within-condition effect sizes. This resulted in the exclusion of studies for which neither pre- or poststatistical tests nor pretreatment means were available.

- Data were reported from a placebo control group.

- Participants were between the ages of 18 and 75.

Of the original 1,500 studies, only 20 met these criteria. Despite the apparent thoroughness of Kirsch and Sapirstein's selection procedure, critics of the paper suggested there were flaws and managed to uncover other relevant studies.

5.3 Publication Bias

Ensuring that a meta-analysis is truly representative can be problematic. It has long been known that journal articles are not a representative sample of work addressed to any particular area of research (see, for example, Sterlin 1959;

Greenwald 1975; Smith 1980). Research with statistically significant results is potentially more likely to be submitted and published than work with null, or nonsignificant, results, particularly if the studies are small (Easterbrook et al. 1991). The problem is made worse by the fact that many medical studies look at multiple outcomes, and there is a tendency for only those outcomes suggesting a significant effect to be mentioned when the study is written up. Outcomes that show no clear treatment effect are often ignored and will not be included in any later review of studies looking at those particular outcomes. Publication bias is likely to lead to an over-representation of positive results.

Clearly, it becomes of some importance to assess the likelihood of publication bias in any meta-analysis reported in the literature. A well-known informal method of examining the possibility of publication bias is the so-called *funnel plot*—usually a plot of a measure of a study's precision (for example, one over the standard error) against effect size. The most precise estimates (e.g., those from the largest studies) will be at the top of the plot and those from less precise or smaller studies at the bottom. The expectation of a 'funnel' shape in the plot relies on two empirical observations:

- The variances of studies in a meta-analysis are not identical, but are distributed in such a way that there are fewer precise studies and rather more imprecise ones.
- At any fixed level of variances, studies are symmetrically distributed about the mean.

Evidence of publication bias is provided by an absence of studies on the left-hand side of the base of the funnel. The assumption is that, whether because of editorial policy or author inaction or another reason, these studies (which are not statistically significant) are the ones that might not be published. Example funnel plots, based on those given in Duval and Tweedie (2000), are shown in Figure 5.1a and b. In the first of these plots, there is little evidence of publication bias; however, in the second, the lack of studies in the bottom left-hand corner of the plot suggests possible publication bias.

Other examples of funnel plots on real data will be given later in the chapter.

5.4 Statistics of Meta-Analysis

Two models that are frequently used in the meta-analysis of medical studies are the *fixed-effects* and *random-effects* models. The former assumes that each observed individual study result is estimating a common, unknown, overall pooled effect. The latter assumes that each individual observed result

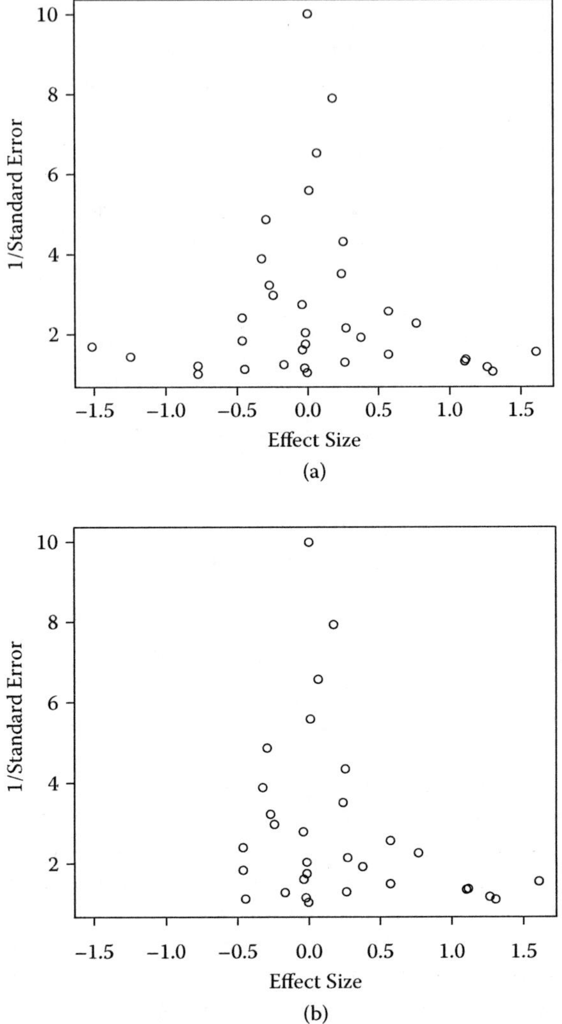

FIGURE 5.1

Example funnel plots from simulated data. The asymmetry in the lower plot gives a hint that publication bias might be a problem.

is estimating its own unknown underlying effect, which in turn is estimating a common population mean. Thus, the random-effects model specifically allows for the existence of *between-study heterogeneity* as well as *within-study variability.*

Demets (1987) and Bailey (1987) discuss the strengths and weaknesses of the two competing models. Bailey suggests that when the research question involves extrapolation to the future—*Will* the treatment have an effect, on the average?—the random-effects model for the studies is the appropriate one. The research question implicitly assumes that there is a population of studies from which those studies analysed in the meta-analysis are sampled and anticipates future studies being conducted or previously unknown studies being uncovered.

When the research question concerns whether treatment *has* produced an effect, on the average, *in the set of studies being analysed*, the fixed-effects model for the studies may be the appropriate one; here, there is no interest in generalising the results to other studies.

Many statisticians believe that random-effects models are more appropriate than fixed-effects models for meta-analysis because between-study variation is an important source of uncertainty that should not be ignored.

5.4.1 Fixed-Effects Model

This model uses as its estimate of the common pooled effect ($\overline{Y}$) a weighted average of the individual study effects, the weights being inversely proportional to the within-study variances. Specifically,

$$\overline{Y} = \frac{\sum_{i=1}^{K} W_i Y_i}{\sum_{i=1}^{K} W_i} \tag{5.1}$$

where

K is the number of the studies in the meta-analysis
Y_i is the effect size estimated in the ith study (this might be a log odds ratio, relative risk, or difference in means, for example)
$W = 1/V_i$, where V_i is the within-study estimate of variance for the ith study

The estimated variance of $\overline{Y}$ is given by

$$\mathrm{Var}\left(\overline{Y}\right) = \frac{1}{\sum_{i=1}^{K} W_i} \tag{5.2}$$

From (5.1) and (5.2), a confidence interval for the pooled effect can be constructed in the usual way.

5.4.2 Random-Effects Model

The random-effects model has the following form:

$$Y_i = \mu_i + \sigma_i \,\epsilon_i \qquad \epsilon_i \sim N(0,1)$$
$$\mu_i \sim N\left(\mu,\tau^2\right) \qquad i = 1, \dots K \tag{5.3}$$

Unlike the fixed-effects model, the individual studies are not assumed to be estimating a true single effect size; rather, the true effects in each study, the μ_i, are assumed to have been sampled from a distribution of effects, assumed to be normal with mean μ and variance τ^2. The estimate of μ is that given in (5.1), but in this case the weights are given by

$$W_i = 1/\left(V_i^2 + \hat{\tau}^2\right) \tag{5.4}$$

where $\hat{\tau}^2$ is an estimate of the between-study variance. DerSimonian and Laird (1986) derive a suitable estimator for $\hat{\tau}^2$, which is as follows:

$$\hat{\tau}^2 = 0 \quad \text{if} \quad Q \leq K - 1$$
$$\hat{\tau}^2 = \left[Q - (K-1)\right]/U \quad \text{if} \quad Q > K - 1 \tag{5.5}$$

where

$$Q = \sum_{i=1}^{K} W_i \left(Y_i - \bar{Y}\right)^2 \tag{5.6}$$

and

$$U = (K - 1)\left[\bar{W} - \frac{S_W^2}{K\bar{W}}\right] \tag{5.7}$$

with $\bar{W}$ and S_W^2 being the mean and variance of the weights, W_i.

A test for homogeneity of studies is provided by the statistic Q given in (5.6). The hypothesis of a common effect size is rejected if Q exceeds χ^2_{k-1} at the chosen significance level. Allowing for this extra between-study variation has the effect of reducing the relative weighting given to the more precise studies. Hence, the random-effects model produces a more conservative confidence interval for the pooled effect size. A Bayesian dimension can be added to the random-effects model by allowing the parameters of the model to have prior distributions. Some examples are given in Sutton et al. (2000).

5.5 An Example of the Application of Meta-Analysis

Cigarette smoking is the leading cause of preventable death in the United States and kills more Americans than AIDS, alcohol, illegal drug use, car accidents, fires, murders, and suicides combined. It has been estimated that 430,000 Americans die from smoking every year. Fighting tobacco use is consequently one of the major public health goals of our time and there are now many programs available to help smokers quit. One of the major aids used in these programs is nicotine chewing gum, which acts as a substitute oral activity and provides a source of nicotine that reduces the withdrawal symptoms experienced when smoking is stopped. But separate randomised clinical trials of nicotine gum have been largely inconclusive, leading Silagy (2003) to consider combining the results from 26 such studies found from an extensive literature search. The results of these trials in terms of numbers of people in the treatment arm and the control arm who stopped smoking for at least 6 months after treatment are given in Table 5.1.

The first step is to calculate an effect size and weight for each study. Here we will use the log of the odds ratio for each study as the corresponding effect size and the inverse of its variance as the weight (see Chapter 4):

TABLE 5.1

Meta-Analysis of Smoking Data on Nicotine Gum

Study	qt	tt	qc	tc
Blondal 1989	37	92	24	90
Campbell 1991	21	107	21	105
Fagerstrom 1982	30	50	23	50
Fee 1982	23	180	15	172
Garcia 1989	21	68	5	38
Garvey 2000	75	405	17	203
Gross 1995	37	131	6	46
Hall 1985	18	41	10	36
Hall 1987	30	71	14	68
Hall 1996	24	98	28	103
Hjalmarson 1984	31	106	16	100
Huber 1988	31	54	11	60
Jarvis 1982	22	58	9	58
Jensen 1991	90	211	28	82
Killen 1984	16	44	6	20
Killen 1990	129	600	112	617
Malcolm 1980	6	73	3	121
McGovern 1992	51	146	40	127
Nakamura 1990	13	30	5	30
Niaura 1994	5	84	4	89
Pirie 1992	75	206	50	211
Puska 1979	29	116	21	113
Schneider 1985	9	30	6	30
Tonnesen 1988	23	60	12	53
Villa 1999	11	21	10	26
Zelman 1992	23	58	18	58

Notes: qt = number of quitters who have been treated; tt = total number of treated; qc = number of quitters in the control group; tc = total number of smokers in the control group.

```
data quitting;
 set quitting;
 nqt=tt-qt;
 nqc=tc-qc;
 lor=log((qt/nqt)/(qc/nqc));
 selor=sqrt(1/qt+1/nqt+1/qc+1/nqc);
 wgt=1/selor**2;
 ss=tt+tc;
run;
```

The fixed-effects estimator of the pooled effect size given in Equation (5.1) is just a weighted mean and this can be calculated with proc means:

```
proc means data=quitting;
 var lor;
 weight wgt;
 output out=mout mean=mes sumwgt=sumwgt css=Q n=k;
run;
```

Output from proc means also includes the sum of the weights, the inverse of which estimates the variance of $\overline{Y}$ in Equation (5.2) and the corrected sums of squares—that is, Q of (5.6). We also save the number of studies, N, for later use.

To calculate U in (5.7), we also need the sum of squared weights. This can be obtained via a second proc means step with wgt as the analysis variable:

```
proc means data=quitting;
 var wgt;
 output out=mout2 uss=ssqwgt;
run;
```

We can then combine the results and calculate $\hat{\tau}^2$:

```
data mout;
   merge mout mout2;
   u=(sumwgt-ssqwgt/sumwgt);
   tau2=max(0,(q-k+1)/u);
run;
```

Next, $\hat{\tau}^2$ is added to the study data set and the DerSimonian and Laird (DSL) weight given in (5.4) is calculated. Then the random-effects estimator of the pooled effect size can be calculated using proc means with the DSL weight:

```
data quitting;
   set quitting;
   if _n_=1 then set mout(keep=tau2);
   DSL_wgt=1/(1/wgt + tau2);
run;
proc means data=quitting;
 var lor;
```

```
  weight DSL_wgt;
  output out=mout3 mean=mes sumwgt=sumwgt;
run;
```

We can then calculate confidence intervals for the fixed- and random-effects estimates along with their *p*-values and that for the chi-squared test for homogeneity:

```
data MA_summary;
  set mout(in=inf) mout3;
  if inf then type='Fixed';
         else type='Random';
  sem=sqrt(1/sumwgt);
  Z=mes/sem;
  cil=mes-1.96*sem;
  ciu=mes+1.96*sem;
  ProbZ = (1-probnorm(abs(z)))*2;
  ProbQ = 1-probchi(q,k-1);
run;
proc print noobs;
  var type mes sem cil ciu z probz q probq;
  format probz probq pvalue6.4;
run;
```

The fact that the preceding code might need to be used repeatedly, changing only the data set used and the effect size and weight variables, makes it a suitable candidate for turning into a SAS macro. We have done this so that the same results can be achieved by the following:

```
%inc "C:\AMSUS\macros\MA_summary.sas";
%MA_summary(data=quitting,es=lor,wgt=wgt)
```

The MA_summary macro takes three parameters: the data set containing the study summaries, the name of the effect size variable, and that of the study weights. The results are shown in Table 5.2. Both models give highly significant effect sizes. For the fixed-effects model, the log odds ratio is estimated to be 0.502 with 95% confidence interval [0.371,0.632], leading to an estimated odds ratio of 1.652 with 95% confidence interval of [1.449,1.881]. For the random-effects model, the corresponding odds ratio estimate and confidence interval are 1.751 [1.482,2.069].

The results from both models give clear evidence that nicotine gum increases the odds of quitting. The random-effects confidence interval is considerably wider than that from the fixed-effects model. In this example, the test of homogeneity of the effect size of the different studies is not significant, apparently implying that we might use the results from the fixed-effects model. But the homogeneity test is not particularly powerful and it is perhaps more sensible to assume a priori that heterogeneity is present and thus use the results from the random-effects model.

TABLE 5.2

Results of Fixed- and Random-Effects Models for the Data in Table 5.1

Test for Homogeneity of effects		
Q	df	ProbQ
34.8740	25	0.0905

Summary effect size						
type	Summary	SE	Lower 95% limit	Upper 95% limit	minimum	maximum
Fixed	0.50171	0.066436	0.37149	0.63192	−0.14073	1.79242
Random	0.56042	0.084842	0.39413	0.72671	−0.14073	1.79242

Next we need investigate whether or not there is any evidence of publication bias by constructing a funnel plot of the studies:

```
proc sgplot data=quitting;
  scatter y=invvar x=lor;
  refline 0 /axis=x lineattrs=(pattern=dash);
  refline .56 /axis=x;
  xaxis label="log(OR)"values=(-1 to 2);
  yaxis label="1/Var(Log(OR))";
run;
```

The result is shown in Figure 5.2. There may be some *slight* evidence of publication bias here with some 'missing' studies is the left-hand corner, but here it is probably not of any real concern.

Next, we examine a forest plot showing the observed effect size for each study along with its 95% confidence interval. The programming to produce a suitable plot is somewhat involved, so we have written a macro, which is invoked as follows:

```
%inc "C:\AMSUS\macros\forest.sas";
%forest(data=quitting,es=lor,se=selor,type=random)
```

The macro has four parameters: the data set containing the study summaries, the effect size variable, the standard error variable, and the type of summary required. The alternative value for this is fixed. The macro uses the summary values calculated by the MA_summary macro and hence assumes that it has been run. It also assumes that the data set contains a variable study, which can be used to identify the studies in the plot. The result is shown in Figure 5.3. The widths of the plotting symbols are proportional to the study weights.

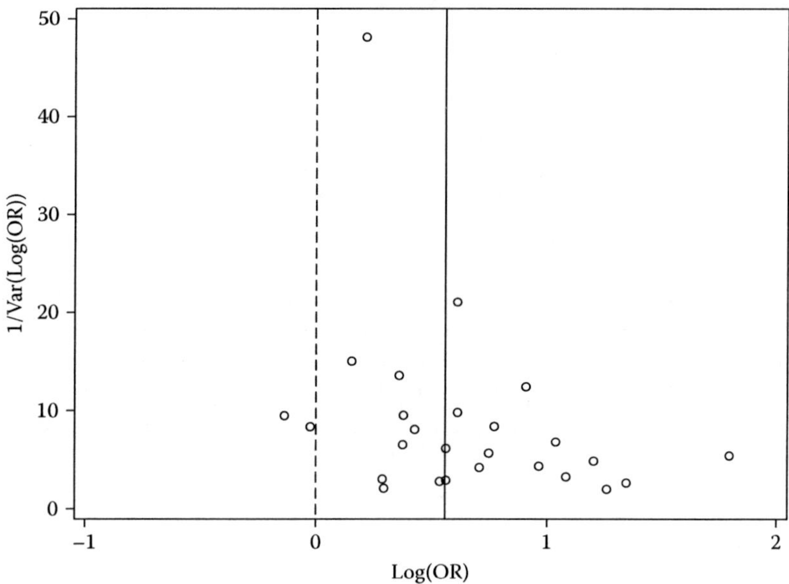

FIGURE 5.2

Funnel plot for nicotine gum data.

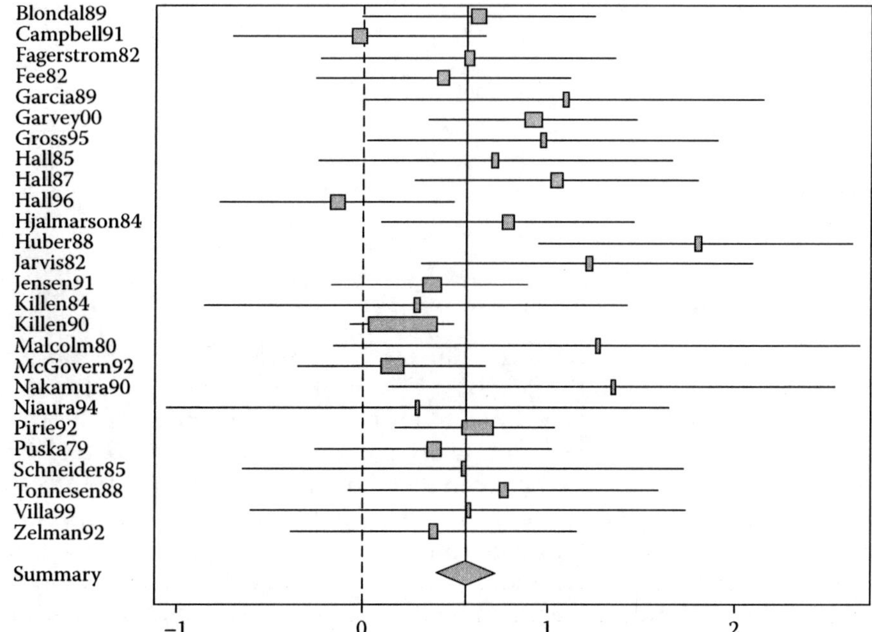

FIGURE 5.3

Forest plot of observed effect sizes and confidence intervals for the nicotine gum data.

5.6 Meta-Analysis on Sparse Data

The data shown in Table 5.3 come from 18 clinical trials comparing the risk of catheter-related bloodstream infection (CRBSI) in patients with an anti-infective catheter and patients with a standard catheter. Very few patients given the anti-infective catheter get CRBSI and, in fact, in several trials there are no patients in this arm of the trial with the condition. This clearly raises problems for a meta-analysis using the log odds as the effect size because, where there are zeroes, the estimate and its standard error are not defined. The simplest way to deal with this problem is to use a continuity correction approach and add 0.5 to all four numbers in the 2×2 table of data for the study.

We apply both fixed- and random-effects models to the CRBSI data using the macro constructed earlier and after applying the continuity correction to the data:

```
data catheters;
   infile 'c:\amsus\data\catheters.dat';
   input study y1 n1 y0 n0;
   if y1=0 then do;
                     y1=.5;
                     n1=n1+.5;
                     end;
   if y0=0 then do;
                     y0=.5;
                     n0=n0+.5;
                     end;
  lor=log(((y1/(n1-y1))/(y0/(n0-y0))));
  selor=sqrt(1/y1+1/(n1-y1)+1/y0+1/(n0-y0));
  wgt=1/selor**2;
run;

%inc "C:\AMSUS\macros\MA_summary.sas";
%MA_summary(data=catheters,es=lor,wgt=wgt)
```

The results are shown in Table 5.4. Here, the results for both models are the same because the value of Q is less than 17 (the number of studies minus one). The estimated 95% confidence interval for the log odds ratio is [−1.39,−0.47]; the corresponding confidence interval for the odds ratio is [0.25,0.63]. The risk of CRBSI is reduced by between 75% and 40% using an anti-infective catheter compared to the use of the standard catheter.

Sweeting, Sutton, and Lambert (2004) consider several alternative continuity corrections, such as adding 0.1 or a number that depends on the extent of the imbalance between the group sizes. Stijnen, Hamza, and Ozdemir (2010) suggest an alternative procedure that uses the exact conditional likelihood given the total number of events in the study and provide SAS code.

TABLE 5.3

Clinical Trials of Anti-Infective Catheters

| | Anti-Infective Catheter | | Standard Catheter | |
Study	No. of CRBSIs	No. of Patients	No. of CRBSIs	No. of Patients
1	0	116	3	117
2	1	44	3	35
3	2	208	9	195
4	0	130	7	136
5	5	151	6	157
6	1	98	4	139
7	1	174	3	177
8	1	74	2	39
9	1	97	19	103
10	1	113	2	122
11	0	66	7	64
12	0	70	1	58
13	3	188	5	175
14	6	187	11	180
15	0	118	0	105
16	0	252	1	262
17	1	345	3	362
18	4	64	1	69

Source: Niel-Weise, B. S., Stijnen, T., and van den Broek, P. J. 2007. *Intensive Care Medicine* 33:2058–2068.

TABLE 5.4

Meta-analysis Results for the Data in Table 5.3

Test for Homogeneity of effects		
Q	df	ProbQ
15.5884	17	0.5532

Summary effect size						
type	Summary	SE	Lower 95% limit	Upper 95% limit	minimum	maximum
Fixed	−0.93089	0.23524	−1.39195	−0.46983	−3.07797	1.51146
Random	−0.93089	0.23524	−1.39195	−0.46983	−3.07797	1.51146

5.7 Meta-Regression

Bacille Calmette Guerin (BCG) is the most widely used vaccination in the world. Developed in the 1930s and made of a live, weakened strain of *Mycobacterium bovis*, the BCG is the only vaccination available against tuberculosis (TBC) today. Colditz et al. (1994) report data from 13 clinical trials of BCG vaccine, each investigating its efficacy in the treatment of tuberculosis. The number of subjects suffering from TB with or without BCG vaccination is given in Table 5.5. In addition, the table contains the values of two other variables for each study—namely, the geographic latitude of the place where the study was undertaken and the year of publication. These two variables will be used to investigate and perhaps explain any heterogeneity among the studies.

The examination of heterogeneity of the effect sizes from the studies in a meta-analysis begins with the formal test for its presence, although in most meta-analyses such heterogeneity can almost be assumed to be present. There will be many possible sources of such heterogeneity and estimating how these various factors affect the observed effect sizes in the studies chosen is often of considerable interest and importance—indeed, usually more important than the relatively simplistic use of meta-analysis to determine a single summary estimate of overall effect size.

TABLE 5.5

Meta-analysis of BCG Vaccine Data

Study	BCGTB	BCGnoTB	noBCGTB	noBCGnoTB	Latitude	Year
1	4	119	11	128	44	1948
2	6	300	29	274	55	1949
3	3	228	11	209	42	1960
4	62	13536	248	12619	52	1977
5	33	5036	47	5761	13	1973
6	180	1361	372	1079	44	1953
7	8	2537	10	619	19	1973
8	505	87886	499	87892	13	1980
9	29	7470	45	7232	27	1968
10	17	1699	65	1600	42	1961
11	186	50448	141	27197	18	1974
12	5	2493	3	2338	33	1969
13	27	16886	29	17825	33	1976

Source: Colditz, G. A., Brewer, T. F., Berkey, C. S., Wilson, M. E., Burdick, E., Fineberg, H. V., and Mosteller, F. 1994. *Journal of the American Medical Association,* 271:698–702.

Notes: BCGTB: the number of TBC cases after a vaccination with BCG = BCGTB; BCGnoTB: the number of people who received BCG but did not contract TB; noBCGTB: the number of TBC cases without vaccination; noBCGnoTB: the number of who did not receive BCG and did not contract TB.

TABLE 5.6

Results from the Fixed- and Random-Effects Models Fitted to the Data in Table 5.5

Test for Homogeneity of effects		
Q	**df**	**ProbQ**
163.165	12	<.0001

Summary effect size						
type	**Summary**	**SE**	**Lower 95% limit**	**Upper 95% limit**	**minimum**	**maximum**
Fixed	−0.43614	0.04227	−0.51898	−0.35330	−1.66619	0.44663
Random	−0.74739	0.19226	−1.12423	−0.37056	−1.66619	0.44663

We can illustrate the process using the BCG vaccine data. We first find the estimate of the overall effect size from applying the fixed- and the random-effects models described previously:

```
data bcg;
  infile 'c:\AMSUS\data\bcg.dat';
  input study BCGTB BCGnoTB noBCGTB noBCGnoTB Latitude Year;
  lor=log((BCGTB/BCGnoTB)/(noBCGTB/noBCGnoTB));
  se=sqrt(1/BCGTB+1/BCGnoTB+1/noBCGTB+1/noBCGnoTB);
  wgt=1/se**2;
run;

%MA_summary(data=bcg,es=lor,wgt=wgt)
```

The results appear in Table 5.6. Both the fixed- and random-effects models give highly significant effect sizes. However, here the test of heterogeneity is highly significant, so we will now investigate whether or not there is any evidence that heterogeneity is related to the year of the study or the latitude where the study took place.

To assess how the two covariates, latitude and year, relate to the observed effect sizes, we shall use multiple linear regression but will weight each observation by $W_i = (\hat{\sigma}^2 + V_i^2)^{-1}$ $i = 1,13$, where $\hat{\sigma}^2$ is the estimated between-study variance and V_i^2 is the estimated variance from the ith study:

```
proc reg data=bcg;
  model lor=latitude year;
  weight dsl_wgt;
run;
```

The main results of the multiple regression are shown in Table 5.7. Clearly, years is not related to effect size, but there is some weak evidence that latitude may be related.

To investigate the possible latitude effect in a little more detail, we will construct a scatter plot of effect size against latitude showing also the fitted

TABLE 5.7

Results of Weighted Multiple Regression of Effect Size on Year and Latitude
for the Data in Table 5.5

		Parameter Estimates			
Variable	DF	Parameter Estimate	Standard Error	t Value	Pr >|t|
Intercept	1	−16.19912	37.60540	−0.43	0.6758
Latitude	1	−0.02581	0.01368	−1.89	0.0886
Year	1	0.00828	0.01897	0.44	0.6718

weighted regression of effect size on latitude. We will also indicate on the
plot, by means of circles with different radii, the precision of each study:

```
proc sgplot data=bcg noautolegend;
   bubble y=lor x=latitude size=wgt;
   reg y=lor x=latitude /nomarkers weight=wgt;
   label lor="log(OR)";
run;
```

The resulting diagram is shown in Figure 5.4. There is some suggestion
that the log odds ratio of a study becomes increasingly negative as latitude
increases.

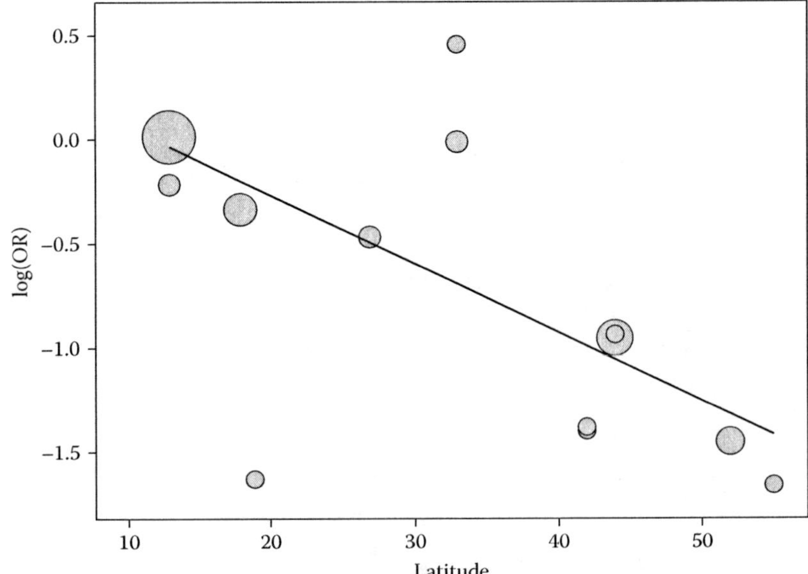

FIGURE 5.4

Plot of observed effect size for the BCG vaccine data against latitude showing the weighted
least squares regression fit.

5.8 Summary

Meta-analysis has had a major impact on medical science in the last decade or so and has been central in the development of evidence-based medical practice. One of the principal reasons that meta-analysis has been so successful is the large number of clinical trials that are now conducted—approximately 10,000 annually. Synthesising results from many studies can be difficult, confusing, and ultimately misleading without some systematic approach. Meta-analysis has the potential to demonstrate treatment effects with a high degree of precision, possibly revealing small, but clinically important effects that may not have been identified in the individual trials.

6

Analysis of Variance and Covariance

6.1 Introduction

As we have seen in our discussion of diagnostic tests in Chapter 2, of clinical trials in Chapter 3, and of epidemiological studies in Chapter 4, many medical investigations involve the comparison of *two* groups of patients and subjects. That is, many but not all, and in this chapter we consider how to analyse data that arise when a continuous (quasicontinuous) outcome variable is measured for subjects who fall into one of the levels of a categorical variable with more than two levels (usually known as the *factor* variable). The appropriate statistical procedure is the *analysis of variance* (ANOVA), which we have already met briefly in Chapter 2. In some situations, the data collected may also contain values of some possible *confounding* (*concomitant*) variable (or variables) thought to be associated with the outcome variable and which, therefore, need to be taken into account in the analysis of this outcome. The relevant technique here is *analysis of covariance,* with which we shall also deal in this chapter.

6.2 A Simple Example of One-Way Analysis of Variance

The data shown in Table 6.1 are steady-state haemoglobin levels for patients with different types of sickle cell disease—namely, HB SS, HB S/-thalassaemia, and HB SC. One question of interest about these data is whether the steady-state haemoglobin levels differ significantly between patients with different types of disease; if so, the haemoglobin level of patients suspected of having a type of sickle cell disease might be able to be used as a diagnostic test (see Chapter 2).

TABLE 6.1

Haemoglobin Levels for Patients with
Different Types of Sickle Cell Disease

HB SS	HB S/-Thalassaemia	HB SC
7.2	8.1	10.7
7.7	9.2	11.3
8.0	10.0	11.5
8.1	10.4	11.6
8.3	10.6	11.7
8.4	10.9	11.8
8.1	11.1	12.0
8.5	11.9	12.1
8.6	12.0	12.3
8.7	12.1	12.6
9.1		12.6
9.1		13.3
9.1		13.3
9.8		13.8
10.1		13.9
10.3		

6.2.1 One-Way Analysis of Variance Model

The formal procedure for analysing the data in Table 6.1 is a *one-way analysis of variance*. If we let y_{ij} represent the jth observation in the ith group, the one-way analysis of variance model is

$$y_{ij} = \mu + \alpha_i + \varepsilon_{ij} \tag{6.1}$$

where
  μ is the overall mean
  α_i is the group effect
  ε_{ij} is a random error term, assumed to be distributed normally with mean
     zero and variance σ^2

Because the model is overparameterised (more parameters than can be uniquely estimated from the data), the group effects need to be constrained in some way, most usually by requiring that $\sum_{i=1}^{k} \alpha_i = 0$, where k is the number of groups. The hypothesis of the equality of group means can be written in terms of the group effects as

$$H_0 : \alpha_1 = \alpha_2 = \ldots = \alpha_k = 0 \tag{6.2}$$

The total variation in the observations is partitioned into that due to differences in the group means and that due to differences among

TABLE 6.2

One-Way Analysis of Variance Table

Source of Variation	DF	Sum of Squares	Mean Square	Mean Square Ratio
Between groups	$k-1$	$\displaystyle\sum_{i=1}^{k} n_i\left(\bar{y}_i - \bar{y}_{..}\right)^2$	$(1) = SS/(k-1)$	$(1)/(2)$
Within groups	$N-k$	$\displaystyle\sum_{i=1}^{k}\sum_{j=1}^{n_i}\left(y_{ij} - \bar{y}_{i.}\right)^2$	$(2) = SS/(N-k)$	
Total	$N-1$	$\displaystyle\sum_{i=1}^{k}\sum_{j=1}^{n_i}\left(y_{ij} - \bar{y}_{..}\right)^2$		

Note: $N = n_1 + n_2 + \ldots + n_k$, where n_i is the number of observations in the ith group. $\bar{y}_{..}$ is the mean of all observations and $\bar{y}_{i.}$ is the mean of the observations in group i.

observations within groups. Under the hypothesis of the equality of group means, both the between-group variance and the within-group variance are estimates of σ^2. Thus, an F-test of the equality of the two variances provides a test of H_0. The necessary terms for calculating the required F-test are usually arranged in an *analysis of variance table* as shown in Table 6.2.

If H_0 is true and the following assumptions are valid, then the MSR has an F-distribution with $k-1$ and $N-k$ degrees of freedom. The assumptions made in a one-way analysis of variance are as follows:

- The observations in each group come from a normal distribution.
- The population variances of each group are the same.
- The observations are independent of one another.

6.2.2 Applying the One-Way Analysis of Variance Model to Sickle Cell Disease Data

In any data analysis, it is good practice to begin by looking at some hopefully informative graphic of the data, and here we choose to look at the three box plots of the haemoglobin observations available for the three types of sickle cell disease. The necessary SAS code to read in the data and construct the box plots is

```
data sickle;
  do type=1 to 3;
  input hglevel 5. @;
  if hglevel~=. then output;
  end;
datalines;
  7.2 8.1 10.7
  7.7 9.2 11.3
. . .
```

```
   8.7 12.1 12.6
   9.1 12.6
   9.1 13.3
   9.1 13.3
   9.8 13.8
  10.1 13.9
  10.3
;

proc sort data=sickle;
  by type;
run;

proc boxplot data=sickle;
  plot hglevel*type / boxstyle=schematic;
run;
```

The data are read using formatted input. Each data value occupies five columns, including the spaces and the decimal point. The trailing @ holds the line for further data to be read from it. For proc boxplot, the data must be sorted in order of the *x*-axis variable. The resulting diagram is shown in Figure 6.1.

The box plots show clear evidence of increasing haemoglobin levels from type HB SS to HB SC, as well as some suggestion of skewness in the distribution of haemoglobin level in disease types 2 and 3. There is no indication of any 'outliers' in the data that may distort their analysis. We shall ignore the indication of some slight departure from the normality assumption given by

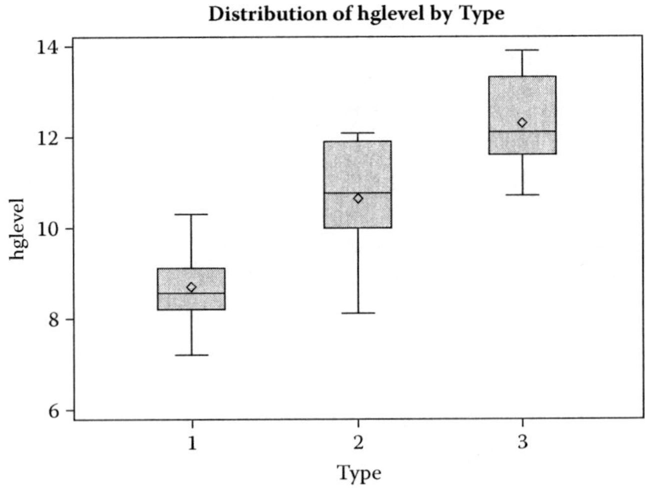

FIGURE 6.1

Box plots of haemoglobin levels for patients with different types of sickle cell disease: 1 = HB SS, 2 = HB S/-thalassaemia, 3 = HB SC.

the box plots and apply a one-way analysis of variance to the data in Table 6.1 using `proc glm` with the following SAS code:

```
ods graphics on;
proc glm data=sickle plots=diagnostics(unpack);
   class type;
   model hglevel=type;
run;
ods graphics off;
```

`Proc glm` can be used to fit the whole class of models that fall within the framework of the *general linear model,* including linear regression and analysis of covariance as well as ANOVA. The `class` statement specifies categorical variables, or factors, which may be numeric or character variables. In this example, the `model` statement simply specifies the outcome variable and the single categorical predictor. When ODS graphics are enabled a panel of diagnostic plots can be produced with the `plots=diagnostics` option. Detailed discussion of the panel as a whole is reserved for Chapter 8, but here we wish to check the distribution of the residuals, so we have 'unpacked' the panel into its separate constituent plots and shown just the Q–Q plot (Figure 6.2).

The results are given in Table 6.3; concentrating on the analysis of variance table part of the results, we see that the p-value associated with the F-statistic for these data is very small, so there is clear evidence of a difference in the average haemoglobin level in the three disease types. (We shall say more about the type I and type III sums of squares that appear in Table 6.3 later in the chapter and the R-square statistic given in Table 6.2 will be explained in Chapter 8, where we deal with *multiple linear regression.*)

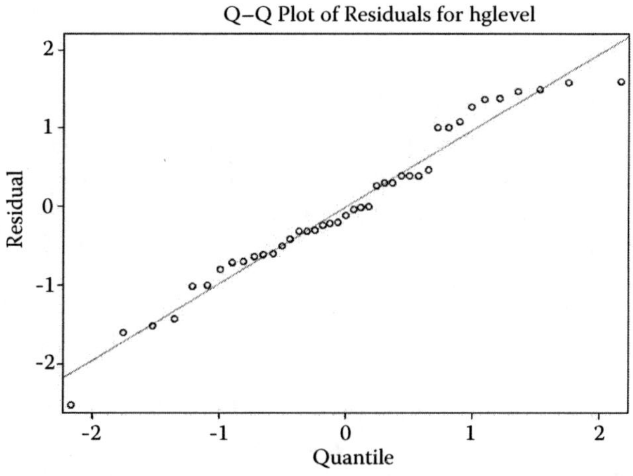

FIGURE 6.2
Q–Q plot of residuals for hglevel.

TABLE 6.3

One-Way Analysis of Variance of Haemoglobin Levels in Three Types of Sickle Cell Disease

Class-Level Information		
Class	Levels	Values
type	3	1 2 3

Number of Observations Read	41
Number of Observations Used	41

Dependent Variable: hglevel					
Source	DF	Sum of Squares	Mean Square	F Value	Pr > F
Model	2	99.8893049	49.9446524	50.00	<.0001
Error	38	37.9585000	0.9989079		
Corrected total	40	137.8478049			

R-Square	Coeff Var	Root MSE	hglevel Mean
0.724635	9.525245	0.999454	10.49268

Source	DF	Type I SS	Mean Square	F Value	Pr > F
type	2	99.88930488	49.94465244	50.00	<.0001

Source	DF	Type III SS	Mean Square	F Value	Pr > F
type	2	99.88930488	49.94465244	50.00	<.0001

6.3 Multiple Comparison Procedures

When the *F*-test in an analysis of variance produces evidence of a difference between the levels of a factor, the investigator usually needs to proceed further to determine the details of the differences and how large they are. There are two different approaches to this problem, both of which are now relatively briefly described.

6.3.1 Planned Comparisons

The first approach to investigating groups' difference in more detail is the use of what are known as *planned comparisons* to test a set of specific hypotheses via specific *contrasts* of group means. In essence, this approach can be formulated in terms of testing a hypothesis involving one (or sometimes more than one) linear combination(s) of the population group means—for example,

$$H_0: c_1\mu_1 + c_2\mu_2 + \ldots c_k\mu_k = 0 \tag{6.3}$$

When the constants $c_1,\ldots,c_k$ sum to zero, this linear combination of the means is known as a *contrast*. An estimate of the contrast is obtained by replacing the population means, $\mu_1,\ldots,\mu_k$, with their sample estimates, $\bar{y}_{1.},\ldots,\bar{y}_{k.}$, to give, say, $L = c_1\bar{y}_{1.} + c_2\bar{y}_{2.} + \ldots + c_k\bar{y}_{k.}$. Two contrasts with defining coefficients $c_{11},\ldots,c_{1k}$ and $c_{21}, c_{22},\ldots, c_{2k}$ are said to be *orthogonal* if $c_{11}c_{21} + c_{12}c_{22} \ldots + c_{1k}c_{2k} = 0$. Such contrasts can be tested independently of each other. The sum of squares for a contrast L is given by

$$SS_{contrast} = \frac{nL^2}{\sum_{i=1}^{k} c_i^2 / n_i} \tag{6.4}$$

This has a single degree of freedom and the F-statistic to test the hypothesis in (6.3) is obtained by dividing this by the within-groups sum of squares from the analysis of variance table for the data.

To illustrate this approach, we shall assume that, in the sickle cell disease example, we want to compare the haemoglobin level of the HB SC group with the average haemoglobin level of the other two types and then to compare types 1 and 2 with each other. The required contrast coefficients are –1, –1, 2 and 1, –1, 0, respectively. The two contrasts are orthogonal.

The sums of squares associated with each contrast can be found simply by rerunning the previous step, adding the following SAS statements:

```
contrast '3 vs 1 & 2' type -1 -1 2;
contrast '1 vs 2' type 1 -1 0;
```

The `contrast` statement comprises some text in quotes to identify the results in the output, the effect or variable to be used for the contrast, and the values of the contrast coefficients. There is no limit to the number of `contrast` statements that can be used, but they must follow the `model` statement. For some procedures, it is possible to submit additional statements in this way, as long as the procedure is still running; this is shown in the title bar of the editor window. A procedure that is still running can be stopped by submitting a `quit` statement.

The results of applying these two contrasts are as follows:

Contrast	DF	Contrast SS	Mean Square	F Value	Pr > F
3 vs 1 & 2	1	64.40692718	64.40692718	64.48	<.0001
1 vs 2	1	22.62650000	22.62650000	22.65	<.0001

Both contrasts are highly significant. The haemoglobin levels of disease types 1 and 2 are different and that of disease type 3 is different from the average of types 1 and 2. In this case, of course, the strong evidence of a difference for types 1 and 2 makes the latter test of little real interest.

6.3.2 Post Hoc Comparisons

When the investigator has no a priori planned comparisons in mind but would still like to investigate the reasons for a significant overall F-statistic, then it is possible to compare *all* pairs of groups. However, care is needed because this approach results in a large number of tests if the number of groups is large. Consequently, the probability of finding at least one pairwise difference when there are no true differences between the groups can become far larger than the nominal significance level being used.

Various safeguards against such false-positive findings are needed. The first is to carry out the pairwise tests *only* if the F-test of the ANOVA is significant. The second is to reduce the significance level of the individual pairwise comparisons in an effort to maintain the overall significance level at its intended value. There are many different ways of adjusting the significance levels, resulting in many different *multiple comparison* procedures. All of these procedures produce intervals or bounds for the difference in (usually) one pair of means of the form (estimate) ± (critical point) × (standard error of estimate). The critical point used depends on the specified multiple comparison method.

Multiple comparison tests aim to retain the nominal significance level at the required value when undertaking tests of mean differences. One of the most commonly used of these procedures is that due to Scheffé (1953); the t-statistic used is given by

$$t = \frac{\text{mean difference}}{s\left(1/n_1 + 1/n_2\right)^{\frac{1}{2}}} \tag{6.5}$$

where s^2 is the error mean square from the analysis of variance table and n_1 and n_2 are the number of observations in the two groups being compared. Each test statistic is compared with the following critical value:

$$\left[(k-1)F_{k-1,N-k}(\alpha)\right]^{\frac{1}{2}} \tag{6.6}$$

where $F_{k-1,N-k}(\alpha)$ is the F-value with $k-1, N-k$ degrees of freedom, corresponding to a significance level α. (Full details are given in Maxwell and Delaney 1990.) The confidence interval for two means is, in this case,

$$\text{mean difference} \pm \text{critical value} \times s\left(\frac{1}{n_1} + \frac{1}{n_2}\right)^{\frac{1}{2}} \tag{6.7}$$

where the critical value is as described before.

TABLE 6.4

Results from Applying Scheffé's Multiple Comparison Test to the Sickle Cell Disease Data

Scheffé's Test for hglevel	
Alpha	0.05
Error Degrees of Freedom	38
Error mean square	0.998908
Critical value of F	3.24482

Comparisons significant at the 0.05 level are indicated by ***.				
type Comparison	Difference Between Means	Simultaneous 95% Confidence Limits		
3 − 2	1.6700	0.6306	2.7094	***
3 − 1	3.5875	2.6724	4.5026	***
2 − 3	−1.6700	−2.7094	−0.6306	***
2 − 1	1.9175	0.8911	2.9439	***
1 − 3	−3.5875	−4.5026	−2.6724	***
1 − 2	−1.9175	−2.9439	−0.8911	***

The Scheffé procedure can be applied to the haemoglobin levels in Table 6.1 by including a `means` statement with the `scheffe` option in the proc glm step as follows:

```
means type / scheffe;
```

The results are shown in Table 6.4 and indicate that, in this case, *all* the pairwise comparisons are significant. The haemoglobin levels of each group differ from those of the other two groups. The confidence intervals quantify the differences.

6.4 A Factorial Experiment

Maxwell and Delaney (1990) report a study designed to investigate the effects of three possible treatments on hypertension. The three treatments were as follows:

drug medication: drug X, drug Y, drug Z

biofeed: physiological feedback, present or absent

diet: present, absent

TABLE 6.5

Blood Pressure Data from Maxwell and Delaney

Biofeedback			No Biofeedback		
Drug X	**Drug Y**	**Drug Z**	**Drug X**	**Drug Y**	**Drug Z**
Diet absent					
170	186	180	173	189	202
175	194	187	194	194	228
165	201	199	197	217	190
180	215	170	190	206	206
160	219	204	176	199	224
158	209	194	198	195	204
Diet present					
161	164	162	164	171	205
173	166	184	190	173	199
157	159	183	169	196	170
152	182	156	164	199	160
181	187	180	176	180	179
190	174	173	175	203	179
Source: Data from Maxwell, S. E., and Delaney, H. D. 1990. *Designing Experiments and Analysing Data.* Belmont, CA: Wadsworth.					

All 12 combinations of treatments were included in the study, so here we are dealing with a $3 \times 2 \times 2$ design. Six subjects were randomly allocated to each cell of the design, and the response variable measured was blood pressure. The data, given in Table 6.5, can be read in as follows:

```
data hyper;
   input n1-n12;
   if _n_<4 then biofeed='P';
         else biofeed='A';
   if _n_ in(1,4) then drug='X';
   if _n_ in(2,5) then drug='Y';
   if _n_ in(3,6) then drug='Z';
   array nall {12} n1-n12;
   do i=1 to 12;
      if i>6 then diet='Y';
            else diet='N';
      bp=nall{i};
      cell=drug||biofeed||diet;
      output;
   end;
   drop i n1-n12;
cards;
170 175 165 180 160 158 161 173 157 152 181 190
186 194 201 215 219 209 164 166 159 182 187 174
```

```
180 187 199 170 204 194 162 184 183 156 180 173
173 194 197 190 176 198 164 190 169 164 176 175
189 194 217 206 199 195 171 173 196 199 180 203
202 228 190 206 224 204 205 199 170 160 179 179
;
```

The 12 blood pressure readings per row, or line, of data are read into variables n1 to n12 and used to create 12 separate observations. The row and column positions in the data are used to determine the values of the factors in the design: drug, biofeedback, and diet.

First, the `input` statement reads the 12 blood pressure values into variables n1 to n12. It uses list input which assumes the data values to be separated by spaces.

The next group of statements uses the SAS automatic variable, _n_ , to determine which row of data is being processed and hence to set the values of `drug` and `biofeed`. Since six lines of data will be read, one line per iteration of the data step, _n_ will increment from one to six, corresponding to the line of data read with the `input` statement.

The key elements in splitting the one line of data into separate observations are the `array`, the `do` loop, and the `output` statement.

The `array` statement defines an array by specifying the name of the array (nall here), the number of variables to be included in it in braces, and the list of variables to be included, n1 to n12 in this case.

In SAS, an array is a shorthand way of referring to a group of variables. In effect, it provides aliases for them so that each variable can be referred to by using the name of the array and its position within the array in braces. For example, in this data step, n12 could be referred to as nall{12} or, when the variable i has the value 12, as nall{i}. However, the array only lasts for the duration of the data step in which it is defined.

The main purpose of an iterative do loop, like the one used here, is to repeat the statements between the do and the end a fixed number of times, with an index variable changing at each repetition. When used to process each of the variables in an array, the do loop should start with the index variable equal to one and end when it equals the number of variables in the array.

Within the do loop, in this example, the index variable, i, is first used to set the appropriate values for `diet`. Then a variable for the blood pressure reading (bp) is assigned one of the 12 input values. A character variable, `cell`, is formed by concatenating the values of the `drug`, `biofeed`, and `diet` variables. The double bar operator (||) concatenates character values.

The `output` statement writes an observation to the output data set with the current value of all variables. An `output` statement is not normally necessary, since without it an observation is automatically written out at the end of the data step. Putting an `output` statement within the do loop results in 12 observations being written to the data set.

Finally, the `drop` statement excludes the index variable i and n1 to n12 from the output data set as they are no longer needed.

As with any relatively complex data manipulation, it is wise to check that the results are as they should be (e.g., by using `proc print`).

As always, before carrying out any formal analysis, it is worth examining the data graphically. One procedure that is often useful in highlighting whether the data should be transformed before analysis is to plot both cell standard deviations against cell means and cell variances against cell means. (The variance should be constant—that is, independent of the mean.) These plots can be constructed from the following SAS instructions:

```
proc means data=hyper noprint;
  class cell;
  var bp;
  output out=cellmeans mean= std= var= /autoname;
run;

proc sgscatter data=cellmeans;
  plot (bp_stddev bp_var)*bp_mean;
run;
```

`Proc means` is used to calculate the summary statistics and write them out, via the `output` statement, to a new data set, `cellmeans`. The `autoname` option on the `output` statement constructs variable names for the summary statistics and can be useful when summary statistics are being computed for several variables. `Proc sgscatter` then produces plots of the standard deviation and variance against the mean, side by side (see Figure 6.3).

There appears to be no obvious relationship between the means and the standard deviations or the means and variances that would indicate the need for a transformation.

A further useful graphic is shown in Figure 6.4; this is a multipanel plot with box plots of blood pressure for each of the levels of each treatment. The distributions appear to be relatively symmetric, and there is no suggestion of any outliers.

Box plots cannot be produced by proc sgscatter, so we have defined a custom graphics template to do it, as follows:

```
proc template;
  define statgraph gridtplt;
    begingraph;
      layout gridded /columns=3 rows=1;
      boxplot y=bp x=drug;
      boxplot y=bp x=diet;
      boxplot y=bp x=biofeed;
      endlayout;
    endgraph;
end;
run;

proc sgrender data=hyper template=gridtplt;
run;
```

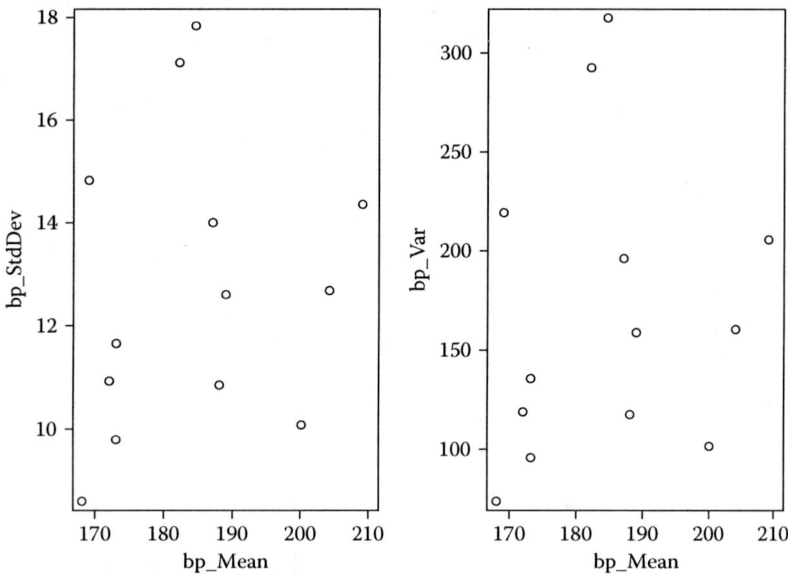

FIGURE 6.3
Plots of means against standard deviations and means against variances for the data in Table 6.5.

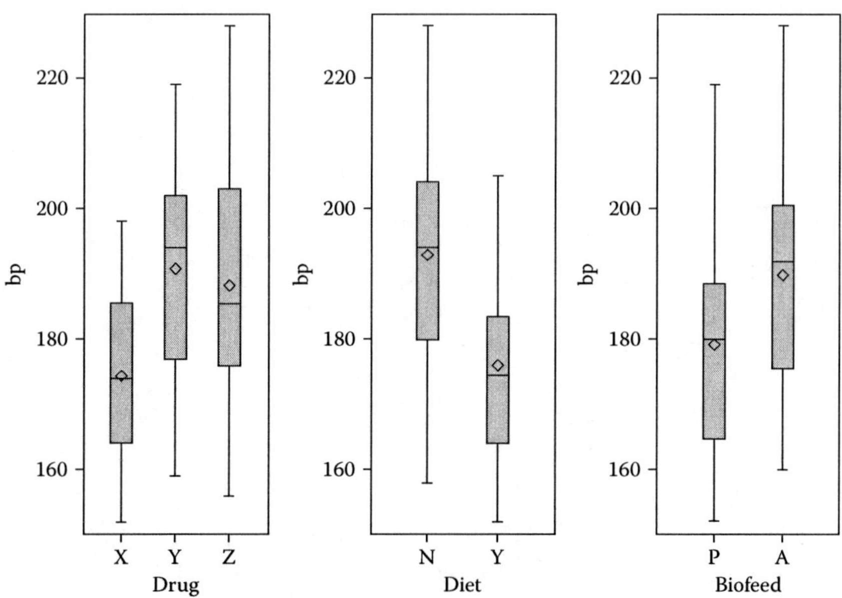

FIGURE 6.4
Box plots of blood pressure for each treatment level for the data in Table 6.5.

The use of the graphics template language is beyond the scope of this book. Nonetheless, this example could be adapted to produce a bespoke grid of graphs simply by changing the numbers of rows and/or columns on the layout statement, including the corresponding number of plot statements before the endlayout statement, and then referencing the appropriate data set on the proc sgrender statement.

6.4.1 Model for Three-Factor Design

A suitable model on which to base the analysis of these data is

$$y_{ijkl} = \mu + \alpha_i + \beta_j + \gamma_k + \delta_{ij} + \tau_{ik} + \omega_{jk} + \theta_{ijk} + \varepsilon_{ijkl} \tag{6.8}$$

where
  y_{ijkl} is the lth observation in the ijkth cell of the design
  α_i, β_j, and γ_k represent main effects
  δ_{ij}, τ_{ik}, and ω_{jk} represent first-order interactions
  θ_{ijk} represents the second-order interaction
  ε_{ijkl} are random error terms assumed to be distributed normally with
    zero mean and variance σ^2

(Once again, the parameters have to be constrained in some way; for details, see Maxwell and Delaney 1990.)

The hypotheses of interest can be written in terms of the parameters of the model as

$$
\begin{aligned}
&H_0^{(1)} : \alpha_1 = \alpha_2 = \cdots = \alpha_a = 0 \\[1.5ex]
&H_0^{(2)} : \beta_1 = \beta_2 = \cdots = \beta_b = 0 \\[1.5ex]
&H_0^{(3)} : \gamma_1 = \gamma_2 = \cdots = \gamma_c = 0 \\[1.5ex]
&H_0^{(4)} : \delta_{11} = \delta_{12} = \cdots = \delta_{ab} = 0 \\[1.5ex]
&H_0^{(5)} : \tau_{11} = \tau_{12} = \cdots = \tau_{ac} = 0 \\[1.5ex]
&H_0^{(6)} : \omega_{11} = \omega_{12} = \cdots = \omega_{bc} = 0 \\[1.5ex]
&H_0^{(6)} : \theta_{111} = \theta_{112} = \cdots = \theta_{abc} = 0
\end{aligned}
\tag{6.9}
$$

where a, b, and c are the numbers of levels of the three factors. The analysis of variance table resulting from this model is given in Table 6.6.

As the design is balanced (same number of observations in each cell), we can use proc anova, although proc glm could, of course, be used again:

TABLE 6.6

Analysis of Variance Table for a Three-Way Factorial Design

Source	SS	DF	MS
A	ASS	$a-1$	$ASS/(a-1)$
B	BSS	$b-1$	$BSS/(b-1)$
C	CSS	$c-1$	$CSS/(c-1)$
A×B	ABSS	$(a-1)(b-1)$	$ABSS/(a-1)(b-1)$
A×C	ACSS	$(a-1)(c-1)$	$ACSS/(a-1)(c-1)$
B×C	BBSS	$(b-1)(c-1)$	$ABSS/(a-1)(b-1)$
A×B×C	ABCSS	$(a-1)(b-1)(c-1)$	$ABSS/(a-1)(b-1)(c-1)$
Within cell (error)	WCSS	$abc(n-1)$	$WCSS/abc(n-1)$

Note: For each term in the table, the appropriate F-statistic for testing the hypothesis about the term is the ratio of the term's mean square divided by the error mean square.

```
proc anova data=hyper;
  class diet biofeed drug;
  model bp=diet|drug|biofeed;
run;
```

The vertical bar operator used on the model statement is a shorthand way of specifying an interaction and including all the lower order interactions and main effects implied by it. The results are shown in Table 6.7.

Several of the main effects are highly significant, but it is the significant second-order interaction term, drug × biofeed × diet, that first requires interpretation. Perhaps the simplest approach to trying to understand the meaning of this interaction is to examine some plots of the cell means. Since proc anova is still running, the cell means for this interaction can be generated and saved in the `cellmeans2` data set by submitting the following statements:

```
  means diet*drug*biofeed;
ods output means=cellmeans2;
run;
```

The resulting means can be plotted stacked in a multipanel plot as follows:

```
proc sgpanel data=cellmeans2;
 panelby drug / columns=1;
 series y=mean_bp x=biofeed /group=diet;
run;
```

The resulting diagram is shown in Figure 6.5. For drug X, there is a large difference in means between biofeedback being present and absent when the diet is not given, but a far smaller difference when the diet is given. For drug Y, the reverse is the case, and for drug Z, the two differences are approximately equal.

TABLE 6.7

Analysis of Variance Results for Blood Pressure Data in Table 6.5

Class-Level Information		
Class	**Levels**	**Values**
diet	2	N Y
biofeed	2	A P
drug	3	X Y Z

Number of Observations Read	72
Number of Observations Used	72

Dependent Variable: bp					
Source	**DF**	**Sum of Squares**	**Mean Square**	**F Value**	**Pr > F**
Model	11	13194.00000	1199.45455	7.66	<.0001
Error	60	9400.00000	156.66667		
Corrected total	71	22594.00000			

R-Square	**Coeff Var**	**Root MSE**	**bp Mean**
0.583960	6.784095	12.51666	184.5000

Source	**DF**	**ANOVA SS**	**Mean Square**	**F Value**	**Pr > F**
diet	1	5202.000000	5202.000000	33.20	<.0001
drug	2	3675.000000	1837.500000	11.73	<.0001
diet*drug	2	903.000000	451.500000	2.88	0.0638
biofeed	1	2048.000000	2048.000000	13.07	0.0006
diet*biofeed	1	32.000000	32.000000	0.20	0.6529
biofeed*drug	2	259.000000	129.500000	0.83	0.4425
diet*biofeed*drug	2	1075.000000	537.500000	3.43	0.0388

The data might now be further analysed by splitting them by drug level and then applying two-way analyses of variance to the resulting tables.

6.5 Unbalanced Designs

The data shown in Table 6.8 are from a study reported in Rifland, Canale, and New (1976) concerned with antipyrine clearance of people suffering from β-thalassemia, a chronic type of anaemia. In this disease, abnormally thick red

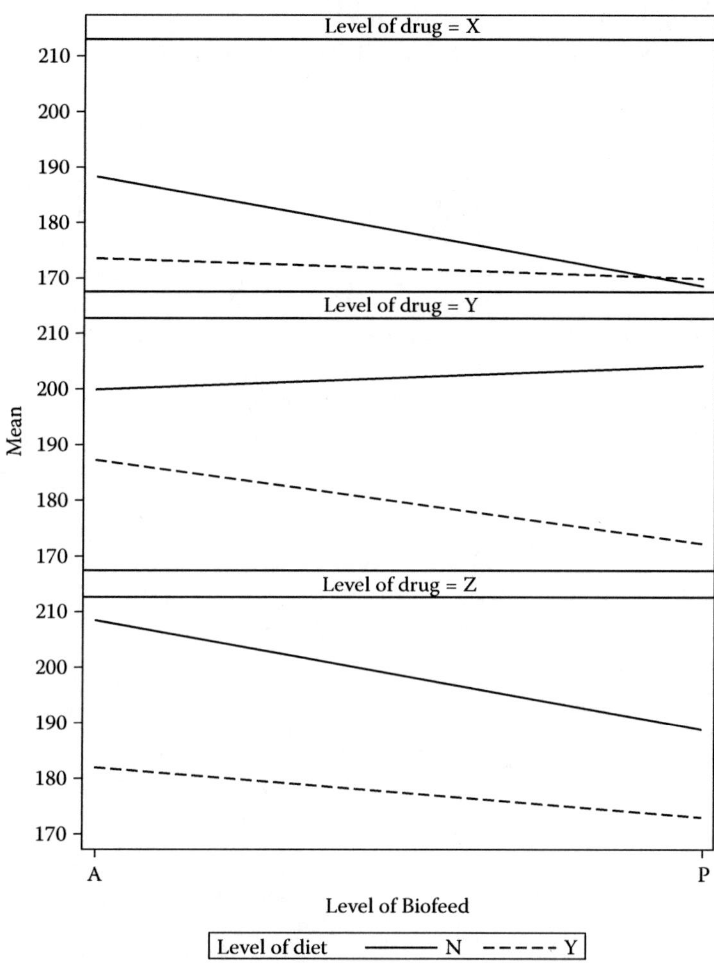

FIGURE 6.5

Plot of factor level means for data in Table 6.5.

TABLE 6.8

Antipyrine Clearance (Half-Life in Hours)

	1			2		3
Males	7.4	5.6	3.7	10.9	11.3	13.3
	6.6	6.0		12.2	10.0	
Females	9.1	6.3	7.1	11.0	8.3	
	11.3	9.4	7.9		4.3	

blood cells are produced. The treatment of the disease has undesirable side effects, including liver damage. Antipyrine is a drug used to assess liver function with a high clearance rate, indicating satisfactory liver function. The main question of interest is whether there is any difference in clearance rate among the pubertal stages (1 = infant, 2 = adolescent, 3 = adult) or between the sexes.

The data in Table 6.8 involve two factors—sex and pubertal stage, but the unbalanced nature of the observations presents considerably more problems for analysis than would a balanced 2×3 design. The main difficulty is that when the data are unbalanced, there is no unique way of finding a 'sum of squares' corresponding to each main effect and its interaction, because these effects are no longer independent of one another. (When the data are balanced, the among-cells sums of squares partition orthogonally into the three component sums of squares—namely, two main effects and an interaction.) Several methods have been suggested for dealing with this problem, each leading to a different type of sums of squares.

6.5.1 Type I Sums of Squares

These sums of squares represent the effect of adding a term to an existing model, in one particular order. For example, a set of type I sums of squares such as the following

Source	Type I SS
A	SSA
B	SSB|A
AB	SSAB|A,B

essentially represents a comparison of the following models:

SSAB|A,B: model including an interaction and main effects, with one including only main effects

SSB|A: model including both main effects, but no interaction, with one including only the main effect of factor A

SSA: model containing only the A main effect, with one containing only the overall mean

The use of these sums of squares in a series of tables in which the effects are considered in different orders (see later discussion) will often provide the most satisfactory way of answering the question as to which model is most appropriate for the observations.

6.5.2 Type II Sums of Squares

These provide sums of squares for a certain term, given all other terms in the model except terms of higher order involving the term being tested. For example, a set of type II sums of squares for the example in the previous subsection would be

Source	Type II SS
A	SSA $\mid$ B
B	SSB $\mid$ A
AB	SSAB $\mid$ A,B

6.5.3 Type III Sums of Squares

Type III sums of squares represent the contribution of each term to a model including all other possible terms. Thus, for a two-factor design, the sums of squares represent the following:

Source	Type III SS
A	SSA $\mid$ B,AB
B	SSB $\mid$ A,AB
AB	SSAB $\mid$ A,B

(SAS also has a type IV sum of squares, which is the same as type III unless the design contains empty cells.)

In a balanced design, type I and type III sums of squares are equal, but for an unbalanced design they are not; there have been numerous discussions over which type is more appropriate for the analysis of such designs. Authors such as Maxwell and Delaney (1990) and Howell (1992) strongly recommend the use of type III sums of squares, and these are the default in SAS. Nelder (1977) and Aitkin (1978), however, are strongly critical of 'correcting' main effects sums of squares for an interaction term involving the corresponding main effect; their criticisms are based on both theoretical and pragmatic grounds. The arguments are relatively subtle but in essence go something like what follows.

When fitting models to data, the principle of *parsimony* is of critical importance. In choosing among possible models, we do not adopt complex models for which there is no empirical evidence. Therefore, if there is no convincing evidence of an AB interaction, we do not retain the term in the model. Thus, additivity of A and B is assumed unless there is convincing evidence to the contrary. The argument proceeds that type III sum of squares for A, in which it is adjusted for AB, makes no sense. First, if the interaction term is necessary in the model, then the experimenter will usually wish to consider simple effects of A at each level of B separately. A test of the hypothesis of no A main effect would not usually be carried out if the AB interaction is significant. If the AB interaction is not significant, then adjusting for it is of no interest, and causes a substantial loss of power in testing the A and B main effects.

The issue does not arise so clearly in the balanced case, for there the sum of squares for A, say, is independent of whether interaction is assumed or not. Thus, in deciding on possible models for the data, the interaction term is not included unless it has been shown to be necessary. In such a case, tests on main effects involved in the interaction are not carried out or, if carried out, are not interpreted (see the biofeedback example in Section 6.4).

The arguments of Nelder and Aitkin against the use of type III sums of squares are powerful and persuasive. Their recommendation to use type I sums of squares (or type II sums of squares), considering effects in a number of orders, as the most suitable way in which to identify a suitable model for a data set is also convincing and strongly endorsed by the authors of this book.

6.5.4 Analysis of Antipyrine Data

We first read in the data and then apply proc glm using the following SAS code:

```
data antipyrine;
input sex$ stage hours;
cards;
M 1 7.4
M 1 5.6

. . .

F 2 11.0
F 3 8.3
F 3 4.3
;

proc glm data=antipyrine;
   class sex stage;
   model hours=sex|stage / ss1 ss2 ss3;
run;
```

The default for proc glm is to produce both type I and type III sums of squares. Here we specify type II sums of squares as well. The results are given in Table 6.9. We see that the interaction sum of squares is the same for type I, type II, and type III sums of squares. But the type III main effects sums of squares are different from those given by type I and type II. The type I and type II sex main effect sums of squares differ because the latter is adjusted for stage whereas the former is not. Running the analysis specifying stage as the first variable would lead to the same type I sum of squares for sex as is given by the type II sum of squares in Table 6.9.

There is some evidence of a sex × stage interaction in the data; the p-value for the associated F-test is 0.049. A plot of the six means may be helpful in

TABLE 6.9

Analysis of Variance Results for Anitipyrine Data

Class-Level Information		
Class	**Levels**	**Values**
Sex	2	F M
Stage	3	1 2 3

Number of Observations Read	19
Number of Observations Used	19

Dependent Variable: hours					
Source	**DF**	**Sum of Squares**	**Mean Square**	**F Value**	**Pr > F**
Model	5	56.6703947	11.3340789	1.88	0.1671
Error	13	78.5275000	6.0405769		
Corrected Total	18	135.1978947			

R-Square	**Coeff Var**	**Root MSE**	**hours Mean**
0.419166	28.87904	2.457759	8.510526

Source	**DF**	**Type I SS**	**Mean Square**	**F Value**	**Pr > F**
sex	1	0.75789474	0.75789474	0.13	0.7289
stage	2	9.59433511	4.79716755	0.79	0.4727
sex*stage	2	46.31816489	23.15908245	3.83	0.0491

Source	**DF**	**Type II SS**	**Mean Square**	**F Value**	**Pr > F**
sex	1	0.43508511	0.43508511	0.07	0.7926
stage	2	9.59433511	4.79716755	0.79	0.4727
sex*stage	2	46.31816489	23.15908245	3.83	0.0491

Source	**DF**	**Type III SS**	**Mean Square**	**F Value**	**Pr > F**
sex	1	4.13281250	4.13281250	0.68	0.4231
stage	2	6.00213652	3.00106826	0.50	0.6196
sex*stage	2	46.31816489	23.15908245	3.83	0.0491

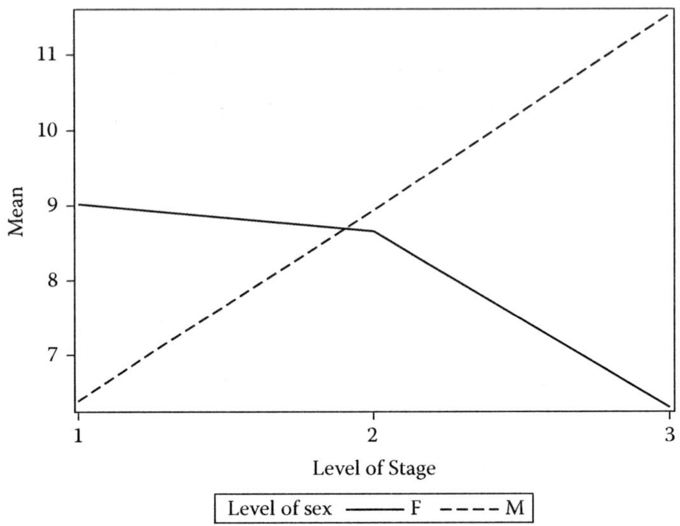

FIGURE 6.6
Plot of mean clearance rate for the three stages and for males and females.

interpreting this interaction. Such a plot can be obtained using the following code:

```
  means sex*stage;
  ods output means=antmns;
run;
proc sgplot data=antmns;
  series y=mean_hours x=stage/ group=sex;
run;
```

The resulting plot is shown in Figure 6.6. Clearly, for males the clearance rate increases with age, but for females it decreases, at first gradually and then more dramatically between adolescence and adult stages.

6.6 Nonparametric Analysis of Variance

Although the F-tests used in the analysis of variance are reasonably robust against departures from normality, there may be occasions where the departure is thought to be so extreme that some alternative method of analysis may be required.

To illustrate, we shall use the data shown in Table 6.10. These data were collected by Kontula et al. (1980) in a study attempting to develop a more

TABLE 6.10

Number of Glucocorticoid Receptor (GR) Sites per Leukocyte Cell

Normal Subjects	Hairy-Cell Anaemia	Chronic Lymphatic Leukaemia	Chronic Myelocytic Leukaemia	Acute Leukaemia
3,500	5,710	2,390	6,320	3,230
3,500	6,110	3,330	6,860	3,880
3,500	8,060	3,580	11,400	7,640
4,000	8,080	3,880	14,000	7,890
4,000	11,400	4,280		8,280
4,000		5,120		16,200
4,300				18,250
4,500				29,900
4,500				
4,900				
5,200				
6,000				
6,750				
8,000				

Source: Kontula, K., Anderrson, L. C., Paavonen, T., Myllyla, G., Terrenharr, L., and Vuopio, P. 1980. *International Journal of Cancer*, 26:177–183.

accurate method for determining the number of glucocortical receptor (GR) sites per cell in patients suffering from leukaemia. The new methodology was used to count the number of GR sites for samples of leukocyte cells from normal subjects as well as patients with hairy-cell leukaemia, chronic lymphatic leukaemia, chronic myelocytic leukaemia, or acute leukaemia.

6.6.1 Kruskal–Wallis Distribution-Free Test for One-Way Analysis of Variance

Rather than use the analysis of variance procedure described in Subsection 6.2.1 for these data, we shall use the Kruskal and Wallis distribution-free procedure for one-way designs. Again, we assume there are k populations to be compared and that a sample of n_j observations is available from population j, $j=1,\ldots,k$. The hypothesis to be tested is that all the populations have the same probability distribution. To apply the Kruskal–Wallis test, the observations are first ranked without regard to group membership and then the sums of the ranks of the observations in each group are calculated. These sums will be denoted by $R_1, R_2, \ldots, R_k$. If the null hypothesis is true, we would expect the R_js to be more or less equal, apart from differences caused by the different sample sizes. A measure of the degree to which the R_js differ from one another is given by

$$H = \frac{12}{N(N+1)} \sum_{j=1}^{k} \frac{R_j^2}{n_j} - 3(N+1) \tag{6.10}$$

where $N = \sum_{j=1}^{k} n_j$

Under the null hypothesis, the statistic H has a chi-squared distribution with $k-1$ degrees of freedom.

6.6.2 Applying the Kruskal–Wallis Test

The data are in a file, grsites.dat, with a letter indicating the group (N, H, C, M, A) and the number of sites. We read the data in and apply the Kruskal–Wallis procedure as follows:

```
data grsites;
   infile 'c:\amsus\data\grsites.dat';
   input group$ ngrs;
run;

proc npar1way data=grsites wilcoxon;
   class group;
   var ngrs;
run;
```

By default, `proc npar1way` produces analyses based on a number of different rank scoring methods. The `wilcoxon` option restricts it to Wilcoxon scores (i.e., rank sums) and the associated Kruskal–Wallis test. The results are shown in Table 6.11.

The p-value associated with the chi-squared test statistic is 0.0022, so there is strong evidence that the average number of GR sites in the leukocyte cells of the different types of subjects differs.

TABLE 6.11

Results of Applying the Kruskal–Wallis Test to the Data in Table 6.10

Wilcoxon Scores (Rank Sums) for Variable ngrs Classified by Variable group				
group	N	Sum of Scores	Expected Under H0	Std Dev Under H0	Mean Score
N	14	202.00	266.0	31.911394	14.428571
H	5	133.50	95.0	22.494577	26.700000
C	6	50.50	114.0	24.253494	8.416667
M	4	114.50	76.0	20.431714	28.625000
A	8	202.50	152.0	27.087058	25.312500
Average scores were used for ties.				

Kruskal–Wallis Test	
Chi-Squared	16.6682
DF	4
Pr > Chi-Squared	0.0022

6.7 Analysis of Covariance

Analysis of covariance is essentially analysis of variance in which differences between levels of a factor are tested after controlling for other variables, termed covariates. The response variable and the covariate are assumed to be related in some way, and from the estimated relationship, the subject's response values are adjusted in an attempt to account for factor level differences in the covariates. Following this adjustment, the usual analysis-of-variance tests are applied to see whether there remains any difference in average response in the different factor levels.

For a single factor design and a single covariate, the appropriate model is

$$y_{ij} = \mu + \alpha_i + \beta\left(x_{ij} - \overline{x}\right) + \varepsilon_{ij} \tag{6.11}$$

where β is the regression coefficient linking response variable and covariate and $\overline{x}$ is the grand mean of the covariate values. The regression coefficient is assumed to be the same in each group. The means of the response variable adjusted for the covariate are obtained simply as adjusted group mean = group mean $+\hat{\beta}(\overline{x}_i - \overline{x})$, where $\overline{x}_i$ is the mean of the ith group.

In ANCOVA, the covariate will most often be a baseline measurement of the outcome variable, although other covariates are also used on occasion. In Chapter 3 we alluded to the advantages of ANCOVA over a change score approach when baseline outcome measures were available, and we shall say no more about change scores here; Senn (2006) puts the final nail into the coffin of change score analysis.

The benefits of analysis of covariance are usually said to be the following:

- If one has an observational study in which the groups have differences in baseline values, ANCOVA can remove a potential bias from the results (but see later discussion).

- If one has a randomised trial where, by virtue of randomisation, any real group differences in baseline values are unlikely, then ANCOVA reduces the amount of unexplained variation in the data. This reduces the error variance and makes the F-test of group difference on the final value of the outcome variable more sensitive; the power of the F-test is increased.

But the following comments of Brown (2005) about analysis of covariance are useful for reminding potential users of the techniques of possible problems:

- The covariates are assumed to be unaffected by treatment; they can be measured before the treatments are assigned, for example.

If the treatment does affect a covariate, then adjusting for differences in this variable may well 'adjust away' the actual treatment difference.

- In a randomised trial, the covariate is used to increase the power of the F-test for the treatment difference. But when ANCOVA is used in an observational study where the covariate may differ considerably in the naturally occurring groups, the investigator is essentially looking for the answer the question, 'What would the group difference on the outcome variable be if the groups had the same level of the covariate?' But this may mean that the groups are compared at a value of the covariate that is not typical of either group. Further, the statistical model will need to *extrapolate* beyond the region where there is most data for both groups and this makes an assumption that the model is correct in that region, for both groups.

- The relationship between the outcome and the covariate must be the same in all groups. In other words, there must be no interaction between the treatments and the covariate. If there is an interaction, it does not make sense to compare the groups at a single value of the covariate because any difference noted will not apply for other values of the covariate. This assumption is equivalent to saying that the relationship between the outcome and the covariate should appear as parallel curves, one for each group. This relationship can be checked, as we shall demonstrate in the following examples.

Thus, application of ANCOVA requires careful consideration of its statistical assumptions about the relationship between outcome and covariate as well as its more subtle aspects. Many reports of ANCOVA report a covariate as having been 'adjusted for' or 'controlled' without producing any convincing argument that the control or adjustment was appropriate.

As an illustration of analysis of covariance, the method will be applied to the data shown in Table 6.12. These data show plasma inorganic phosphate measurements obtained from 13 controls and 20 obese patients taken 10 minutes (labelled 0 hours in Table 6.12) and 3 hours after an oral glucose challenge (data adapted from Zerbe 1979). Here, interest centres on whether there is a difference in average plasma inorganic phosphate level between control and obese patient population 3 hours after the challenge after controlling for the difference after 10 minutes.

Before applying analysis of covariance, it will be helpful to examine the data graphically. Here we can plot a scattergram of 10-minute level against 3-hour level, identifying control and obese patients and also showing the simple linear regression line for the two variables, calculated separately in each group. The required SAS code is

TABLE 6.12

Plasma Inorganic Phosphate Levels from
13 Control and 20 Obese Patients

		Hours after Glucose Challenge	
Group	**Patient**	**0**	**3**
Control	1	4.3	2.5
	2	3.7	3.2
	3	4.0	3.1
	4	3.6	3.9
	5	4.1	3.4
	6	3.8	3.6
	7	3.8	3.4
	8	4.4	3.8
	9	5.0	3.6
	10	3.7	2.3
	11	3.7	2.2
	12	4.4	4.3
	13	4.7	4.2
Obese	1	4.3	2.5
	2	5.0	4.1
	3	4.6	4.2
	4	4.3	3.1
	5	3.1	1.9
	6	4.8	3.1
	7	3.7	3.6
	8	5.4	3.7
	9	3.0	26
	10	4.9	4.1
	11	4.8	3.7
	12	4.4	3.4
	13	4.9	4.1
	14	5.1	4.2
	15	4.8	4.0
	16	4.2	3.1
	17	6.6	3.8
	18	3.6	2.4
	19	4.5	2.3
	20	4.6	3.6

```
data pip;
 input pip1 pip2;
 group='C';
 if _n_>13 then group='O';
cards;
```

```
4.3    2.5
3.7    3.2


. . .


3.6    2.4
4.5    2.3
4.6    3.6
;

proc sgplot data=pip;
  reg y=pip2 x=pip1 / group=group;
run;
```

The data step reads in the two plasma inorganic phosphate measurements. We know that the first 13 observations belong to control subjects and the remainder to obese subjects, so we can use the automatic SAS variable_n_ to assign values to a group variable. The `reg` plot type within `proc sgplot` can be used for the plot and the result is shown in Figure 6.7.

Figure 6.6 gives little evidence that the regression lines of each group of patients differ in slope, which is reassuring because this is one of the assumptions of the analysis of covariance.

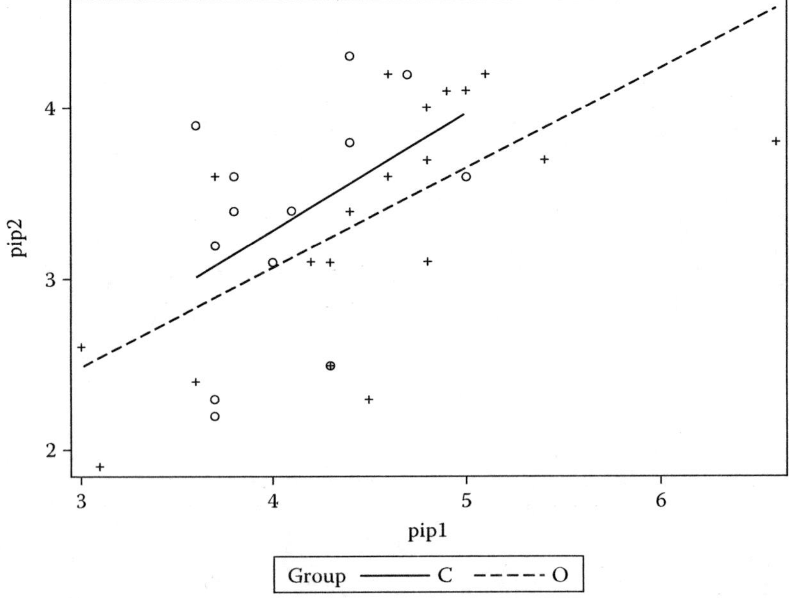

FIGURE 6.7
Plot of the data in Table 6.12.

Analysis of covariance can be applied to the data using `proc glm`:

```
proc glm data=pip;
  class group;
  model pip2=pip1 group pip1*group;
run;
```

As the variable `pip1` is not mentioned on the `class` statement, it is assumed to be continuous. The results are shown in Table 6.13.

Using the type I sums of squares in Table 6.13, we can conclude that the regression coefficient of the 3-hour phosphate measurement on the 10-minute measurement is significantly different from zero and that, after adjusting for

TABLE 6.13

Analysis of Covariance Results for the Data in Table 6.12

Class-Level Information		
Class	**Levels**	**Values**
Group	2	C O

Number of Observations Read	33
Number of Observations Used	33

Dependent Variable: pip2s					
Source	**DF**	**Sum of Squares**	**Mean Square**	**F Value**	**Pr > F**
Model	3	5.28062622	1.76020874	5.15	0.0056
Error	29	9.91573742	0.34192198		
Corrected Total	32	15.19636364			

R-Square	**Coeff Var**	**Root MSE**	**pip2 Mean**
0.347493	17.38419	0.584741	3.363636

Source	**DF**	**Type I SS**	**Mean Square**	**F Value**	**Pr > F**
pip1	1	4.86961807	4.86961807	14.24	0.0007
group	1	0.39083650	0.39083650	1.14	0.2938
pip1*group	1	0.02017164	0.02017164	0.06	0.8098

Source	**DF**	**Type III SS**	**Mean Square**	**F Value**	**Pr > F**
pip1	1	3.13693492	3.13693492	9.17	0.0051
group	1	0.00398906	0.00398906	0.01	0.9147
pip1*group	1	0.02017164	0.02017164	0.06	0.8098

the 10-minute level, there is no difference between the control and obese patients. The p-value of the F-statistic for the interaction demonstrates that there is no evidence of a difference in the regression slopes of 3-hour value on 10-minute level in the two groups.

6.8 Summary

In this chapter we have described the application of both ANOVA and ANCOVA to a number of data sets and pointed out some features of the latter that need careful thought and consideration when applying the method in practice. Both ANOVA and ANCOVA can be formulated in a regression framework, as we shall illustrate in Chapter 8, and further subsumed within a more general approach known as generalised linear models, which we shall discuss in Chapter 10.

7

Scatter Plots, Correlation, Simple Regression, and Smoothing

7.1 Introduction

In many medical investigations, measurements and observations are taken on two variables of interest for a sample of patients or subjects. In part, of course, this has been true of the data sets discussed in earlier chapters—for example, the two categorical variables, 'risk factor present' or 'risk factor absent' and disease or illness present, 'yes' or 'no'. But in this chapter, our interest will be in the situation where the two variables measured are continuous or quasicontinuous. For such *bivariate data,* answers to a number of questions may be of interest. For example, are the variables related in some way? Can one variable be predicted from the other and, if so, what form of mathematical equation is it best to use? The starting point for the investigation of bivariate data is almost always the humble *scatter plot* and it is this we discuss and illustrate in the next section.

7.2 Scatter Plot and Correlation Coefficient

According to Martin and Welsh (2005), the simplest and one of the most powerful graphics for describing the relationship between two variables is the scatter plot, which represents each pair of data values using (x, y) coordinates in a Cartesian plan. The 'shape' of the scatter plot is used to describe the relationship between the two variables. Two elements of the shape of a scatter plot that are most useful in describing relationships between variables are measures of 'location' and 'spread'. For example, location might be measured as a line or a curve that runs through the bulk of the data, while spread might be measured in terms of deviations of (x, y) points from the estimated location.

The simple *xy* scatter plot has certainly been in use for a long time—at least from the eighteenth century, and it has many virtues, indeed, according to Tufte (1983):

> The relational graphic—in its barest form the scatterplot and its variants—is the greatest of all graphical designs. It links at least two variables encouraging and even imploring the viewer to assess the possible causal relationship between the plotted variables. It confronts causal theories that *x* causes *y* with empirical evidence as to the actual relationship between *x* and *y*.

Now let's have a look at an example of a scatter plot. For this we will use the data shown in Table 7.1, which were collected in a study investigating the possible link between alcohol consumption and the death rate per 100,000 of the population from cirrhosis and alcoholism (data collected before West Germany ceased to exist as a separate country). A scatter plot of the data that includes appropriate labels for each bivariate observation can be constructed using the following SAS code, which also produces the value of *Pearson's correlation coefficient* for the two variables (see later for the definition of this coefficient):

```
data drinking;
  input country $ 1-12 alcohol cirrhosis;
cards;
France        24.7       46.1
Italy         15.2       23.6
W.Germany     12.3       23.7
Austria       10.9        7.0
Belgium       10.8       12.3
USA            9.9       14.2
Canada         8.3        7.4
E&W            7.2        3.0
Sweden         6.6        7.2
Japan          5.8       10.6
Netherlands    5.7        3.7
Ireland        5.6        3.4
Norway         4.2        4.3
Finland        3.9        3.6
Israel         3.1        5.4
;

proc corr; run;

proc sgplot data=drinking;
   scatter y=cirrhosis x=alcohol /datalabel=country;
run;
```

Some of the country names are longer than the default of eight for character variables, so column input is used to read them in. The values of the two numeric variables can then be read in with list input. This is an example of mixing different forms of input on one `input` statement. Proc corr produces

TABLE 7.1

Average Alcohol Consumption and Death Rate

Country	Alcohol Consumption (litres/person/year)	Cirrhosis and Alcoholism (death rate/100,000)
France	24.7	46.1
Italy	15.2	23.6
W. Germany	12.3	23.7
Austria	10.9	7.0
Belgium	10.8	12.3
United States	9.9	14.2
Canada	8.3	7.4
England and Wales	7.2	3.0
Sweden	6.6	7.2
Japan	5.8	10.6
Netherlands	5.7	3.7
Ireland	5.6	3.4
Norway	4.2	4.3
Finland	3.9	3.6
Israel	3.1	5.4

Pearson correlations by default. A `var` statement would normally be used as the default is to include all numeric variables.

The scatter plot produced by SAS is shown in Figure 7.1. The scatter plot indicates that there is a very strong relationship between death rate from cirrhosis and alcohol consumption, with cirrhosis deaths increasing with alcohol consumption. The relationship shown in Figure 7.1 can be summarised in the value of a correlation coefficient, here Pearson's correlation coefficient, r (there are others; for example, *Spearman's rho* and *Kendall's tau*—see Bland 2011) given for a sample of bivariate data (x_i, y_i), $i = 1 \ldots n$ by

$$r = \frac{\sum_{i=1}^{n} (y_i - \bar{y})(x_i - \bar{x})}{\sqrt{\sum_{i=1}^{n} (y_i - \bar{y})^2 \sum_{i=1}^{n} (x_i - \bar{x})^2}} \tag{7.1}$$

where n is the sample size and $\bar{y}$ and $\bar{x}$ are the sample means of the y and x variables. The correlation coefficient is a measure of the *linear relationship* between the two variables and measures how closely the points lie to a straight line. The correlation coefficient takes a value between –1 and 1, with the two extreme values being obtained for a perfect linear relationship between the variables in different directions. The linear part in the previous sentence needs to be emphasised; for nonlinear relationships, the correlation coefficient is not of any great use. That this is the case is demonstrated by the example in Figure 7.2, where the correlation is zero and in Figure 7.3, where

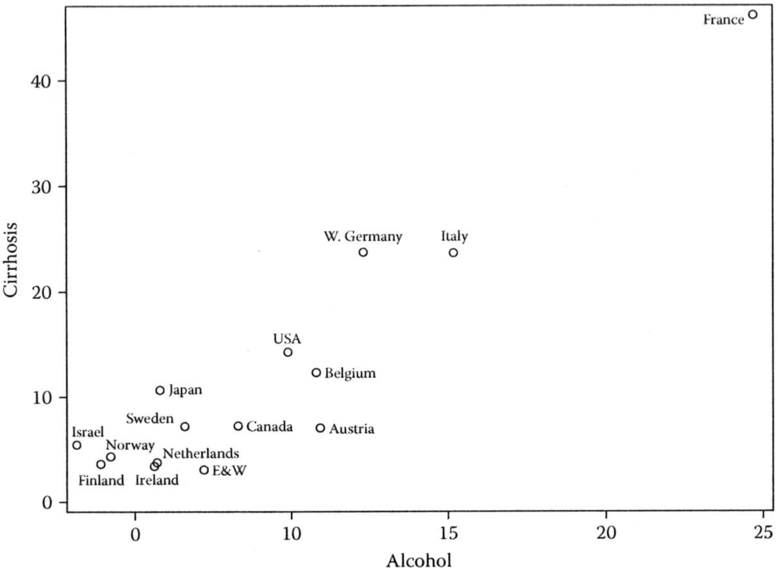

FIGURE 7.1

Scatter plot of cirrhosis death rates against alcohol consumption for a number of countries.

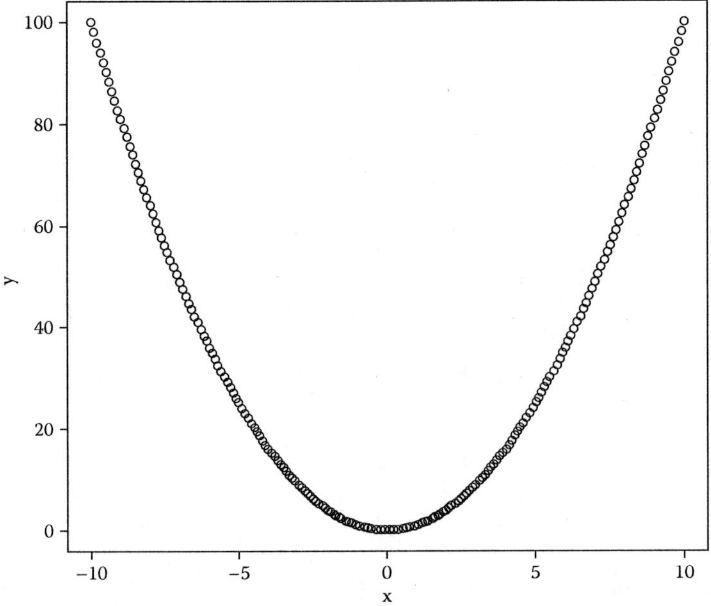

FIGURE 7.2

Bivariate data where the relationship between the two variables is exact but the correlation is zero.

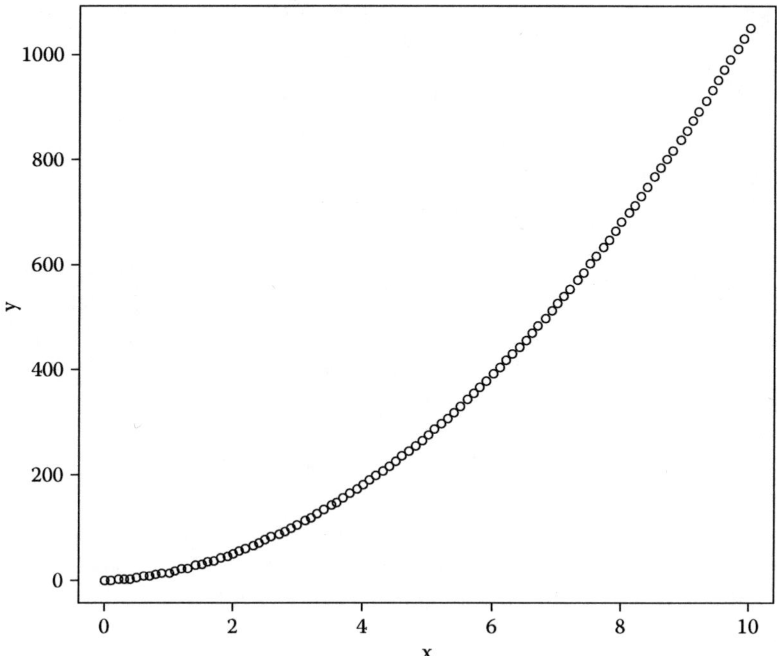

FIGURE 7.3
Bivariate data where the relationship between the two variables is exact but the correlations are less than 1 (0.97).

TABLE 7.2

Correlation Coefficient for Cirrhosis Death Rate and Alcohol Data

				Pearson Correlation Statistics (Fisher's z Transformation)		
Variable	With Variable	N	Sample Correlation	Fisher's z	Bias Adjustment	Correlation Estimate
alcohol	cirrhosis	15	0.93883	1.72809	0.03353	0.93473

	Pearson Correlation Statistics (Fisher's z Transformation)		
Variable	With Variable	95% Confidence Limits	p Value for H0:Rho=0
alcohol	cirrhosis	0.810597 0.978472	<.0001

it is 0.97, although in both cases the relationship between the two variables is exact, it is not linear.

Returning to the alcohol and cirrhosis data, we see from Table 7.2 that the value of Pearson's correlation coefficient is 0.939, confirming the conclusion from Figure 7.1 that the relationship between the two variables is very strong.

Also given in Table 7.2 is an associated *p*-value for the correlation coefficient of '<.0001'. This is simply the result of testing the hypothesis that the population correlation coefficient is zero using the test statistic $t = r\sqrt{\dfrac{n-2}{1-r^2}}$, which if the null hypotheses is true (and the data are sampled from a bivariate normal distribution—an assumption we shall not dwell upon here), has a Student's *t*-distribution with $n-2$ degrees of freedom. In the case of the alcohol/cirrhosis data, there is extremely strong evidence that the null hypothesis is incorrect. In medical papers, estimated values of correlations are almost always followed by a *p*-value resulting from testing for a zero population correlation, whether or not this value is plausible or not. Usually, it would be more informative if *Fisher's z-transformation* of the correlation coefficient—that is,

$$z = \frac{1}{2}\log\left(\frac{1+r}{1-r}\right) \tag{7.2}$$

were used to find a confidence interval for the population correlation by first finding a confidence interval for z from its known standard error of $1/\sqrt{n-3}$ and then transforming back to the correlation scale. In SAS, this can be done using the following code:

```
proc corr data=drinking fisher;
 var alcohol cirrhosis;
run;
```

The results are shown in Table 7.2. The 95% confidence interval for the population correlation coefficient is [0.81,0.98]. (This approach is based on the assumption that both variables have normal distributions—a stronger assumption than that required for the test that the population correlation is zero.)

Thus, for the alcohol/cirrhosis data, we have an estimated correlation of 0.94 and 95% confidence interval of [0.81,0.98]; however, this needs to be interpreted in association with the scatter plot in Figure 7.1 (correlation coefficients *always* need to be used along with the scatter plot). The scatter plot certainly indicates that the assumption of a linear relationship seems a reasonable one, but it also indicates one possible problem—namely, the *outlier* that is France (only, of course, in the limited sense of this graph!). Correlation coefficients can often (but not always) be badly affected by outliers, so it might be sensible to recalculate the correlation after excluding France.

The necessary SAS code is

```
data drinking2;
 set drinking;
 if country~='France';
run;

proc corr; run;
```

The new value of the correlation coefficient found from the resulting output is 0.832, which, although lower than the previous value, is again highly significant.

7.3 Simple Linear Regression and Locally Weighted Regression

The correlation coefficient calculated for the alcohol consumption and death rate data in the previous section indicates the strength of the linear relationship between a pair of variables. But there may be other questions of interest about bivariate data, and the one that will be of concern in this section is, 'How can one of the variables be best predicted from the other?' One answer to this question is to fit a simple *linear regression model* to the data. We assume that there are n data pairs, (x_i, y_i), $i = 1 \ldots n$, where the ys are the values of the variable to be predicted (the *response* variable) and the xs are the corresponding values of the variable used for prediction (the *explanatory* variable). The simple linear regression model is

$$y_i = \beta_0 + \beta_i x_i + \varepsilon_i \tag{7.3}$$

where β_0 is the *intercept* and β_1 is the *slope* of the linear relationship, and ε_i is an error or residual term accounting for the difference between the observed value of y_i and the linear regression model. The residuals are assumed to be independent random variables having a normal distribution with mean zero and constant variance σ^2. The *regression coefficients* β_0 and β_1 may be estimated as $\hat{\beta}_0$ and $\hat{\beta}_1$ using *least squares*. Here, the sum of squared differences between the observed values of the response variable y_i and the values 'predicted' by the regression equation $\hat{y}_i = \hat{\beta}_0 + \hat{\beta}_1 x_i$ is minimised, leading to the estimates

$$\hat{\beta}_0 = \bar{y} - \hat{\beta}_1 \bar{x} \tag{7.4}$$

$$\hat{\beta}_1 = \frac{\sum_{i=1}^{n}(x_i - \bar{x})(y_i - \bar{y})}{\sum_{i=1}^{n}(x_i - \bar{x})^2} \tag{7.5}$$

The model predicted values of the response variable are given by

$$\hat{y}_i = \hat{\beta}_0 + \hat{\beta}_1 x_i \tag{7.6}$$

The variance σ^2 is estimated as s^2, given by

$$s^2 = \sum_{i=1}^{n} (y_i - \hat{y}_i)^2 / (n-2) \tag{7.7}$$

The estimated variance of the estimate of the slope parameter is

$$\text{Var}(\hat{\beta}_1) = \frac{s^2}{\sum_{i=1}^{n} (x_i - \bar{x})^2} \tag{7.8}$$

The estimated variance of a predicted value y_{pred} at a given value of x—say, x_0—is

$$\text{Var}(y_{\text{pred}}) = s^2 \left[1 + \frac{1}{n} + \frac{(x_0 - \bar{x})^2}{\sum_{i=1}^{n} (x_i - \bar{x})^2} \right] \tag{7.9}$$

As our first example of applying the simple linear regression model, we will return to the data used in the previous section but leave out France because its inclusion could distort estimates of the parameters in the model for the bulk of the data. To fit the model, we use proc reg as follows:

```
ods graphics on;
proc reg data=drinking2 plot(only)=fitplot;
   model cirrhosis=alcohol;
run;
```

Basic use of `proc reg` need only involve the `model` statement. With ODS graphics on, a number of plots are produced by default. Here we have used the `plot` option on the `proc` statement to request only the fitplot, which is shown in Figure 7.4.

The tabular SAS output is shown in Table 7.3. The regression coefficient of cirrhosis death rate on alcohol consumption is highly significant. The value of R-squared (where R is the multiple correlation coefficient; see Chapter 8) indicates that 69% of the variation in death rates amongst the countries is due to variation in alcohol consumption.

Our second example (given in Daly et al. 1995) arises from the year 1975, when the British government set up a Resources Allocation Working Party to 'review the arrangement for distributing National Health Service (NHS) capital and revenue'. It was decided to base regional resource

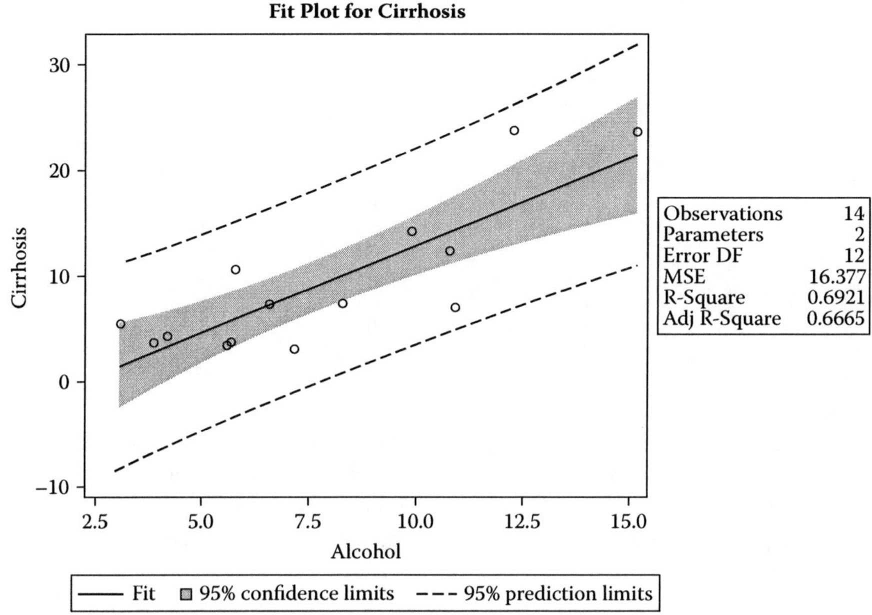

FIGURE 7.4
Linear regression fit and confidence interval for cirrhosis death rate against alcohol consumption.

allocation on death rate within regions (or, more precisely, on a 'standardised mortality rate'). But NHS resources need to reflect regional variations in 'chronic sickness'—long-standing health problems that require medical treatment. The question then, which was a controversial one at the time, was 'Are death rates a good predictor of sickness rates?' Data that can be used to address this question are shown in Table 7.4. These data show standardised mortality rates per 10,000 and standardised morbidity rates per 1000 for 10 regions of England and Wales, for the 1972–1973 period.

The data can be read in and linear regression applied using the following SAS code:

```
data SMRMorb;
input region $15 SMR Morbidity;
datalines;
North           132.7   228.2
Yorkshire       126.8   235.2
North West      132.8   218.6
East Midlands   119.2   222.0
West Midlands   124.8   210.5
East Anglia     108.2   205.0
```

```
Greater London   116.3   202.6
South East       109.5   189.6
South West       112.2   186.6
Wales            128.6   249.9
;

proc sgplot data=SMRMorb;
  scatter y=Morbidity x=SMR / datalabel=region;
run;

ods graphics on;
proc reg data=SMRMorb plot(only)=fitplot;
  model Morbidity=SMR;
run;
```

The scatter plot of morbidity against SMR is shown in Figure 7.5 and the fitted regression and confidence intervals in Figure 7.6. The numerical results are shown in Table 7.5. The estimate of the slope parameter is 1.64, which is highly significant; there is strong evidence that death rates *are* predictive of sickness rates.

TABLE 7.3

Linear Regression Results for Cirrhosis and Alcohol Consumption Data

Model: MODEL1	
Dependent Variable: cirrhosis	
Number of Observations Read	14
Number of Observations Used	14

Analysis of Variance					
Source	**DF**	**Sum of Squares**	**Mean Square**	**F Value**	**Pr > F**
Model	1	441.84624	441.84624	26.98	0.0002
Error	12	196.52804	16.37734		
Corrected Total	13	638.37429			

Root MSE	4.04689	R-Square	0.6921	
Dependent Mean	9.24286	Adj R-Sq	0.6665	
Coeff Var	43.78400			

Parameter Estimates					
Variable	**DF**	**Parameter Estimate**	**Standard Error**	**t Value**	**Pr > |t|**
Intercept	1	−3.61154	2.70081	−1.34	0.2060
alcohol	1	1.64348	0.31641	5.19	0.0002

TABLE 7.4

Standardised Mortality Rates and Morbidity Rate in the UK, 1972–1973

Region	Mortality Rate (per 10,000)	Morbidity Rate (per 1000)
North	132.7	228.2
Yorkshire	126.8	235.2
Northwest	132.8	218.6
East Midlands	119.2	222.0
West Midlands	124.8	210.5
East Anglia	108.2	205.0
Greater London	116.3	202.6
Southeast	109.5	189.6
Southwest	112.2	186.6
Wales	128.6	249.9

Source: Daly, D., Hand, D. J., Jones, M. C., Lunn, A. D., and McConway, K. J. 1995. *Elements of Statistics.* Reading, MA: Addison-Wesley.

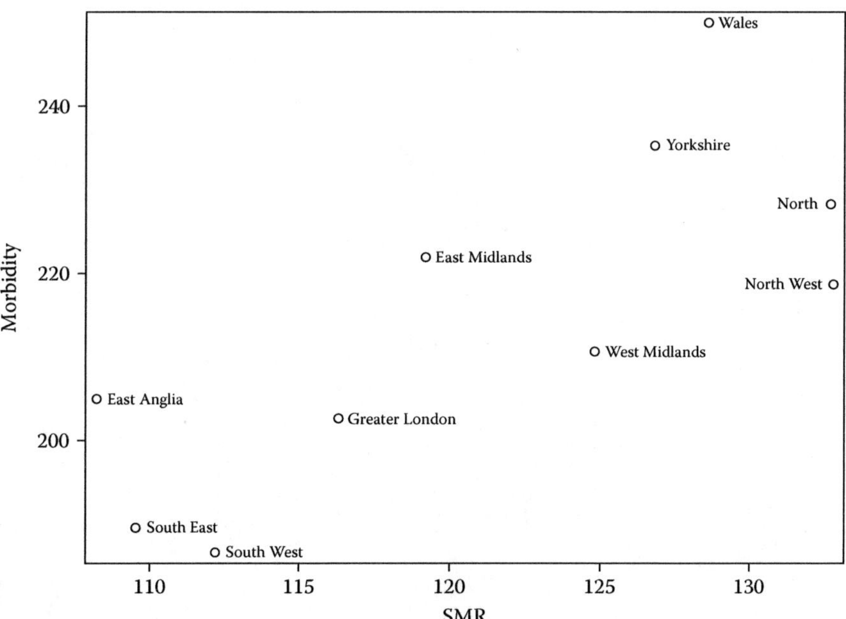

FIGURE 7.5
Scatter plot of SMR against morbidity for the data in Table 7.4.

For our final example of simple linear regression, we shall use data from an experiment in *kinesiology,* a natural care system that uses gentle muscle testing to evaluate many functions of the body in the structural, chemical, neurological, and biological realms. A subject performed a standard exercise at a gradually increasing level. Two measurements were made: (1) oxygen

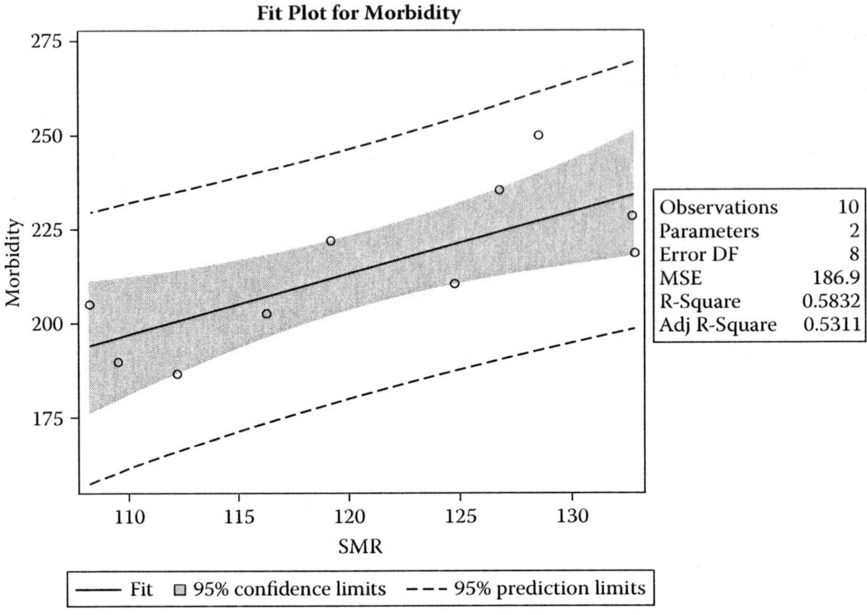

FIGURE 7.6
Fitted regression and confidence intervals for data in Table 7.4.

TABLE 7.5

Linear Regression Results for the Data in Table 7.4

Model: MODEL1	
Dependent Variable: Morbidity	
Number of Observations Read	10
Number of Observations Used	10

Analysis of Variance					
Source	DF	Sum of Squares	Mean Square	F Value	Pr > F
Model	1	2092.43857	2092.43857	11.20	0.0101
Error	8	1495.21743	186.90218		
Corrected Total	9	3587.65600			

Root MSE	13.67122	R-Square	0.5832
Dependent Mean	214.82000	Adj R-Sq	0.5311
Coeff Var	6.36403		

TABLE 7.5 (*Continued*)

Linear Regression Results for the Data in Table 7.4

Parameter Estimates					
Variable	**DF**	**Parameter Estimate**	**Standard Error**	**t Value**	**Pr > |t|**
Intercept	1	16.54783	59.41489	0.28	0.7877
SMR	1	1.63712	0.48929	3.35	0.0101

TABLE 7.6

Data on Oxygen Uptake and Expired Volume

Subject	Oxygen Uptake (litres)	Expired Ventilation (litres)
1	574	21.9
2	592	18.6
3	664	18.6
4	667	19.1
5	718	19.2

uptake and (2) expired ventilation, which is related to exchange of gases in the lungs. Part of the data is shown in Table 7.6 (there are 53 subjects in the full data set, which is given in Hand et al. 1994).

The required scatter plots and numerical results can be found from the following SAS code:

```
data anaerob;
   infile 'c:\amsus\data\anaerob.dat' expandtabs;
   input o2in exp @@;
run;

proc sgplot data=anaerob;
   scatter y=exp x=o2in;
run;

ods graphics on;
proc reg data=anaerob;
 model exp=o2in;
run;
```

The results are shown in Figures 7.7 and 7.8 and in Table 7.7 (the SAS output also produces other plots, which we will discuss in the next chapter).

The estimated regression coefficient given in Table 7.7 is highly significant, but the plot in Figure 7.8 makes it very clear that the simple linear regression model in Equation (7.3) is not appropriate for these data; we need to consider a more complicated model. An obvious choice here is to consider a model that, in addition to the linear effect of oxygen uptake, includes a quadratic term in this variable—that is, the following model:

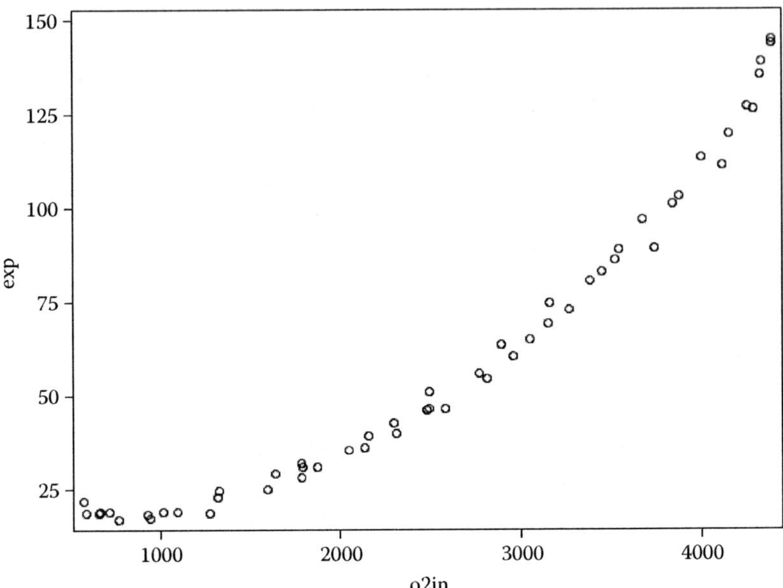

FIGURE 7.7
Scatter plot of data in Table 7.6.

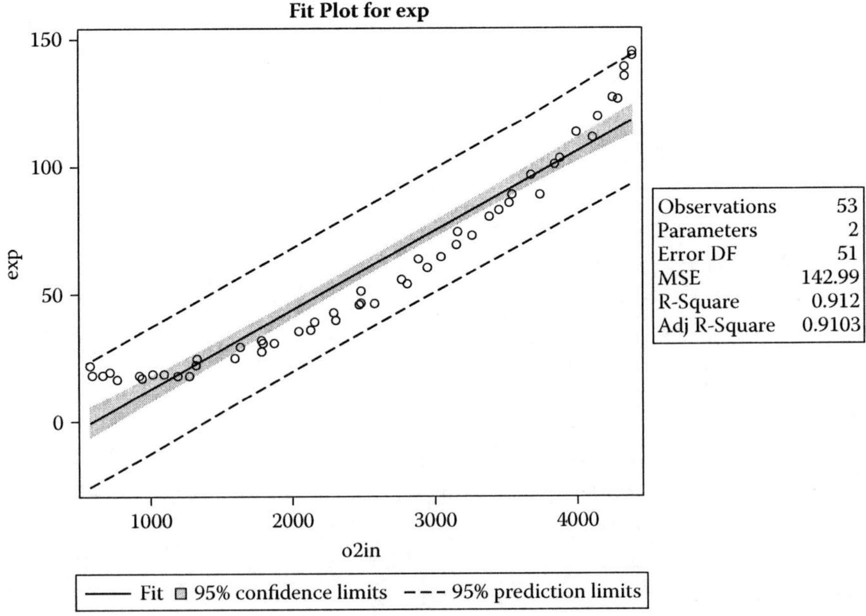

FIGURE 7.8
Fitted linear regression and confidence interval for the data in Table 7.6.

TABLE 7.7

Linear Regression Results for the Data in Table 7.6

Number of Observations Read	53
Number of Observations Used	53

Analysis of Variance					
Source	DF	Sum of Squares	Mean Square	F Value	Pr > F
Model	1	75555	75555	528.40	<.0001
Error	51	7292.38118	142.98787		
Corrected Total	52	82848			

Root MSE	11.95775	R-Square	0.9120
Dependent Mean	60.70755	Adj R-Sq	0.9103
Coeff Var	19.69731		

Parameter Estimates					
Variable	DF	Parameter Estimate	Standard Error	t Value	Pr > |t|
Intercept	1	−18.44873	3.81520	−4.84	<.0001
o2in	1	0.03114	0.00135	22.99	<.0001

$$y_i = \beta_0 + \beta_1 x_i + \beta_2 x_i^2 + \varepsilon_i \tag{7.10}$$

This model can be fitted using the following SAS code:

```
data anaerob;
  set anaerob;
  o2sq=o2in*o2in;
run;

proc reg data=anaerob;
 model exp=o2in o2sq;
 output out=regout p=pr uclm=citop lclm=cibot;
run;

proc sort data=regout; by o2in; run;
proc sgplot data=regout;
  band upper=citop lower=cibot x=o2in;
  series y=pr x=o2in;
  scatter y=exp x=o2in;
run;
```

The results are shown in Table 7.8 and in Figure 7.9.

Clearly, the quadratic term in Equation (7.10) is needed, as shown by the very small *p*-value in Table 7.8 associated with this term. And the model provides a very good fit for the data, as is clearly seen in Figure 7.9.

TABLE 7.8

Results for Regression Model Including a Quadratic Term Fitted to Data in Table 7.6

Model: MODEL1	
Dependent Variable: exp	
Number of Observations Read	53
Number of Observations Used	53

Analysis of Variance					
Source	DF	Sum of Squares	Mean Square	F Value	Pr > F
Model	2	82340	41170	4054.90	<.0001
Error	50	507.65646	10.15313		
Corrected Total	52	82848			

Root MSE	3.18640	R-Square	0.9939
Dependent Mean	60.70755	Adj R-Sq	0.9936
Coeff Var	5.24877		

Parameter Estimates					
Variable	DF	Parameter Estimate	Standard Error	t Value	Pr > |t|
Intercept	1	24.27040	1.94023	12.51	<.0001
o2in	1	−0.01344	0.00176	−7.63	<.0001
o2sq	1	0.00000890	3.443676E-7	25.85	<.0001

One point to note about the model in Equation (7.10) is that it remains a linear model despite the presence of the quadratic term because the 'linear' in linear models refers to the model's parameters rather than to the explanatory variables. An example of a nonlinear model is

$$y_i = \beta_1 x_i + \exp(\beta_2 x_i) + \varepsilon_i \tag{7.11}$$

We shall not deal with such models in this book. It is worth mentioning here that including polynomial terms, for example, x and x^2, in a linear regression model can sometimes lead to a problem known as *collinearity*, which will be discussed in Chapter 8. This can often be overcome by what is known as centring the explanatory variable—that is, using the original variable with its mean subtracted as the explanatory variable. Kleinbaum, Kupper, and Muller (1988) provide an example of the effectiveness of such an approach for correcting collinearity.

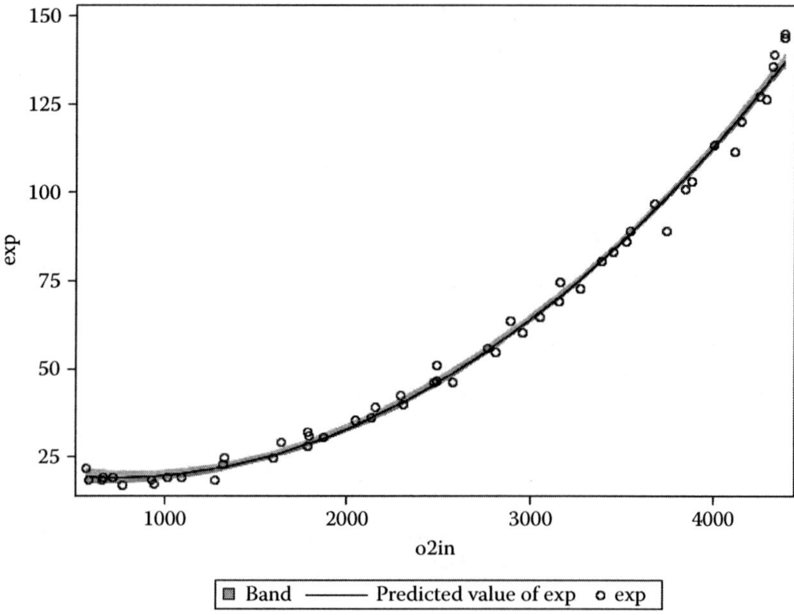

FIGURE 7.9
Fitted regression model including a quadratic term for data in Table 7.6.

7.4 Locally Weighted Regression

The simple linear regression model in (7.3) is an example of a *parametric model* depending as it does on the values of two parameters, β_0, the intercept, and β_1, the slope, of the regression line. Parametric models are very useful but they are not adequate for all data sets. The patterns in many bivariate relationships are too complex to be described by a simple parametric family. An alternative approach to dealing with such data is to fit a curve to the observations *locally* so that, at any point, the curve at that point depends only on the observations at that point and some specified neighbouring points. Because such a fit produces an estimate of the response that is less variable than the originally observed response, the result is often called a *smooth,* and procedures for producing such fits are called *scatter plot smoothers.* We assume we have observations on a response variable y and an explanatory variable x and we assume that observations on the two variables are related as follows:

$$y_i = g(x_i) + \varepsilon_i \tag{7.12}$$

where g is a 'smooth' function and the ε_i are random variables with mean zero and a constant scale.

Fixed values are used to estimate the response y_i at each x_i by fitting poly-nomials using weighted least squares with large weights for points close to x_i and smaller weights otherwise. Two parameters need to be chosen to fit a lowess curve; the first is a smoothing parameter with larger values leading to smoother curves, and the second is the degree of certain polynomials that are fitted by the method.

A lowess curve can be fitted to the alcohol consumption and cirrhosis data in Table 7.1 and then plotted along with the simple refitted regression line on a scatter plot of the data as follows:

```
proc sgplot data=drinking2;
   reg y=cirrhosis x=alcohol;
   loess y=cirrhosis x=alcohol/nomarkers;
run;
```

The resulting plot is shown in Figure 7.10. There is some deviation of the locally weighted regression line from the simple linear regression fit, but with such a small number of observations, this is not convincing evidence that the relationship between death rate and alcohol consumption is not linear.

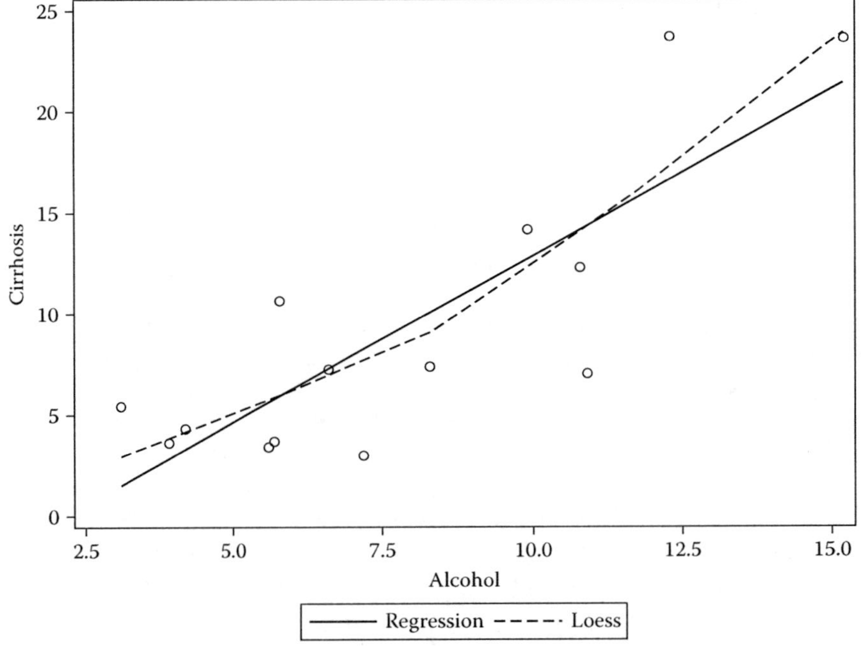

FIGURE 7.10
Scatter plot of death rate against alcohol consumption showing both the fitted linear regression and the locally weighted regression fit.

We shall have more to say about scatter plot smoothers and how they they can be used in more complex models in Chapter 11.

7.5 Aspect Ratio of a Scatter Plot

An important parameter of a scatter plot that can greatly influence our ability to recognise patterns is the *aspect ratio*—the physical length of the vertical axis divided by that of the horizontal axis. By default, SAS scales plots and other graphics to fill the available graphics area. This will typically result in an aspect ratio of 3:4, which may not be the most useful. To illustrate how changing this characteristic of a scatter plot can help understand what the data are trying to tell us, we shall use the example given by Cook and Weisberg (1982) involving the monthly US births, per thousand population, for the years 1940–1948. The data are given in Table 7.9 and a scatter plot of the birthrates against month with the default aspect ratio can be obtained using the following SAS instructions:

```
data USbirth;
  retain obs 0;
  do year=1940 to 1947;
    do month=1 to 12;
    input rate @@;
    obs=obs+1;
    datestr=('15'||put(month,z2.)||put(year,4.));
    obsdate=input(datestr,ddmmyy8.);
    output;
    end;
  end;
cards;
1890 1957 1925 1885 1896 1934 2036 2069 2060
1922 1854 1852 1952 2011 2015 1971 1883 2070
2221 2173 2105 1962 1951 1975 2092 2148 2114
2013 1986 2088 2218 2312 2462 2455 2357 2309
2398 2400 2331 2222 2156 2256 2352 2371 2356
2211 2108 2069 2123 2147 2050 1977 1993 2134
2275 2262 2194 2109 2114 2086 2089 2097 2036
1957 1953 2039 2116 2134 2142 2023 1972 1942
1931 1980 1977 1972 2017 2161 2468 2691 2890
2913 2940 2870 2911 2832 2774 2568 2574 2641
2691 2698 2701 2596 2503 2424
;

ods graphics / height=480 width=640;
proc sgplot data=usbirth;
  scatter y=rate x=obsdate;
  format obsdate year.;
run;
```

TABLE 7.9

US Monthly Birthrates between 1940 and 1943

1890	1957	1925	1885	1896	1934	2036	2069	2060
1922	1854	1852	1952	2011	2015	1971	1883	2070
2221	2173	2105	1962	1951	1975	2092	2148	2114
2013	1986	2088	2218	2312	2462	2455	2357	2309
2398	2400	2331	2222	2156	2256	2352	2371	2356
2211	2108	2069	2123	2147	2050	1977	1993	2134
2275	2262	2194	2109	2114	2086	2089	2097	2036
1957	1953	2039	2116	2134	2142	2023	1972	1942
1931	1980	1977	1972	2017	2161	2468	2691	2890
2913	2940	2870	2911	2832	2774	2568	2574	2641
2691	2698	2701	2596	2503	2424			

Note: Read along rows for temporal sequence.

The data are read in using two do loops to set values of `year` and `month` and each observation is, somewhat arbitrarily, given a date of the 15th of the month. Formatted values of this date variable can then be used to label the *x*-axis of the plots. We begin with the default aspect ratio of 480 by 640. We specify the unit in pixels, but inches (in) or centimetres (cm) could be used.

The resulting plot in Figure 7.11 shows that the US birthrate was increasing between 1940 and 1943, decreasing between 1943 and 1946, rapidly increasing during 1946, and then decreasing again during 1947 and 1948. As Cook and Weisberg (1986) comment: 'These trends seem to deliver an interesting history lesson since the U.S. involvement in World War II started in 1942 and troops began returning home during the part of 1945, about nine months before the rapid increase in the birth rate'.

Now let us see what happens when we alter the aspect ratio of the plot to 0.3.

```
ods graphics / height=300 width=1000;
proc sgplot data=usbirth;
  scatter y=rate x=obsdate;
  format obsdate year.;
run;
```

The resulting graph appears in Figure 7.12. The new plot displays many peaks and troughs and suggests perhaps some minor within-year trends in addition to the global trends apparent in Figure 7.11. A clearer picture is obtained by plotting only a part of the data; here we will plot the observations for the years 1940–1943 using the SAS code:

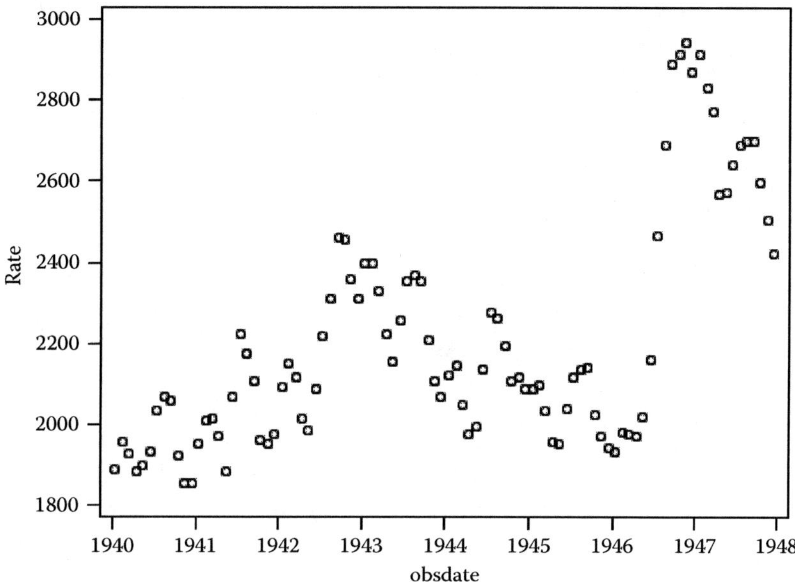

FIGURE 7.11
US birthrate against year with default aspect ratio.

```
proc sgplot data=usbirth;
  scatter y=rate x=obsdate;
  format obsdate monyy7.;
  where year<1943;
run;
```

This plot is shown in Figure 7.13. Now, a within-year cycle is clearly apparent, with the lowest within-year birthrate at the beginning of the summer and the highest occurring in the autumn. This pattern can be made clearer by connecting adjacent points in the plot with a line; the necessary SAS instructions are

```
proc sgplot data=usbirth;
  series y=rate x=obsdate;
  format obsdate monyy7.;
  where year<1943;
run;
```

The new plot appears in Figure 7.14. By reducing the aspect ratio to 0.2, replotting all 96 observations, and again joining adjacent points with a line, both the within-year and global trends become clearly visible. The relevant SAS code is

```
ods graphics / height=200 width=1000;
proc sgplot data=usbirth;
 series y=rate x=obsdate;
 format obsdate year.;
run;
```

The plot appears in Figure 7.15.

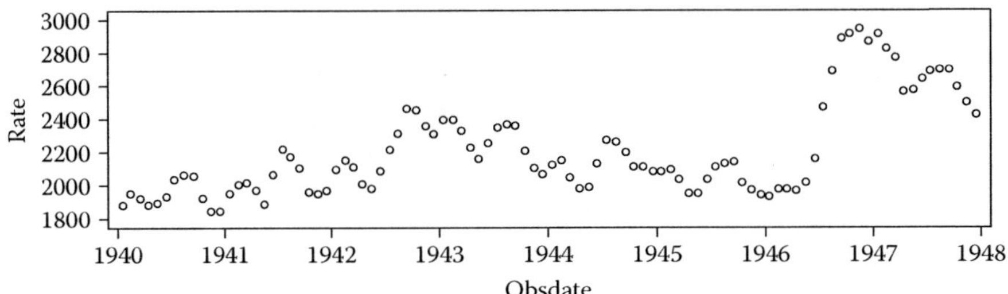

FIGURE 7.12
US birthrate against year with aspect ratio 0.3.

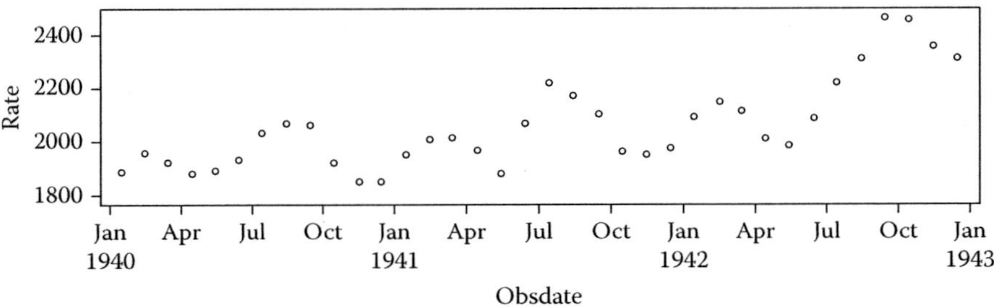

FIGURE 7.13
US birthrate against year (1940–1943) with aspect ratio 0.3.

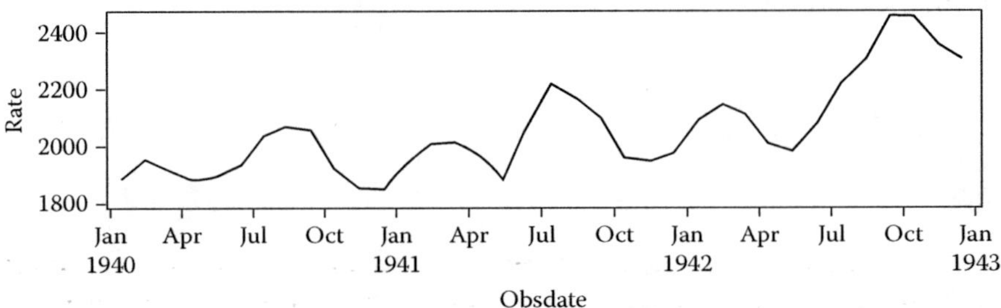

FIGURE 7.14
US birthrate against year (1940–1943) with observations joined and aspect ratio 0.3.

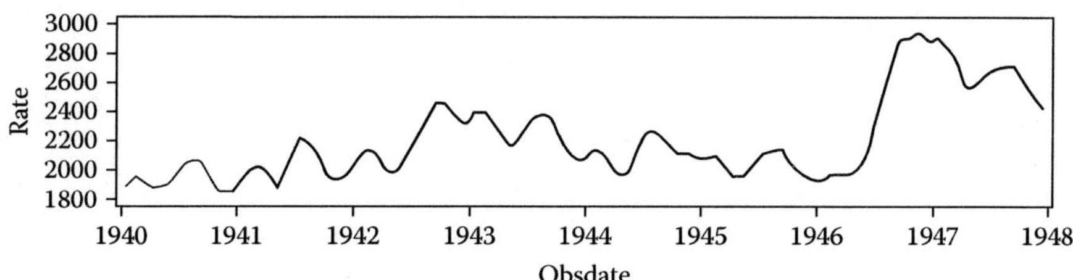

FIGURE 7.15
US birthrate against year with observations joined and aspect ratio 0.2.

7.6 Estimating Bivariate Densities

Examination of scatter plots often centres on assessing density patterns such as clusters, gaps, or outliers. But humans are not particularly good at visually examining point density, and some type of density estimate added to the scatter plot will frequently be very helpful. There is now a vast literature on density estimation (see, for example, Silverman 1986) and here we give only a very brief summary.

We assume that we have n bivariate data points represented by $\mathbf{X}_1, \mathbf{X}_2, \ldots, \mathbf{X}_n$ and we wish to estimate the underlying bivariate density of the data. The bivariate kernel density estimator with kernel K and window width h is defined by

$$\hat{f}(\mathbf{x}) = \frac{1}{nh^2} \sum_{i=1}^{n} K\left\{\frac{1}{h}(\mathbf{x} - \mathbf{X}_i)\right\} \tag{7.13}$$

The kernel function $K(\mathbf{x})$ is a function, defined for bivariate $\mathbf{x}$, satisfying $\int K(\mathbf{x})d\mathbf{x} = 1$. Usually, $K(\mathbf{x})$ will be a radially symmetric unimodal probability density function—for example, the standard bivariate normal density function:

$$K(\mathbf{x}) = \frac{1}{2\pi}\exp\left(-\frac{1}{2}\mathbf{x}'\mathbf{x}\right) \tag{7.14}$$

To illustrate how bivariate density estimation can be used to enhance a scatter plot, we shall use data on birth and death rates for 69 countries; the data for 10 countries are given in Table 7.10.

The SAS code for reading in the data and calculating the required bivariate density estimate is

TABLE 7.10

Birth and Death Rates for 10 Countries

Country	Births	Deaths
Algeria	36.4	14.6
Congo	37.3	8.0
Egypt	42.1	15.3
Ghana	55.8	25.6
Ict	56.1	33.1
Mag	41.8	15.8
Morocco	46.1	18.7
Tunisia	41.7	10.1
Cameroon	41.4	19.7
Cey	35.8	8.5

```
data fertility;
  infile 'c:\amsus\data\fertility.dat';
  input country$ birth death;
run;

ods graphics / reset=all;
proc kde data=fertility;
  bivar birth death / plots=contourscatter noprint;
run;
```

Proc kde produces univariate and bivariate density estimates using normal kernels. The bivar statement requests a bivariate density (univar for univariate density). With ODS graphics on, a number of plots are available. Here, we select a contour plot overlaid with a scatter plot. The ODS graphics statement restores the default aspect ratio. The resulting plot is shown in Figure 7.16.

As the default bandwidths tend to oversmooth the data, the bwm=option can be used to control the bandwidth separately for each variable. Values less than one produce a rougher estimate than the default and those greater than one produce a smoother estimate. To change the bandwidths and replot requires the SAS code that follows:

```
proc kde data=fertility;
  bivar birth death / bwm=.5 plots=contourscatter noprint;
run;
```

Figure 7.17, in particular, gives some evidence that there are two modes in the data, perhaps indicating the presence of two 'clusters' of countries, one of which largely corresponds to the 'West' and the other to the developing countries.

The density estimates can also be presented in the form of perspective plots, as shown in Figures 7.18 and 7.19, obtained using

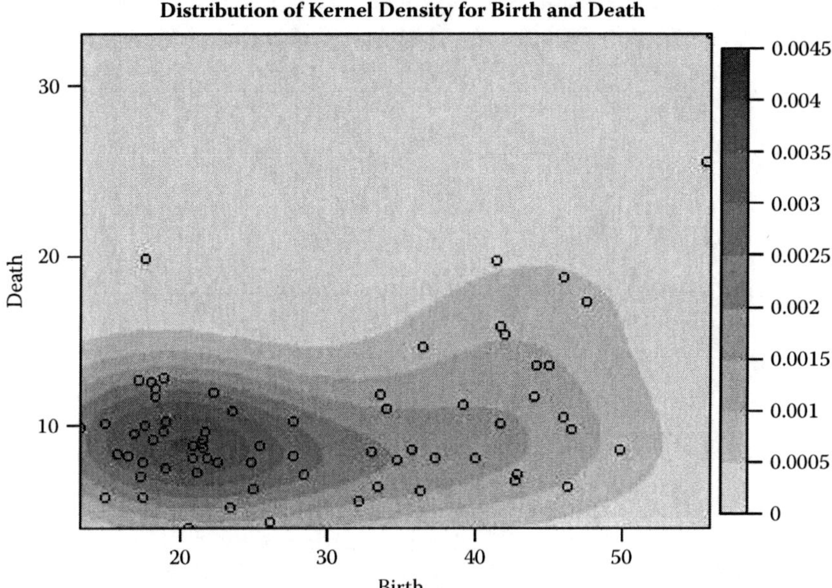

FIGURE 7.16
Estimated bivariate density for birth and death rate data in Table 7.10.

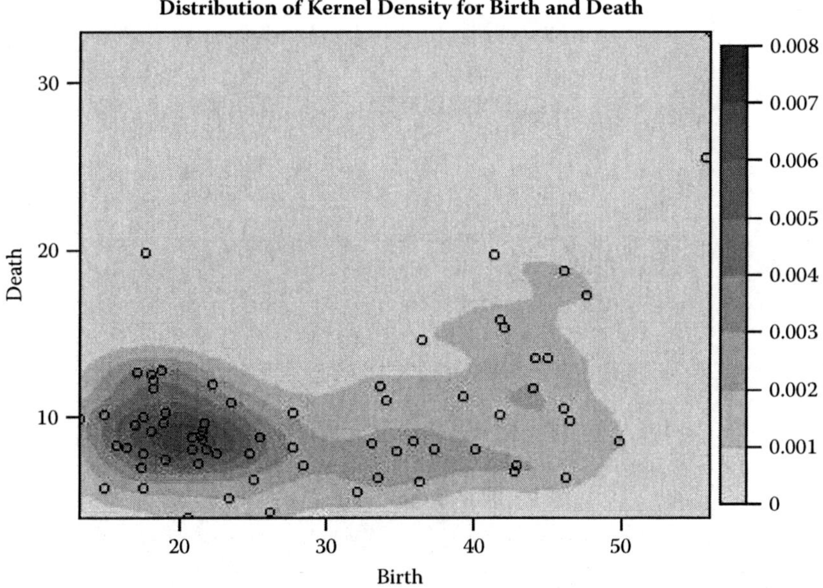

FIGURE 7.17
Estimated bivariate density for the birth and death rate data.

                                    Applied Medical Statistics Using SAS

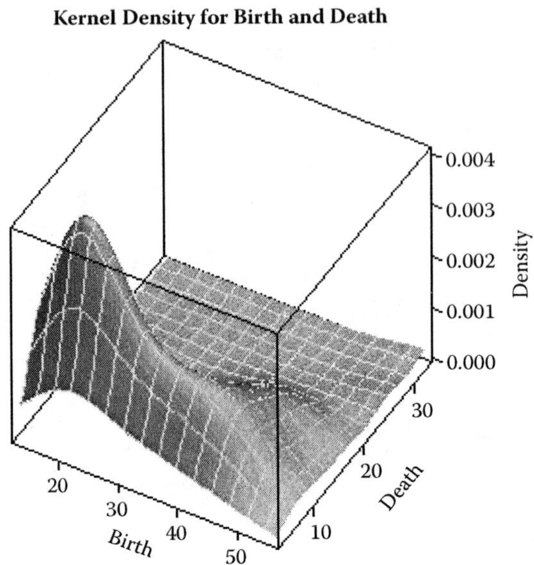

FIGURE 7.18
Perspective plot of estimated bivariate density for birth and death rate data.

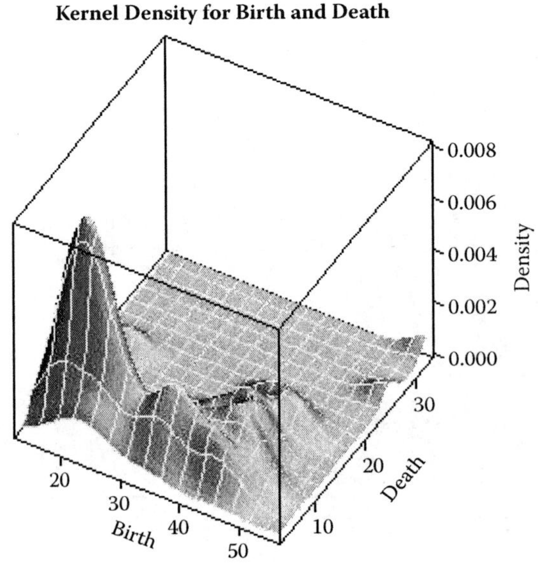

FIGURE 7.19
Perspective plot of estimated bivariate density for birth and death rate data.

```
proc kde data=fertility;
  bivar birth death / plots=surface(rotate=30 tilt=45) noprint;
run;

proc kde data=fertility;
  bivar birth death / bwm=.5 plots=surface(rotate=30 tilt=45)
noprint;
run;
```

We have used the `rotate` and `tilt` options to give a better view of the plots. With the default values, too much detail was hidden behind the main peak. The `rotate` option turns the y-axis the specified number of degrees anticlockwise from the vertical. The `tilt` option tilts the graph away from you, starting from the viewpoint directly above.

7.7 Scatter Plot Matrices

The observations in Table 7.11 are part of a set of data reported in Begg and Hearns (1966) which were collected in an investigation of the relative contributions of haematocrit (packed cell volume, PCV), fibrinogen, and other proteins (albutin and globulen) to the viscosity of blood; the complete data set contains observations on 32 patients. The four observed variables generate between them six possible scatter plots, and it is very important that the separate bivariate displays be presented in a way that aids in overall comprehension and understanding of the data. The scatter plot matrix is intended to accomplish exactly this objective.

A scatter plot matrix is defined as a square, symmetric grid of bivariate scatter plots. This grid has p rows and columns, each one corresponding to a different variable. Each of the grid's cells shows a scatter plot of two variables. Variable j is plotted against variable i in the ijth cell, and the same variables appear in cell ji with the x- and y-axes of the scatter plots interchanged.

TABLE 7.11

Data on Blood Viscosity, Packed Cell Volume (PCV), Plasma Fibrinogen, and Other Proteins from Five Hospital Patients

Patient	Blood Viscosity (cP)	PCV (100%)	Plasma Fibrinogen (mg/100 mL)	Plasma Protein (g/100 mL)
1	3.71	40	344	6.27
2	3.78	40	330	4.86
3	3.85	42.5	280	5.09
4	3.88	42	418	6.79
5	3.98	45	744	6.40

Source: Begg, T. B., and Hearns, J. B. 1966. *Clinical Science* 31:87–93.

The reason for including both the upper and lower triangles of the grid, despite the seeming redundancy, is that it enables a row and column to be scanned visually to see one variable against all others, with the scales of the one variable lined up along the horizontal axis or the vertical axis:

```
data blood;
  infile 'c:\amsus\data\blood_viscosity.dat' firstobs=2;
  input patid viscosity PCV fibrinogen protein;
run;
proc sgscatter data=blood;
  matrix viscosity -- protein / diagonal=(histogram kernel);
run;
```

The resulting scatter plot matrix is shown in Figure 7.20. Histograms and univariate density estimates of the distribution of each of the four variables are shown on the main diagonal.

The scatter plot matrix is a useful (and almost essential) graphic to be used when looking at the correlation matrix of a set of variables. Such a matrix can be found for the data in Table 7.11 using proc corr. A scatter plot matrix will also be produced by proc corr when ODS graphics is on:

```
proc corr data=blood;
  var viscosity--protein;
run;
```

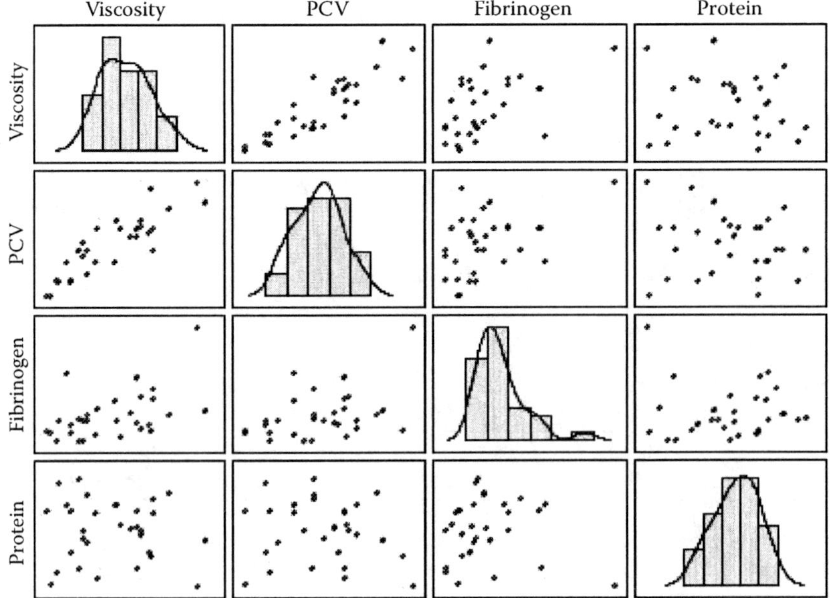

FIGURE 7.20
Scatter plot matrix of blood viscosity data.

The resulting output is shown in Table 7.12 and indicates that there are substantial correlations between several pairs of variables—for example, fibrinogen and viscosity.

When three or more variables are measured, as in Table 7.11, it is often of interest to calculate *partial correlation coefficients*. For three variables x, y, and z, with correlation coefficients for a sample of n observations of r_{xy}, r_{xz}, and r_{yz}, the partial correlations are calculated as follows:

$$r_{xy|z} = \frac{r_{xy} - r_{xz}r_{yz}}{\sqrt{\left(1 - r_{xz}^2\right)\left(1 - r_{yz}^2\right)}}$$

$$r_{xz|y} = \frac{r_{xz} - r_{xy}r_{yz}}{\sqrt{\left(1 - r_{xy}^2\right)\left(1 - r_{yz}^2\right)}} \tag{7.15}$$

$$r_{yz|x} = \frac{r_{yz} - r_{xy}r_{xz}}{\sqrt{\left(1 - r_{xy}^2\right)\left(1 - r_{xz}^2\right)}}$$

TABLE 7.12

Correlation Matrix for the Data in Table 7.11

4 Variables:	viscosity	PCV	fibrinogen	protein

Simple Statistics					
Variable	**N**	**Mean**	**Std Dev**	**Sum**	**Minimum**	**Maximum**
viscosity	32	4.64563	0.62088	148.66000	3.71000	5.90000
PCV	32	47.93750	4.45678	1534	40.00000	57.00000
fibrinogen	32	465.96875	169.43292	14911	276.00000	1070
protein	32	5.89406	0.56861	188.61000	4.82000	6.89000

Pearson Correlation Coefficients, N=32 **Prob > |r| Under H0: Rho=0**				
	viscosity	**PCV**	**fibrinogen**	**protein**
viscosity	1.00000	0.87882	0.46791	–0.10107
		<.0001	0.0069	0.5820
PCV	0.87882	1.00000	0.42332	–0.15749
	<.0001		0.0158	0.3893
fibrinogen	0.46791	0.42332	1.00000	–0.05680
	0.0069	0.0158		0.7575
protein	–0.10107	–0.15749	–0.05680	1.00000
	0.5820	0.3893	0.7575	

TABLE 7.13

Partial Correlation Coefficients for Data in Table 7.11

Pearson Partial Correlation Coefficients, N = 32 Prob > |r| under H0: Partial Rho = 0		
	viscosity	fibrinogen	protein
viscosity	1.00000	0.22180	0.07922
		0.2304	0.6718
fibrinogen	0.22180	1.00000	0.01103
	0.2304		0.9530
protein	0.07922	0.01103	1.00000
	0.6718	0.9530	

The test that a population partial correlation coefficient is zero can be applied using the appropriate sample partial correlation in the test statistic used for the usual correlation correlation described earlier in this chapter, except that there are now $n-3$ degrees of freedom rather than $n-2$. For example, to test the hypothesis $\rho_{xy|z}=0$, the test statistic is $r_{xy|z}\sqrt{\dfrac{n-3}{1-r_{xy|z}^2}}$ tested against a t-distribution with $n-3$ degrees of freedom.

For the data in Table 7.11, it is of most interest to see if the association of blood viscosity and fibrinogen remains after allowing for the association with PCV. The SAS code needed to get the relevant coefficients is

```
proc corr data=blood nosimple;
 var viscosity fibrinogen protein;
 partial pcv;
run;
```

The output is shown in Table 7.13. Note that the partial correlation between viscosity and fibrinogen is now reduced to 0.222, which is not significantly different from zero. This suggests that the association between blood viscosity and fibrinogen can be largely explained by variation in PCV.

7.8 Summary

The scatter plot is one of the basic tools for an initial investigation of bivariate data. From it, the form of the relationship between two variables is often apparent, as are outliers that may interfere with later analyses. Using the scatter plot when interpreting the value of a correlation coefficient is essential; drawing conclusions about the relationship between two variables simply from the numerical value of a correlation coefficient is poor data analysis practice and can lead to misjudgements and errors. A scatter plot enhanced with an estimate of the bivariate density of the two variables may suggest more complex structure in the data—for example, the presence of clusters of similar observations—and suggest that the application of *cluster analysis* (see Everitt et al. 2011) to the data might be useful.

Consideration of a locally weighted regression fit alongside the fitting of a simple linear regression model is often a useful exercise. Lastly, checking the assumptions of the model fitted is always essential. However, we will leave consideration of how to do this until the next chapter, in which we consider the extension of the simple linear model to the case where there is more than a single explanatory variable.

8

Multiple Linear Regression

8.1 Introduction

Multiple linear regression represents a generalisation, to more than a single explanatory variable, of the simple linear regression procedure described in Chapter 7. It is now that the relationship between a response variable and several explanatory variables becomes of interest. (Note that in many accounts of multiple linear regression, what we term *explanatory variables* are called *independent variables*; however, this is a misleading term because the variables are only rarely independent of one another.) The adjective 'multiple' indicates that at least two explanatory variables are involved in the modelling exercise. At the onset, it is important to note that the explanatory variables are strictly assumed to be fixed and under the control of the investigator. That is, they are not considered to be random variables; only the response variable is considered to be a random variable.

In practice, of course, this assumption is unlikely to be true; in this case, the results from a multiple linear regression are interpreted as being *conditional* on the observed values of the explanatory variables, and the inherent variation in the explanatory variables is ignored. Because there are no distributional assumptions about the explanatory variables, they may be nominal, categorical with more than two categories (such variables need to be coded in an appropriate way), ordered categorical, or interval. The goals of a multiple regression may be to determine whether the response variable and one or more explanatory variables are associated in some systematic way or to predict values of the response variables from values of the explanatory variables, or both.

Details of the model, including the estimation of its parameters by least squares and the calculation of standard errors, are given in the next section.

8.2 Multiple Linear Regression Model

The multiple linear regression model relates a response variable to a set of explanatory variables. The relationship assumed is linear (in terms of the parameters rather than in terms of the explanatory variables; see Chapter 7), and the parameters in the model (usually known as *regression coefficients*) are generally estimated by least squares. An inferential framework is added by making specific distributional assumptions about the error terms in the model. Details of the structure of the model, estimation and testing of its parameters, and assessing its fit are all described in this section.

We start by letting y_i represents the value of the response variable on the ith individual, and $x_{i1}, x_{i2}, \ldots, x_{ip}$ represent the individual's values on p explanatory variables, with $i = 1,2\ldots n$. As usual, n represents the sample size. The multiple linear regression model is given by

$$y_i = \beta_0 + \beta_1 x_{i1} + \ldots + \beta_p x_{ip} + \varepsilon_i \tag{8.1}$$

The residual or error terms ε_i, $i = 1, \ldots, n$ are assumed to be independent random variables having a normal distribution with mean zero and constant variance σ^2.

Consequently, the distribution of the random response variable, y, is also normal with expected value

$$E(y \mid x_1, x_2, \ldots, x_p) = \beta_0 + \beta_1 x_1 + \ldots + \beta_p x_p \tag{8.2}$$

and variance σ^2.

The parameters of the model β_k, $k = 1, 2, \ldots, p$ are known as *regression coefficients*. They represent the expected change in the response variable associated with a unit change in the corresponding explanatory variable, when the remaining explanatory variables are held constant. As explained in Chapter 7, the 'linear' in multiple linear regression applies to the regression parameters—not to the response or explanatory variables. Consequently, models in which, for example, the logarithm of a response variable is modelled in terms of quadratic functions of some of the explanatory variables would be included in this class of models.

The multiple regression model can be written most conveniently for all n individuals by using matrices and vectors as

$$\mathbf{y} = \mathbf{X}\boldsymbol{\beta} + \boldsymbol{\varepsilon} \tag{8.3}$$

where $\mathbf{y}' = \left[y_1, y_2, \ldots, y_n\right]$, $\boldsymbol{\beta}' = \left[\beta_0, \beta_1, \ldots, \beta_p\right]$, $\boldsymbol{\varepsilon}' = \left[\varepsilon_1, \varepsilon_2, \ldots, \varepsilon_n\right]$ and

$$\mathbf{X} = \begin{bmatrix} 1 & x_{11} & x_{12} & \cdots & x_{1p} \\ 1 & x_{21} & x_{22} & \cdots & x_{2p} \\ \vdots & \vdots & \vdots & \vdots & \vdots \\ 1 & x_{n1} & x_{n2} & \cdots & x_{np} \end{bmatrix} \tag{8.4}$$

Each row in $\mathbf{X}$ (sometimes known as the *design matrix*) represents the values of the explanatory variables for one of the individuals in the sample, with the addition of unity, which takes care of the parameter, β_0, needed in the model for each individual in the sample. Assuming that $\mathbf{X'X}$ is nonsingular (i.e., can be inverted), then the least squares estimator of the parameter vector $\boldsymbol{\beta}$ is

$$\hat{\boldsymbol{\beta}} = \left(\mathbf{X'X}\right)^{-1}\mathbf{X'y} \tag{8.5}$$

This estimator $\hat{\boldsymbol{\beta}}$ has the following properties:

$$E\left(\hat{\boldsymbol{\beta}}\right) = \boldsymbol{\beta} \tag{8.6}$$

and

$$\mathrm{cov}\left(\hat{\boldsymbol{\beta}}\right) = \sigma^2\left(\mathbf{X'X}\right)^{-1} \tag{8.7}$$

The diagonal elements of the matrix $\mathrm{cov}\left(\hat{\boldsymbol{\beta}}\right)$ give the variances of the $\hat{\beta}_j$, whereas the off-diagonal elements give the covariances between pairs $\hat{\beta}_j, \hat{\beta}_k$. The square roots of the diagonal elements of the matrix are thus the standard errors of the $\hat{\beta}_j$. The fit of the regression model can be partially assessed, at least, by using the analysis of variance table shown in Table 8.1, which partitions the total sum of squares of the response variable into a part due to regression on the explanatory variables and in part due to the errors in the model. In this table, $\hat{y}_i$ is the predicted value of the response variable for the ith individual $\left(\hat{y}_i = \hat{\beta}_0 + \hat{\beta}_1 x_{ij} + \cdots + \hat{\beta}_p x_{ip}\right)$ and $\bar{y}$ is the mean value of the response variable.

The mean square ratio MSR/MSE provides an F-test of the null hypothesis that the regression coefficients of all p explanatory variables take the value zero—that is,

$$H_0 : \beta_1 = \beta_2 = \cdots \beta_p = 0$$

TABLE 8.1

Analysis of Variance Table for the Multiple Linear Regression Model

Source of Variation	Sum of Squares (SS)	Degrees of Freedom (DF)	Mean Square
Regression	$\sum_{i=1}^{n}\left(\hat{y}_i - \bar{y}\right)^2$	p	MSR = SS/DF
Residual	$\sum_{i=1}^{n}\left(y_i - \hat{y}_i\right)^2$	$n - p - 1$	MSE = SS/DF
Total	$\sum_{i=1}^{n}\left(y_i - \bar{y}\right)^2$	$n - 1$	

Under H_0, the mean square ratio has an F-distribution with $p, n-p-1$ degrees of freedom. (Testing this very general hypothesis is usually of limited interest, as we shall see later in the chapter.)

An estimate of σ^2 is provided by s^2, given by

$$s^2 = \frac{1}{n-p-1} \sum_{i=1}^{n} (y_i - \hat{y}_i)^2 \qquad (8.8)$$

The correlation between the observed values y_i and the predicted values $\hat{y}_i$, R, is known as the *multiple correlation coefficient*. The value of R^2 gives the proportion of variance of the response variable accounted for by the explanatory variables. Individual regression coefficients can be assessed by using the ratio $\hat{\beta}_j / SE\left(\hat{\beta}_j\right)$, although these ratios should only be used as rough guides to the 'significance' or otherwise of the coefficients for reasons discussed later in the chapter.

8.3 Some Examples of the Application of the Multiple Linear Regression Model

8.3.1 Effect of the Amount of Anaesthetic Agent Administered during an Operation

This example is described in full in Cullen and van Belle (1975). The main interest in the study was the degree of trauma on the immune system, as measured by the decreasing ability of lymphocytes to transform in the presence of mitogen (a substance that enhances cell division). The explanatory variables measured were the duration of anaesthesia (in hours) and the trauma factor rated on a five-point scale of increasing seriousness of the operation as follows:

0 *Diagnostic or therapeutic regional anaesthesia;* examination under general anaesthesia

1 *Joint manipulation; minor orthopaedic procedures;* cystoscopy; dilation and curettage

2 *Extremity, genitourinary, rectal, and eye procedures;* hernia repair; laparoscopy

3 *Laparotomy; craniotomy; laminectomy;* peripheral vascular surgery

4 *Pelvic exterteration; jejuna interposition;* total cystectomy

TABLE 8.2

Depression of Lymphocyte Transformation
during Operation

Duration	Trauma	Depression
4.0	3	36.7
6.0	3	51.3
1.5	2	40.8
4.0	2	58.3
2.5	2	42.2

Source: Cullen, B. F. and van Belle, G. 1975.
Anaesthesiology, 43:577–583.

(In what follows, we will assume that the last variable is a quasicontinuous rather than a categorical scale; if we had decided to consider the variable as categorical, it would need to be recast as a series of four *dummy variables*—see later in the chapter for a brief explanation.)

The response variable in this example is the percentage depression of lymphocyte transformation following anaesthesia. It is assumed that the amount of anaesthetic agent administered is directly proportional to the duration of anaesthesia. The data for the first 5 of the 35 patients in the data are shown in Table 8.2.

The multiple linear regression model can be fitted to the anaesthesia data using the following SAS code:

```
data anaesthetic;
   infile 'c:\AMSUS\data\anaesthetic.dat' expandtabs;
   input duration trauma dlt;
run;


proc reg data=anasthetic;
   model dlt=duration trauma;
run;
```

The output is shown in Table 8.3. Here, the F-test that the regression coefficients β_1 and β_2 are both zero has an associated p-value of 0.055, and the t-statistics given by the ratios of the estimated regression coefficients to their estimated standard errors have associated p-values of 0.76 and 0.17. It appears that neither duration of anaesthesia nor degree of trauma is useful for predicting the percentage depression of lymphocyte transformation following anaesthesia, although jointly they do approach significance at the 5% level. The R-squared value of just 0.17 underlines that the two explanatory variables have little predictive power for the response variable, accounting as they do for only 17% of the variance in the latter. The number of observations in this example is, however, rather small, so inferences are not particularly powerful.

TABLE 8.3

Results of Applying Multiple Linear Regression to the Data in Table 8.2

Model: MODEL1	
Dependent Variable: dlt	
Number of Observations Read	35
Number of Observations Used	35

Analysis of Variance					
Source	DF	Sum of Squares	Mean Square	F Value	Pr > F
Model	2	4163.43495	2081.71747	3.19	0.0547
Error	32	20901	653.17162		
Corrected Total	34	25065			

Root MSE	25.55722	R-Square	0.1661	
Dependent Mean	25.54571	Adj R-Sq	0.1140	
Coeff Var	100.04505			

Parameter Estimates					
Variable	DF	Parameter Estimate	Standard Error	t Value	Pr > |t|
Intercept	1	−2.50201	12.34502	−0.20	0.8407
duration	1	1.11313	3.60534	0.31	0.7595
trauma	1	10.31859	7.42995	1.39	0.1745

8.3.2 Mortality and Water Hardness

The data shown in Table 8.4 were collected in an investigation of environmental causes of disease. The data give the annual mortality rate per 100,000 for males, averaged over the years 1958–1964, and the calcium concentration (in parts per million) in the drinking water supply for 61 large towns in England and Wales. (The higher the calcium concentration is, the harder is the water.) Towns at least as far north as Derby are identified in Table 8.4. The questions of interest for these data are whether water hardness is predictive of mortality and whether there is a geographical factor in the relationship.

In this example, one of the explanatory variables is binary (north/south), making the multiple regression model equivalent to the analysis of covariance model encountered in Chapter 6. The presence of the categorical variable raises no real problems because, in the multiple regression model, no distributional assumptions are made about the explanatory variables (strictly speaking, they are not considered to be random variables). However, `proc reg` expects all variables to be numeric, so the character

TABLE 8.4

Mortality and Water Hardness

Town	Mortality per 100,000	Calcium (ppm)
S	1247	105
N	1668	17
S	1466	5
N	1800	14
N	1609	18
N	1558	10
N	1807	15
S	1299	78
N	1637	10
S	1359	84
S	1392	73
S	1519	21
N	1755	12
S	1307	78
S	1254	96
N	1491	20
N	1555	39
N	1428	39
S	1318	122
S	1260	21
N	1723	44
N	1379	94
N	1742	8
N	1574	9
N	1569	91
S	1096	138
N	1591	16
S	1402	n
N	1702	44
S	1581	14
S	1309	59
S	1259	133
N	1427	27
N	1724	6
S	1175	107
S	1486	5
S	1456	90
N	1696	6
S	1236	101
N	1711	13

(Continued)

TABLE 8.4 (*Continued*)

Mortality and Water Hardness

Town	Mortality per 100,000	Calcium (ppm)
N	1444	14
N	1591	49
N	1987	8
N	1495	14
S	1369	68
S	1257	50
N	1587	75
N	1713	71
N	1557	13
N	1640	57
N	1709	71
S	1625	13
N	1625	20
S	1527	60
S	1627	53
S	1486	122
N	1772	15
N	1828	8
N	1704	26
S	1485	81
N	1378	71

variable `location` is recoded into a 0/1 numeric variable `region` in the data step, as follows:

```
data water;
   infile 'c:\AMSUS\data\water.dat';
   input location$ mortality calcium;
   if location='N' then region=1;
     else region=0;
run;

proc sort data=water; by calcium; run;

proc reg data=water;
   model mortality= calcium region;
   output out=regout p=pred uclm=cihi lclm=cilo;
run;
```

The results of this analysis are shown in Table 8.5.

The global test that both regression coefficients in the model are zero has an associated p-value less than 0.0001. Clearly, at least one of the regression coefficients differs from zero. Examination of the t-statistics for the individual regression coefficients suggests that calcium concentration is of greatest importance in predicting mortality rate. The R^2 value is 0.43 so, together, the

TABLE 8.5

Results from Applying Multiple Linear Regression to the Data in Table 8.4

Model: MODEL1
Dependent Variable: Mortality
Number of Observations Read   61
Number of Observations Used   61

Analysis of Variance					
Source	DF	Sum of Squares	Mean Square	F Value	Pr > F
Model	2	914803	457402	22.14	<.0001
Error	58	1198371	20662		
Corrected Total	60	2113174			

Root MSE	143.74130	R-Square	0.4329
Dependent Mean	1524.14754	Adj R-Sq	0.4133
Coeff Var	9.43093		

Parameter Estimates					
Variable	DF	Parameter Estimate	Standard Error	t Value	Pr > |t|
Intercept	1	1660.82438	38.01682	43.69	<.0001
calcium	1	−3.19101	0.49016	−6.51	<.0001
region	1	24.18383	37.44636	0.65	0.5209

two explanatory variables account for over 40% of the variation in mortality rates. The estimated regression coefficient for calcium concentration suggests that a 1 ppm increase in calcium concentration reduces mortality by about 3 per 100,000 conditional on region, with a 95% confidence interval of approximately [2,4] per 100,000.

With just two explanatory variables in this example, it becomes possible to show the fitted model graphically; this can be done using the following statements:

```
proc sgplot data=regout;
 band x=calcium upper=cihi lower=cilo /group=location;
 scatter y=mortality x=calcium / markerchar=location;
 series y=pred x=calcium /group=location;
run;
```

When combining the band plot with other plots, the band statement should usually come first. Otherwise, the bands will overwrite the line and the points that lie within them.

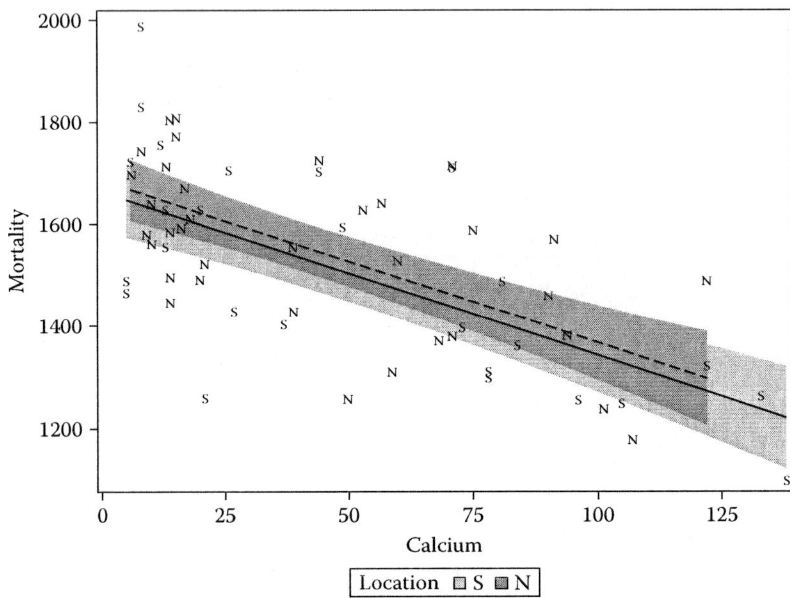

FIGURE 8.1
Multiple regression model for the water hardness data displayed graphically; the regression lines for each region are assumed to have the same slope.

The resulting diagram, shown in Figure 8.1, consists of a scatter plot of mortality and calcium concentration together with the fitted *parallel* regression lines (i.e., lines with equal slopes that are assumed in this model for the two regions).

A more complex model that might be considered for these data is one that allows for a possible interaction between location and hardness. Unlike `proc glm`, `proc reg` does not allow interactions to be specified on the `model` statement in the form `region*calcium`. Instead, a separate variable needs to be calculated to represent the interaction, as follows:

```
data water;
  set water;
  reg_calc=region*calcium;
run;

proc reg data=water;
  model mortality= calcium region reg_calc;
  output out=regout p=pred uclm=cihi lclm=cilo;
run;
```

The results are given in Table 8.6. Again, the overall *F*-test provides clear evidence of at least one nonzero regression coefficient. The individual *t*-tests

TABLE 8.6

Multiple Linear Regression Model Including Region × Mortality Interaction

Model: MODEL1
Dependent Variable: mortality
Number of Observations Read   61
Number of Observations Used   61

Analysis of Variance					
Source	DF	Sum of Squares	Mean Square	F Value	Pr > F
Model	3	931321	310440	14.97	<.0001
Error	57	1181852	20734		
Corrected Total	60	2113174			

Root MSE	143.99392	R-Square	0.4407
Dependent Mean	1524.14754	Adj R-Sq	0.4113
Coeff Var	9.44751		

Parameter Estimates					
Variable	DF	Parameter Estimate	Standard Error	t Value	Pr > |t|
Intercept	1	1681.96605	44.84877	37.50	<.0001
calcium	1	−3.59728	0.66954	−5.37	<.0001
region	1	−17.55734	59.95146	−0.29	0.7707
reg_calc	1	0.87905	0.98486	0.89	0.3758

again suggest that only calcium concentration is predictive of mortality. In particular, it appears that the interaction term is not needed. This is confirmed by examining the R^2 values for the two models: 0.43 for the first, with no interaction term, and 0.44 for the second, which includes the interaction term. The increase corresponding to the addition of the interaction term to the first model is very small.

The plot illustrating the second model is shown in Figure 8.2. In this case, the two regression lines are not assumed to be parallel. But it is clear from our previous discussion that the parallel lines model is adequate for these data; indeed, since there is no evidence that region is predictive of mortality, a simple fit of mortality on calcium concentration is probably all that is required for an adequate account of the data.

The shading in Figures 8.1 and 8.2 shows the boundaries of the confidence limits of the regression lines of mortality on calcium concentration for the two regions (see Chapter 7). (This is a convenient point to note that categorical explanatory variables with more than two variables can also be used in

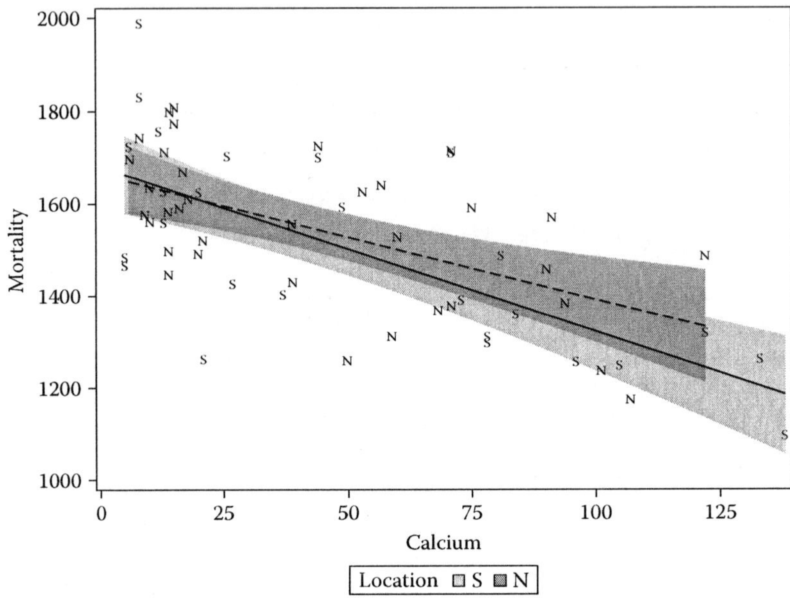

FIGURE 8.2
Graphical illustration of a multiple linear regression model including a region x mortality interaction fitted to water hardness data.

multiple linear regression modelling as long as they are represented by a series of dummy variables. To 'dummy-code' a categorical variable with k categories, $k - 1$ binary dummy variables are created. Each of the dummy variables relates to a single category of the original variable and takes the value '1' when the subject falls into the category and '0' otherwise. The category that is ignored in the dummy coding represents what is known as the *reference category*.)

8.3.3 Weight and Physical Measurements in Men

Larner (1996) measured the weight and various physical measurements for 22 males aged 16–30. Subjects were randomly chosen volunteers and all were in reasonably good health. Subjects were requested to tense each muscle being measured slightly to ensure measurement consistency. The data are shown in Table 8.7. (These data are useful for illustrating various aspects of multiple regression, as we shall attempt to demonstrate in what follows. But in practice, one would probably be ill advised to fit multiple regression models to a data set with only 22 observations and 10 explanatory variables; in general, the number of observations should be at least 10 times the number of variables.)

The question of interest for these data is how weight can best be predicted from the other measurements. To begin, it is useful to examine the scatter

TABLE 8.7

Weight and Physical Measurements in Men

Mass	Fore	Bicep	Chest	Neck	Shoulder	Waist	Height	Calf	Thigh	Head
77	28.5	33.5	100	38.5	114	85	178	37.5	53	58
85.5	29.5	36.5	107	39	119	90.5	187	40	52	59
63	25	31	94	36.5	102	80.5	175	33	49	57
80.5	28.5	34	104	39	114	91.5	183	38	50	60
79.5	28.5	36.5	107	39	114	92	174	40	53	59
94	30.5	38	112	39	121	101	180	39.5	57.5	59
66	26.5	29	93	35	105	76	177.5	38.5	50	58.5
69	27	31	95	37	108	84	182.5	36	49	60
65	26.5	29	93	35	112	74	178.5	34	47	55.5
58	26.5	31	96	35	103	76	168.5	35	46	58
69.5	28.5	37	109.5	39	118	80	170	38	50	58.5
73	27.5	33	102	38.5	113	86	180	36	49	59
74	29.5	36	101	38.5	115.5	82	186.5	38	49	60
68	25	30	98.5	37	108	82	188	37	49.5	57
80	29.5	36	103	40	117	95.5	173	37	52.5	58
66	26.5	32.5	89	35	104.5	81	171	38	48	56.5
54.5	24	30	92.5	35.5	102	76	169	32	42	57
64	25.5	28.5	87.5	35	109	84	181	35.5	42	58
84	30	34.5	99	40.5	119	88	188	39	50.5	56
73	28	34.5	97	37	104	82	173	38	49	58
89	29	35.5	106	39	118	96	179	39.5	51	58.5
94	31	33.5	106	39	120	99.5	184	42	55	57

Notes: Mass = weight in kilograms; fore = maximum circumference of forearm; bicep = maximum circumference of bicep; chest = distance around chest directly under the armpits; neck = distance around neck, approximately halfway up; waist = distance around waist, approximately at trouser line; thigh = circumference of thigh, measured halfway between the knee and the top of the leg; calf = maximum circumference of calf; height = height from top to toe; shoulders = distance around shoulders, measured around the peak of the shoulder blades. All measurements are in centimetres.

plot matrix of the data (see Chapter 7). The following SAS code reads in the data and constructs the matrix of scatter plots, in this case including a histogram for each variable on the main diagonal:

```
data PhysicalMeasures;
   infile 'c:\AMSUS\data\PhysicalMeasures.dat';
input Mass Fore Bicep Chest Neck Shoulder Waist Height Calf
Thigh Headcards;
run;

proc sgscatter data=PhysicalMeasures;
 matrix mass--head /diagonal=(histogram kernel);
run;
```

   Applied Medical Statistics Using SAS

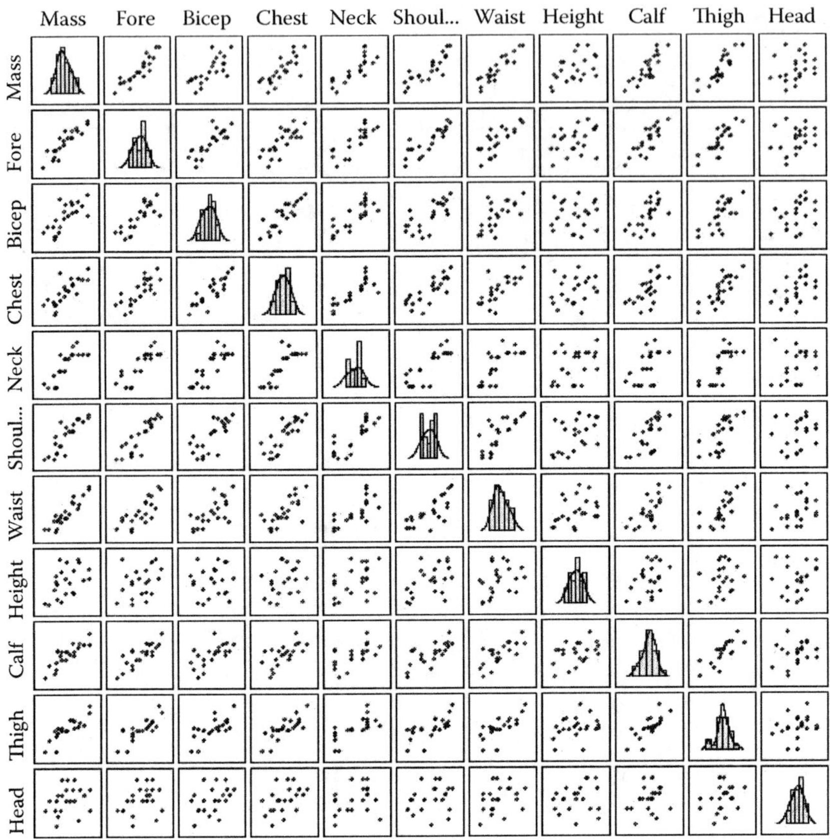

FIGURE 8.3
Scatter plot matrix of physical measurements of young men.

The resulting diagram is shown in Figure 8.3.

The scatter plot matrix clearly highlights the very strong relationship between most pairs of variables in Table 8.7. Highly correlated explanatory variables may be an indication of approximate *multicollinearity*, a phenomenon that can cause several problems when applying the multiple regression model, including:

- Severely limiting the size of the multiple correlation coefficient, R, because the explanatory variables are largely attempting to explain much of the same variability in the response variable (see Dizney and Gromen 1967 for an example)

- Making the assessment of the importance of a given explanatory variable (see later discussion) difficult because the effects of explanatory variables are confounded due to their intercorrelations

- Increasing the variances of the regression coefficients, thus making the model for prediction less stable for prediction—the parameter estimates become unreliable

Spotting multicollinearity amongst a set of explanatory variables may not be easy. The obvious course of action is simply to examine the correlations between these variables, but whilst this *is* often helpful, it is by no means foolproof because more subtle forms of multicollinearity may be missed. An alternative and generally far more useful approach is to examine what are known as the *variance inflation factors* of the explanatory variables. The variance inflation factor for the *j*th variable, VIF_j, is given by

$$VIF_j = \frac{1}{1 - R_j^2} \qquad (8.9)$$

where R_j^2 is the square of the multiple correlation coefficient from the regression of the *j*th explanatory variable on the remaining explanatory variables.

The variance inflation factor of an explanatory variable indicates the strength of the linear relationship between the variable and the remaining explanatory variables. A rough rule of thumb is that variance inflation factors greater than 10 give some cause for concern.

How can multicollinearity be combated? One way is to combine in some way explanatory variables that are highly correlated. An alternative is simply to select one of the set of correlated variables. Two more complex possibilities are *regression on principal components* and *ridge regression,* both of which are described in Chatterjee and Price (2000).

We can look at the variance inflation factors for the data in Table 8.7 using the following SAS instructions:

```
proc reg data=PhysicalMeasures;
  model mass=fore--head /vif;
run;
```

The output is shown in Table 8.8.

Concentrating for the moment on the variance inflation factors, we see that some are quite large; for example, the factor for forearm is a little greater than 10. It might be advisable to consider dropping this variable, but here we will retain it and interpret the results of the multiple regression as they are given in Table 8.8. The overall *F*-test indicates that not all the regression coefficients are zero and the R^2 value of 0.98 shows that, jointly, the 10 explanatory variables account for 98% of the variation in the weight. For what they are worth here—with so many explanatory variables, some of which are highly correlated—the *t*-tests suggest that waist and height are the best predictors of mass.

But the problem is that the values of the *t*-statistics are *conditional* on which explanatory variables are included in the current model. The values of these

TABLE 8.8

Variance Inflation Factors for the Explanatory Variables in the Data in Table 8.7

Model: MODEL1
Dependent Variable: Mass
Number of Observations Read   22
Number of Observations Used   22

Analysis of Variance					
Source	DF	Sum of Squares	Mean Square	F Value	Pr > F
Model	10	2466.62407	246.66241	47.17	<.0001
Error	11	57.52366	5.22942		
Corrected Total	21	2524.14773			

Root MSE	2.28679	R-Square	0.9772
Dependent Mean	73.93182	Adj R-Sq	0.9565
Coeff Var	3.09311		

Parameter Estimates						
Variable	DF	Parameter Estimate	Standard Error	t Value	Pr > |t|	Variance Inflation
Intercept	1	−69.51714	29.03739	−2.39	0.0356	0
Fore	1	1.78182	0.85473	2.08	0.0612	10.80790
Bicep	1	0.15509	0.48530	0.32	0.7553	7.98620
Chest	1	0.18914	0.22583	0.84	0.4201	9.28524
Neck	1	−0.48184	0.72067	−0.67	0.5175	7.03335
Shoulder	1	−0.02931	0.23943	−0.12	0.9048	9.38106
Waist	1	0.66144	0.11648	5.68	0.0001	3.31098
Height	1	0.31785	0.13037	2.44	0.0329	2.62357
Calf	1	0.44589	0.41251	1.08	0.3029	3.99248
Thigh	1	0.29721	0.30510	0.97	0.3509	4.83034
Head	1	−0.91956	0.52009	−1.77	0.1047	1.71458

statistics will change, as will the values of the estimated regression coefficients and their standard errors as other variables are included and excluded from the model. Consequently, using these *t*-statistics to decide which of the explanatory variables are most predictive of the response and thus to decide on a more parsimonious model for the data (i.e., one with fewer explanatory variables but still adequate to describe the variation on the response) is rarely satisfactory. Other, more involved procedures are needed to search for the required more parsimonious model and a number of these are described in the next section.

8.4 Identifying a Parsimonious Model

A multiple regression analysis begins with a set of observations on a response variable and a number of explanatory variables. After an initial analysis has established that some, at least, of the explanatory variables are predictive of the response, the question arises as to whether a subset of the explanatory variables might provide a simpler model that is essentially as useful as the full model in predicting or explaining the response.

As pointed out at the end of the previous section, because the t-statistics associated with each regression coefficient provide only a partial answer to this question, we need to consider other possible approaches. The best approach is to build a model based on theory—for example, by first considering the most important predictors and confounders and then sequentially considering inclusion of further variables believed to be associated with the response variable.

Often, however, this approach is not possible and then the investigator may consider using one of the automatic procedures that are available. These rely on testing many different combinations of variables and therefore suffer from all of the problems of multiple testing; spurious results (false positives) are likely, and the analysis must be considered exploratory. Nevertheless, we shall briefly examine two automatic selection procedures.

8.4.1 All Possible Subsets Regression

Consider a p-parameter multiple regression model in which there is a parameter for the intercept and $p - 1$ explanatory variables; for such a model, there are $2^{p-1} - 1$ possible regression models. Each variable can be in or out of the model, and the model containing no explanatory variables is excluded. In all possible subsets, regression of *all* these models is estimated and then compared using some numerical criterion designed to indicate which models are the 'best'. The most commonly used of the criteria that have been proposed is Mallows' C_p statistic, which is defined as

$$C_p = (RSS_p \, / \, s^2) - (n - 2p) \tag{8.10}$$

where RSS_p is the residual sum of squares from a regression model with a particular set of $p - 1$ of the explanatory variables, plus an intercept, and s^2 is the estimate of σ^2 from the model, including *all* explanatory variables under consideration. (Note that we are using p here for the number of variables in the putative model, *not* for the number of available explanatory variables, which we shall denote by t.)

It can be shown that C_p is an unbiased estimate of the mean square error, $E\left[\sum \hat{y}_i - E(y_i)\right]^2 / n$, of the model's fitted values as estimates of the true expectations of the observations. 'Low' values of C_p are those that indicate the best models to consider. One way to use C_p is to plot its value against p. In such a plot, the subsets of variables worth considering in searching for a parsimonious model are those lying close to the line $C_p = p$; the model with the lowest C_p value approximately equal to p is considered to be the 'best' model for the data.

In this plot, the value of p is (roughly) the contribution to C_p from the variance of the estimated parameters, whereas the remaining $C_p - p$ is (roughly) the contribution from the bias of the model. This feature makes the plot a useful device for a broad assessment of the C_p values of a range of models, although its use should not necessarily rule out choice of the model with the lowest value of C_p. (The C_p criterion is described in more detail in Mallows 1973, 1995 and Burman 1996.)

All possible subsets' regression using the C_p criterion can be performed using the `selection=cp` option on the `model` statement. For the purposes of illustration, we use the `best=` option to limit the output and plot to the best 20 models:

```
ods graphics on;
proc reg data=PhysicalMeasures plots(only)=cpplot;
  model mass=fore--head / selection=cp best=20;
run;
```

The output in Table 8.9 lists the resulting models in ascending order of C_p.

The plot of C_p values is shown in Figure 8.4. The continuous line is $C_p = p$ (remember that p here is the number of *parameters* in the model—that is, the number of explanatory variables plus the intercept). Although the model that includes the explanatory variables forearm, waist, height, thigh, and head has the lowest value of C_p, the model including only forearm, waist, height, and thigh has a value only slightly larger and lies closer to the line. Both of these models are worth considering as parsimonious models that describe the data adequately. The noncontinuous line is $C_p = 2p - t$ and arises from the suggestion made in Hocking (1976) that models for which $C_p \leq 2p - t$ are most suitable for estimation and extrapolation. Use of this approach would lead to choosing the model containing the seven explanatory variables: forearm, chest, waist, height, calf, thigh, and head, for which the C_p value is less than 6 (i.e., $2 \times 8 - 10$).

8.4.2 Stepwise Methods

Perhaps the most common approach to selecting informative subsets of explanatory variables in a multiple regression is to use a method that relies on a significance test to select a particular explanatory variable for inclusion

TABLE 8.9

Results from Applying Mallows' C_p Statistic to the Data of Physical Measurements in Young Men

Model: MODEL1
Dependent Variable: Mass
C_p Selection Method
Number of Observations Read   22
Number of Observations Used   22

Model Index	Number in Model	C(p)	R-Square	Variables in Model
1	5	4.1421	0.9707	Fore Waist Height Thigh Head
2	6	4.3765	0.9744	Fore Waist Height Calf Thigh Head
3	4	4.4405	0.9659	Fore Waist Height Thigh
4	6	4.8125	0.9735	Fore Chest Waist Height Calf Head
5	5	4.8188	0.9693	Fore Waist Height Calf Thigh
6	5	5.3519	0.9682	Fore Waist Height Calf Head
7	7	5.4685	0.9762	Fore Chest Waist Height Calf Thigh Head
8	6	5.4969	0.9720	Fore Chest Waist Height Thigh Head
9	6	5.9143	0.9712	Fore Bicep Waist Height Thigh Head
10	6	5.9904	0.9710	Fore Neck Waist Height Thigh Head
11	7	6.0719	0.9750	Fore Bicep Waist Height Calf Thigh Head
12	6	6.0811	0.9708	Fore Shoulder Waist Height Thigh Head
13	4	6.1028	0.9625	Fore Waist Height Calf
14	7	6.1184	0.9749	Fore Shoulder Waist Height Calf Thigh Head
15	5	6.1465	0.9665	Fore Neck Waist Height Thigh
16	5	6.1922	0.9665	Fore Chest Waist Height Head
17	5	6.2265	0.9664	Fore Shoulder Waist Height Thigh
18	6	6.2985	0.9704	Fore Shoulder Waist Height Calf Thigh
19	7	6.3277	0.9745	Fore Chest Neck Waist Height Calf Head
20	7	6.3757	0.9744	Fore Neck Waist Height Calf Thigh Head

in, or deletion from, the current regression model. There are three main possibilities:

- Forward selection
- Backward elimination
- Stepwise regression

The forward selection approach begins with an initial model that contains only a constant term and successively adds explanatory variables to the model from the pool of candidate variables until a stage is reached where none of the candidate variables, if added to the current model, would contribute

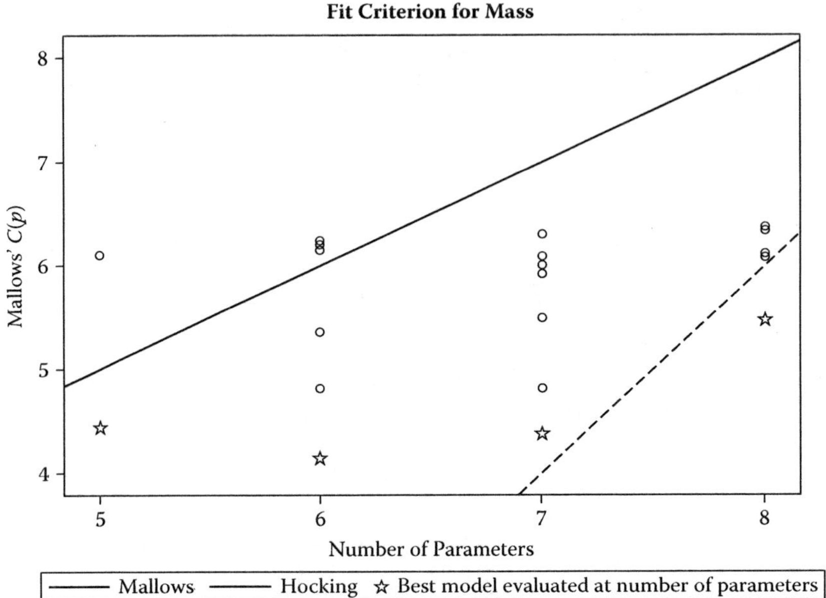

FIGURE 8.4
Plot of number of variables in a model against the value of Mallows' C_p criterion.

information that is statistically important concerning the expected value of
the response. The variable considered for inclusion at any step (say, variable
i) is the one having the largest single degree of freedom F-ratio among those
variables eligible for inclusion where

$$F_i = \max\left(\frac{RSS_p - RSS_{p+i}}{s^2_{p+i}} \right) \qquad (8.11)$$

where the subscript $p + i$ refers to quantities computed when variable i is added
to the current p-term model and RSS stands for residual sum of squares. The
variable i is added to the model if $F_i > F_{in}$, with the quantity F_{in} being a threshold value specified by the user; see Draper and Smith (1998) for details.

The backward elimination method begins with an initial model that contains all explanatory variables and then identifies the single variable that
contributes the least information concerning the expected value of the
response. At any step, the variable (say, variable i) with the smallest F-ratio,
as calculated from the current model, is eliminated if the value of this F-ratio
does not exceed a specified threshold value (F_{out}), where now

$$F_i = \min\left(\frac{RSS_{p-i} - RSS_p}{s^2_p} \right) \qquad (8.12)$$

where RSS_{p-i} denotes the residual sum of squares obtained when variable i is deleted from the current p-term model. Successive iterations of the method result in a 'final' model from which no variables can be eliminated without adversely affecting, in a statistical sense, the predicted value of the expected response. (The threshold values F_{in} and F_{out} can be specified in terms of the equivalent p-values, which is what we use in the following example.)

The stepwise regression method combines elements of both forward selection and backward elimination. The initial model for stepwise regression is one that contains only a constant term. Variables are then considered for inclusion as for forward selection, but in each step, variables included previously are also considered for possible elimination as in the backward method; this will occur if they no longer make any contribution to predicting the expected response.

The three procedures described depend crucially on the thresholds set by the investigator, an obvious danger when seeking a convincing simplified model. A separate factor that influences the results of all such automatic methods in an unpredictable fashion is the underlying correlation of the data. It is highly unlikely, for example, that any of the procedures would produce a final model that included both of two highly correlated explanatory variables. This is, of course, appropriate because including both variables might lead to *collinearity* problems. It does, however, mask the fact that the variable not selected might, if selected, lead to a somewhat different, but equally acceptable, final model. Caution is needed in using any automatic technique for variable selection and users might take heed of the following warning from Agresti (1996):

> Computerized variable selection procedures should be used with caution. When one considers a large number of terms for potential inclusion in a model, one or two of them that are not of real importance may look impressive simply due to chance. For instance, when all true effects are weak, the largest sample effect may substantially overestimate its true effect. In addition it often makes sense to include certain variables of special interest in a model and report their estimated effects even if they are not statistically significant at some level.

Bearing such warnings in mind, we will now investigate the use of all three selection procedures on the physical measurements data. The three methods can all be specified as values for the `selection=` option on the `model` statement, as follows:

```
proc reg data=PhysicalMeasures;
forward: model mass=fore--head / selection=f sle=.05;
backward: model mass=fore--head / selection=b sls=.05;
```

```
stepwise: model mass=fore--head / selection=stepwise sle=.05
sls=.05;
run;
```

This example also illustrates the fact that several models can be fitted within a single `proc reg` step. To distinguish the output from each of
them, it is useful to give each model a label. Note that the label must be the
first word on the `model` statement and must end in a colon. The `sle=` and
`sls=` options specify the significance levels for variables to enter and stay
in the models, respectively. The output from forward selection is shown in
Table 8.10 and from backward elimination in Table 8.11. The output stepwise
regression is shown in Table 8.12. All three tables list the explanatory variables chosen by the corresponding selection method.

TABLE 8.10

Results from Forward Selection

Model: forward					
Dependent Variable: Mass					
Forward Selection: Step 1					
Variable	**Parameter Estimate**	**Standard Error**	**Type II SS**	**F Value**	**Pr > F**
Intercept	−36.19109	10.89480	226.49185	11.03	0.0034
Waist	1.28696	0.12682	2113.64322	102.98	<.0001

Model: forward					
Dependent Variable: Mass					
Forward Selection: Step 2					
Variable	**Parameter Estimate**	**Standard Error**	**Type II SS**	**F value**	**Pr > F**
Intercept	−68.71836	9.19914	471.48633	55.80	<.0001
Fore	2.75462	0.50644	249.96884	29.58	<.0001
Waist	0.77303	0.12469	324.72983	38.43	<.0001

Model: forward					
Dependent Variable: Mass					
Forward Selection: Step 3					
Variable	**Parameter Estimate**	**Standard Error**	**Type II SS**	**F Value**	**Pr > F**
Intercept	−107.48776	15.99818	281.25379	45.14	<.0001
Fore	2.57923	0.43942	214.65503	34.45	<.0001
Waist	0.73194	0.10809	285.70246	45.86	<.0001
Height	0.26422	0.09481	48.38708	7.77	0.0122

TABLE 8.10 (*Continued*)

Results from Forward Selection

	Model: forward				
	Dependent Variable: Mass				
	Forward Selection: Step 4				
Variable	Parameter Estimate	Standard Error	Type II SS	F Value	Pr > F
Intercept	−113.31204	14.63911	302.99990	59.91	<.0001
Fore	2.03558	0.46243	97.99698	19.38	0.0004
Waist	0.64688	0.10431	194.49518	38.46	<.0001
Height	0.27175	0.08548	51.10714	10.11	0.0055
Thigh	0.54008	0.23740	26.17429	5.18	0.0361

	Model: forward					
	Dependent Variable: Mass					
	Summary of Forward Selection					
Step	Variable Entered	Number Vars In	Partial R-Square	Model R-Square	C(p)	F Value	Pr > F
1	Waist	1	0.8374	0.8374	60.4990	102.98	<.0001
2	Fore	2	0.0990	0.9364	14.6985	29.58	<.0001
3	Height	3	0.0192	0.9556	7.4457	7.77	0.0122
4	Thigh	4	0.0104	0.9659	4.4405	5.18	0.0361

TABLE 8.11

Results from Backward Elimination

	Model: backward				
	Dependent Variable: Mass				
	Backward Elimination: Step 0				
Variable	Parameter Estimate	Standard Error	Type II SS	F Value	Pr > F
Intercept	−69.51714	29.03739	29.97245	5.73	0.0356
Fore	1.78182	0.85473	22.72597	4.35	0.0612
Bicep	0.15509	0.48530	0.53409	0.10	0.7553
Chest	0.18914	0.22583	3.66801	0.70	0.4201
Neck	−0.48184	0.72067	2.33767	0.45	0.5175
Shoulder	−0.02931	0.23943	0.07838	0.01	0.9048
Waist	0.66144	0.11648	168.62682	32.25	0.0001
Height	0.31785	0.13037	31.08457	5.94	0.0329
Calf	0.44589	0.41251	6.10990	1.17	0.3029
Thigh	0.29721	0.30510	4.96258	0.95	0.3509
Head	−0.91956	0.52009	16.34775	3.13	0.1047

(*Continued*)

TABLE 8.11 (*Continued*)

Results from Backward Elimination

	Model: backward				
	Dependent Variable: Mass				
	Backward Elimination: Step 1				
Variable	Parameter Estimate	Standard Error	Type II SS	F Value	Pr > F
Intercept	−70.53857	26.64703	33.63662	7.01	0.0213
Fore	1.71790	0.64838	33.69700	7.02	0.0212
Bicep	0.16155	0.46220	0.58643	0.12	0.7328
Chest	0.17286	0.17491	4.68850	0.98	0.3425
Neck	−0.48458	0.69012	2.36669	0.49	0.4960
Waist	0.65846	0.10913	174.76132	36.41	<.0001
Height	0.31082	0.11216	36.86259	7.68	0.0169
Calf	0.45289	0.39141	6.42642	1.34	0.2698
Thigh	0.31225	0.26756	6.53796	1.36	0.2659
Head	−0.89324	0.45370	18.60586	3.88	0.0725

	Model: backward				
	Dependent Variable: Mass				
	Backward Elimination: Step 2				
Variable	Parameter Estimate	Standard Error	Type II SS	F Value	Pr > F
Intercept	−71.95027	25.43433	35.81935	8.00	0.0142
Fore	1.79678	0.58696	41.94304	9.37	0.0091
Chest	0.19282	0.15965	6.52939	1.46	0.2486
Neck	−0.37432	0.59271	1.78520	0.40	0.5386
Waist	0.65393	0.10463	174.82730	39.06	<.0001
Height	0.28849	0.08902	47.01218	10.50	0.0064
Calf	0.47487	0.37305	7.25297	1.62	0.2253
Thigh	0.30508	0.25761	6.27806	1.40	0.2575
Head	−0.85259	0.42348	18.14303	4.05	0.0653

	Model: backward				
	Dependent Variable: Mass				
	Backward Elimination: Step 3				
Variable	Parameter Estimate	Standard Error	Type II SS	F Value	Pr > F
Intercept	−76.05013	24.05809	42.80654	9.99	0.0069
Fore	1.62588	0.50955	43.61405	10.18	0.0065
Chest	0.13796	0.13103	4.74838	1.11	0.3103
Waist	0.63648	0.09873	178.03754	41.56	<.0001
Height	0.26875	0.08154	46.53822	10.86	0.0053

TABLE 8.11 (*Continued*)

Results from Backward Elimination

Model: backward					
Dependent Variable: Mass					
Backward Elimination: Step 3					
Variable	**Parameter Estimate**	**Standard Error**	**Type II SS**	**F Value**	**Pr > F**
Calf	0.54684	0.34751	10.60732	2.48	0.1379
Thigh	0.32121	0.25077	7.02813	1.64	0.2211
Head	−0.82210	0.41159	17.09086	3.99	0.0656

Model: backward					
Dependent Variable: Mass					
Backward Elimination: Step 4					
Variable	**Parameter Estimate**	**Standard Error**	**Type II SS**	**F Value**	**Pr > F**
Intercept	−79.72624	23.88925	48.05720	11.14	0.0045
Fore	1.79485	0.48536	59.00469	13.67	0.0021
Waist	0.65671	0.09719	196.98777	45.65	<.0001
Height	0.25388	0.08059	42.81545	9.92	0.0066
Calf	0.50718	0.34671	9.23324	2.14	0.1641
Thigh	0.43298	0.22801	15.55932	3.61	0.0770
Head	−0.65722	0.38200	12.77197	2.96	0.1059

Model: backward					
Dependent Variable: Mass					
Backward Elimination: Step 5					
Variable	**Parameter Estimate**	**Standard Error**	**Type II SS**	**F Value**	**Pr > F**
Intercept	−80.45330	24.72024	48.95889	10.59	0.0050
Fore	2.12319	0.44541	105.02769	22.72	0.0002
Waist	0.66561	0.10040	203.16460	43.95	<.0001
Height	0.27704	0.08179	53.03117	11.47	0.0038
Thigh	0.52317	0.22720	24.50837	5.30	0.0351
Head	−0.63714	0.39512	12.01901	2.60	0.1264

Model: backward					
Dependent Variable: Mass					
Backward Elimination: Step 6					
Variable	**Parameter Estimate**	**Standard Error**	**Type II SS**	**F Value**	**Pr > F**
Intercept	−113.31204	14.63911	302.99990	59.91	<.0001
Fore	2.03558	0.46243	97.99698	19.38	0.0004

(*Continued*)

TABLE 8.11 (*Continued*)

Results from Backward Elimination

		Model: backward			
		Dependent Variable: Mass			
		Backward Elimination: Step 6			
Variable	**Parameter Estimate**	**Standard Error**	**Type II SS**	**F Value**	**Pr > F**
Waist	0.64688	0.10431	194.49518	38.46	<.0001
Height	0.27175	0.08548	51.10714	10.11	0.0055
Thigh	0.54008	0.23740	26.17429	5.18	0.0361

			Model: backward				
			Dependent Variable: Mass				
			Summary of Backward Elimination				
Step	**Variable Removed**	**Number Vars in**	**Partial R-Square**	**Model R-Square**	**C(p)**	**F Value**	**Pr > F**
1	Shoulder	9	0.0000	0.9772	9.0150	0.01	0.9048
2	Bicep	8	0.0002	0.9769	7.1271	0.12	0.7328
3	Neck	7	0.0007	0.9762	5.4685	0.40	0.5386
4	Chest	6	0.0019	0.9744	4.3765	1.11	0.3103
5	Calf	5	0.0037	0.9707	4.1421	2.14	0.1641
6	Head	4	0.0048	0.9659	4.4405	2.60	0.1264

TABLE 8.12

Results from Stepwise Selection

		Model: stepwise			
		Dependent Variable: Mass			
		Stepwise Selection: Step 1			
Variable	**Parameter Estimate**	**Standard Error**	**Type II SS**	**F Value**	**Pr > F**
Intercept	−36.19109	10.89480	226.49185	11.03	0.0034
Waist	1.28696	0.12682	2113.64322	102.98	<.0001

		Model: stepwise			
		Dependent Variable: mass			
		Stepwise selection: Step 2			
Variable	**Parameter Estimate**	**Standard Error**	**Type II SS**	**F Value**	**Pr > F**
Intercept	−68.71836	9.19914	471.48633	55.80	<.0001
Fore	2.75462	0.50644	249.96884	29.58	<.0001
Waist	0.77303	0.12469	324.72983	38.43	<.0001

TABLE 8.12 (*Continued*)

Results from Stepwise Selection

Model: stepwise					
Dependent Variable: mass					
Stepwise selection: Step 3					
Variable	Parameter Estimate	Standard Error	Type II SS	F Value	Pr > F
Intercept	−107.48776	15.99818	281.25379	45.14	<.0001
Fore	2.57923	0.43942	214.65503	34.45	<.0001
Waist	0.73194	0.10809	285.70246	45.86	<.0001
Height	0.26422	0.09481	48.38708	7.77	0.0122

Model: stepwise					
Dependent Variable: Mass					
Stepwise Selection: Step 4					
Variable	Parameter Estimate	Standard Error	Type II SS	F Value	Pr > F
Intercept	−113.31204	14.63911	302.99990	59.91	<.0001
Fore	2.03558	0.46243	97.99698	19.38	0.0004
Waist	0.64688	0.10431	194.49518	38.46	<.0001
Height	0.27175	0.08548	51.10714	10.11	0.0055
Thigh	0.54008	0.23740	26.17429	5.18	0.0361

Model: stepwise							
Dependent Variable: Mass							
Summary of Stepwise Selection							
Step	Variable Entered	Variable Removed	Number Vars In	Partial R-Square	Model R-Square	C(p)	F Value	Pr > F
1	Waist		1	0.8374	0.8374	60.4990	102.98	<.0001
2	Fore		2	0.0990	0.9364	14.6985	29.58	<.0001
3	Height		3	0.0192	0.9556	7.4457	7.77	0.0122
4	Thigh		4	0.0104	0.9659	4.4405	5.18	0.0361

8.5 Checking Model Assumptions: Residuals and Other Regression Diagnostics

A regression analysis should not end without an attempt to check assumptions such as those of constant variance and normality of the error terms. Violation of these assumptions may invalidate conclusions based on the regression analysis. The estimated residuals $r_i = y_i - \hat{y}_i$ play an essential role in diagnosing a fitted model, although because these do not have the same variance (the precision of $\hat{y}_i$ depends upon x_i), they are sometimes standardised before use. There are two possibilities: the *standardised residual* and the *Studentised residual*, which are defined as follows:

- *Standardised residual:*

$$r_{sta} = \frac{y_i - \hat{y}_i}{s\sqrt{1 - h_i}}$$

(8.13)

- *Studentised residual:*

$$r_{stu} = \frac{y_i - \hat{y}_i}{s_{(-i)}\sqrt{1 - h_i}}$$

(8.14)

where h_i is the ith diagonal element of the so-called 'hat matrix', $\mathbf{H}$, given by $\mathbf{H} = \mathbf{X}(\mathbf{X}'\mathbf{X})^{-1}\mathbf{X}$, and $s^2_{(-i)}$ is the estimated residual variance from fitting the model after the exclusion of the ith observation. See Cook and Weisberg (1982) for full details.

The following diagnostic plots using one or other of the residual terms are generally helpful when assessing model assumptions:

- Residuals versus fitted values: if the fitted model is appropriate, the plotted points should lie in an approximately horizontal band across the plot. Departures from this appearance may indicate that the functional form of the assumed model is incorrect or, alternatively, that there is nonconstant variance.

- Residuals versus explanatory variables: systematic patterns in these plots can indicate violations of the constant variance assumption or an inappropriate model form.

- Normal probability plot of the residuals: the plot checks the normal distribution assumptions on which all statistical inference procedures are based.

Figure 8.5 shows some idealised plots that indicate particular points about models. Figure 8.5(a) is what is looked for to confirm that the fitted model meets the assumptions of the regression model. Figure 8.5(b) suggests that the assumption of constant variance is not justified, so a transformation of the response variable before fitting might be a sensible option to consider. Figure 8.5(c) implies that the model requires a quadratic term in the explanatory variables used in the plot.

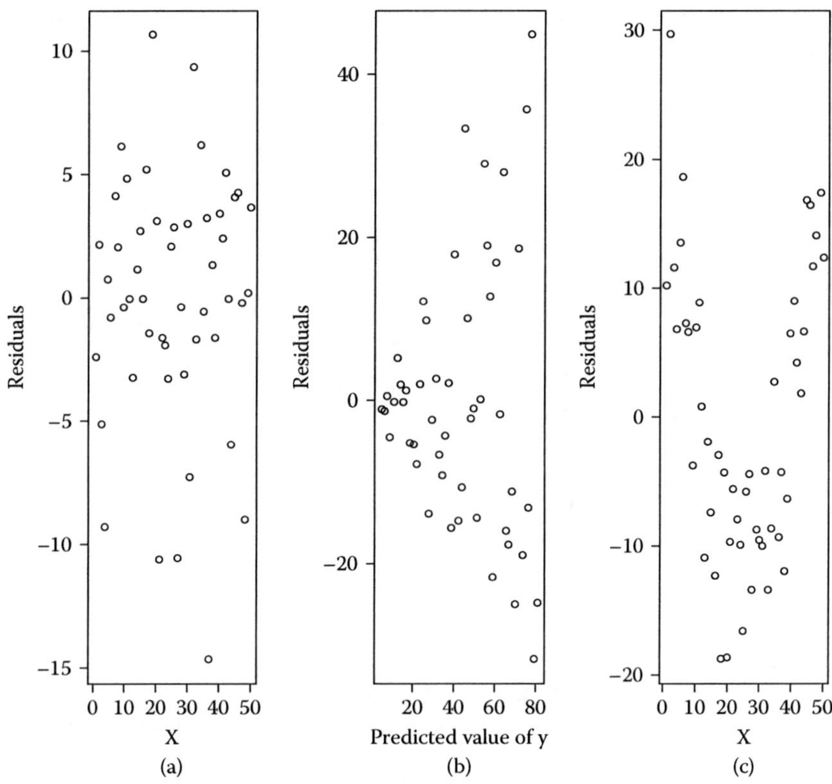

FIGURE 8.5
Idealized residual plots.

A further diagnostic that is often very useful is an index plot of the Cook's distances for each observation. This statistic is defined as follows:

$$D_k = \frac{1}{(p+1)s^2} \sum_{i=1}^{n} \left[\hat{y}_{i(k)} - \hat{y}_i \right]^2 \tag{8.15}$$

where $\hat{y}_{i(k)}$ is the fitted value of the ith observation when the kth observation is omitted from the model. The values of D_k assess the impact of the kth observation on the estimated regression coefficients. Values of D_k greater than one are suggestive that the corresponding observation has undue influence on the estimated regression coefficients (see Cook and Weisberg 1982).

We can obtain all the required plots for the residuals from the 'final model' selected for the physical measurements data (i.e., the one that has the four explanatory variables: fore, waist, height, and thigh) by default simply by switching ODS graphics on, as shown in Table 8.12.

In this example, all three selection methods arrive at the same final model, which contains the explanatory variables: forearm, waist, height, and thigh. This is the third best model as judged by the size of the Mallows' C_p criterion, but one for which the corresponding C_p value is close to p. We will consider this model further in the next section and leave interpretation until then.

```
ods graphics on;
proc reg data=PhysicalMeasures;
  model mass=fore waist height thigh;
run;
```

The plots are shown in two panels in Figure 8.6. The first panel contains the following eight plots:

- Raw residuals versus predicted values
- Studentised residuals (RSTUDENT) versus predicted values
- Studentised residuals versus the leverage
- Q–Q plot of the residuals
- Observed values versus the predicted values
- Cook's D versus observation number
- Histogram of the residuals
- Side-by-side quantile plots of the centred fit and the residuals

The second panel gives the plots of residuals against each explanatory variable. With so few data points, it is difficult to draw very firm conclusions from these plots except to reflect that, overall, they give little cause for concern that the fitted model is suspect in any obvious way. There may be some slight indication of non-normality in Figure 8.6 and observation 11 has a rather high value of Cook's distance, but not above the generally recommended 'cause for concern' value of one.

As the residual plots are generally satisfactory we can move on to interpret the parameters in the fitted mode:

- *Forearm:* the estimated increase in weight for a 1 cm increase in forearm is 2.04 kg conditional on the other three explanatory variables, with an approximate 95% confidence interval of [1,3] kg.
- *Waist:* the estimated increase in weight for a 1 cm increase in waist is 0.65 kg conditional on the other three explanatory variables with an approximate 95% confidence interval of [0.45,0.85] kg.
- *Height:* the estimated increase in weight for a 1 cm increase in height is 0.27 kg conditional on the other three explanatory variables with an approximate 95% confidence interval of [0.09,0.45] kg.
- *Thigh:* the estimated increase in weight for a 1 cm increase in thigh is 0.54 kg conditional on the other three explanatory variables with an approximate 95% confidence interval of [0.06,1.00] kg.

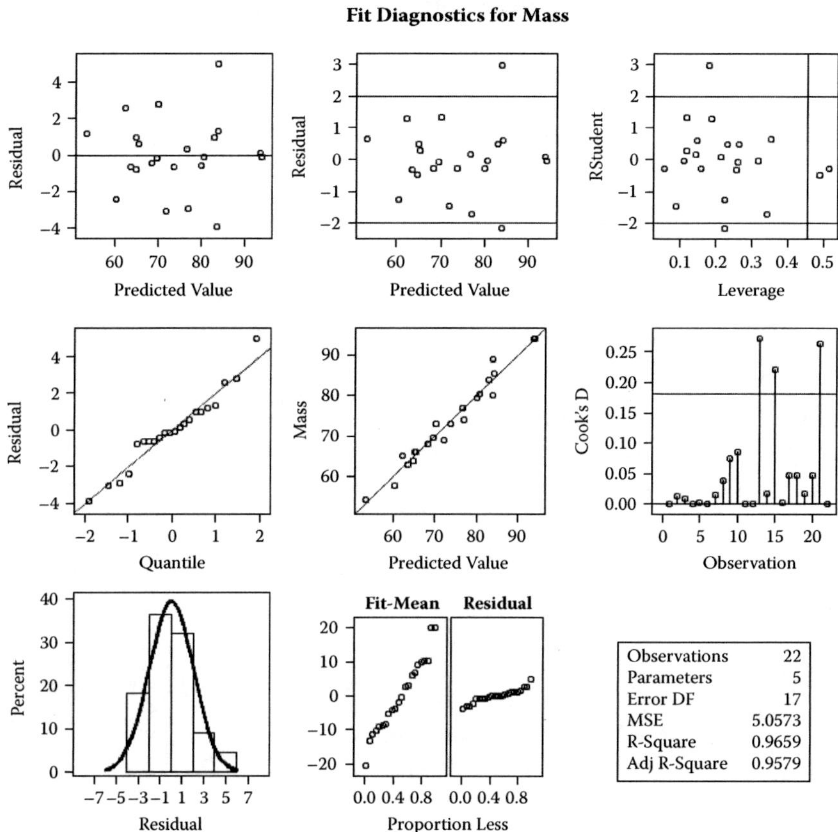

FIGURE 8.6
Some plots of residuals from the final model chosen for the physical measurements data.

(It should perhaps be pointed out that the 'conditional' part of these interpretations is somewhat suspect here because of the high correlations between the explanatory variables.)

8.6 General Linear Model

We have so far discussed ANOVA, ANCOVA, and linear regression as though they were separate models. In fact, all of these models are equivalent and can be viewed as special cases of a general linear model in which the residuals have a normal distribution with constant variance, σ^2. The only difference between ANOVA, ANCOVA, and linear regression models as described in this and previous chapters is that ANOVA uses categorical explanatory variables, linear regression uses continuous (or binary) explanatory variables,

TABLE 8.13

Balanced 2 × 2 Data Set

	A1	A2
B1	23	22
	25	23
	27	21
	29	21
B2	26	37
	32	38
	30	40
	31	35

and ANCOVA uses a mixture of the two. But such apparent differences can easily be accommodated by a general formulation in which a continuous response variable is modelled as a linear function of explanatory variables. We will illustrate this equivalence using the small set of data for a 2 × 2 factorial design shown in Table 8.13.

The usual ANOVA model for such a design is

$$y_{ijk} = \mu + \alpha_i + \beta_j + \gamma_{ij} + \varepsilon_{ijk} \tag{8.16}$$

where

y_{ijk} represents the kth observation in the ijth cell of the design

α_i represents the effect of the ith level of factor A

β_j represents the effect of the jth level of factor B

γ_{ij} represents the interaction of A and B

as always, ε_{ijk} represents random error terms with the usual distributional assumptions of normality with zero mean and constant variance, σ^2.

The usual constraints on the parameters of the model to deal with overparameterisation in this case are

$$\sum_{i=1}^{2} \alpha_i = \sum_{j=1}^{2} \beta_j = \sum_{i=1}^{2} \gamma_{ij} = \sum_{j=1}^{2} \gamma_{ij} = 0$$

These constraints imply that the parameters in the model are such that $\alpha_1 = -\alpha_2$, $\beta_1 = -\beta_2$, $\gamma_{1j} = -\gamma_{2j}$, $\gamma_{i1} = -\gamma_{i2}$, with the last two of these equations implying that $\gamma_{12} = -\gamma_{11}$, $\gamma_{21} = -\gamma_{11}$, and $\gamma_{22} = \gamma_{11}$—showing that there is only a single parameter describing the interaction between factors A and B. The model for the expected values of the observations in each of the four cells of the design can now be written explicitly as follows:

	A1	A2
B1	$\mu + \alpha_1 + \beta_1 + \gamma_{11}$	$\mu - \alpha_1 + \beta_1 - \gamma_{11}$
B2	$\mu + \alpha_1 - \beta_1 - \gamma_{11}$	$\mu - \alpha_1 - \beta_1 + \gamma_{11}$

Now we define two variables as follows:

$x_1 = 1$ if first level of A, $x_1 = -1$ if second level of A

$x_2 = 1$ if first level of B, $x_2 = -1$ if second level of B

The original ANOVA model for the design can now be written as

$$y_{ijk} = \mu + \alpha_1 x_1 + \beta_1 x_2 + \gamma_{11} x_3 + \varepsilon_{ijk} \text{ where } x_3 = x_1 \times x_2 \tag{8.17}$$

We can now recognise this as a multiple linear regression model with three explanatory variables, and we can fit it in the usual way. Note that all observations in cell A1, B1 have $x_1 = 1$ and $x_2 = 1$; all observations in cell A1, B2 have $x_1 = 1$, $x_2 = -1$, and so on for the remaining observations in Table 8.13. To begin, we will fit the model with the single explanatory variable x_1 using the SAS code:

```
data factorial;
do a=1 to 2;
input resp @;
b=1;
if _n_>4 then b=2;
output;
end;
cards;
23 22
25 23
27 21
29 21
26 37
32 38
30 40
31 35
;

data factorial;
  set factorial;
  if a=1 then x1=1;
         else x1=-1;
  if b=1 then x2=1;
         else x2=-1;
  x3=x1*x2;
run;

proc reg data=factorial;
x1: model resp=x1;
x12: model resp=x1 x2;
x123: model resp=x1-x3;
run; quit;
```

TABLE 8.14

Multiple Regression Results for Data in Table 8.13

Model: x1					
Dependent Variable: resp					
Analysis of Variance					
Source	**DF**	**Sum of Squares**	**Mean Square**	**F Value**	**Pr > F**
Model	1	12.25000	12.25000	0.30	0.5954
Error	14	580.75000	41.48214		
Corrected Total	15	593.00000			

Parameter Estimates					
Variable	**DF**	**Parameter Estimate**	**Standard Error**	**t Value**	**Pr > |t|**
Intercept	1	28.75000	1.61017	17.86	<.0001
x1	1	−0.87500	1.61017	−0.54	0.5954

TABLE 8.15

More Multiple Regression Results for Data in Table 8.13

Model: x12					
Dependent Variable: resp					
Analysis of Variance					
Source	**DF**	**Sum of Squares**	**Mean Square**	**F Value**	**Pr > F**
Model	2	392.50000	196.25000	12.72	0.0009
Error	13	200.50000	15.42308		
Corrected Total	15	593.00000			

Parameter Estimates					
Variable	**DF**	**Parameter Estimate**	**Standard Error**	**t Value**	**Pr > |t|**
Intercept	1	28.75000	0.98181	29.28	<.0001
x1	1	−0.87500	0.98181	−0.89	0.3890
x2	1	−4.87500	0.98181	−4.97	0.0003

The results are shown in Table 8.14.

The regression sum of squares 12.25 is what would be the between levels of A sum of squares in an ANOVA table. Now fit the regression with x_1 and x_2 as explanatory variables using the code to give the results shown in Table 8.15.

The difference between the regression sums of squares for the two-variable and one-variable models gives the sum of squares for factor B that would be obtained in an ANOVA. Note that the corresponding parameter estimates in

TABLE 8.16

Further Multiple Regression Results for Data in Table 8.13

Model: x123					
Dependent Variable: resp					
Analysis of Variance					
Source	**DF**	**Sum of Squares**	**Mean Square**	**F Value**	**Pr > F**
Model	3	536.50000	178.83333	37.98	<.0001
Error	12	56.50000	4.70833		
Corrected Total	15	593.00000			

Parameter Estimates					
Variable	**DF**	**Parameter Estimate**	**Standard Error**	**t Value**	**Pr > |t|**
Intercept	1	28.75000	0.54247	53.00	<.0001
x1	1	−0.87500	0.54247	−1.61	0.1327
x2	1	−4.87500	0.54247	−8.99	<.0001
x3	1	3.00000	0.54247	5.53	0.0001

both models fitted remain the same. Now we can add in the interaction term to get Table 8.16.

The difference between the regression sums of squares for the three-variable and two-variable models gives the sum of squares for the A × B interaction that would be obtained in an analysis of variance. The residual sum of squares in the final step corresponds to the error sum of squares in the usual ANOVA table. (Readers might like to confirm the results in Table 8.16 by running an analysis of variance on the data.)

Note that, unlike the estimated regression coefficients in the examples considered earlier in this chapter, the estimated regression coefficients for the balanced 2 × 2 design do not change as extra explanatory variables are introduced into the regression model. The factors in a balanced design are independent; a more technical term is that they are *orthogonal*. When the explanatory variables are orthogonal, adding variables to the regression model in any order will alter nothing; the corresponding sums of squares and regression coefficient estimates will be the same. (Readers are encouraged to repeat this exercise using a small *unbalanced* data set.)

8.7 Summary

Multiple regression is one of the most used (one is tempted to say 'overused') statistical techniques. It can be helpful for assessing the relationship between a response variable and a number of explanatory variables, but researchers using the technique should take care to check assumptions using a variety of regression diagnostics, and they should not accept blindly the results of the automatic techniques for selecting subsets of explanatory variables. The multiple regression model and the ANOVA and ANCOVA models described in previous chapters are all essentially the same model—one that can be further subsumed into an even more general setting of generalised linear models, as we shall see in the next two chapters.

9

Logistic Regression

9.1 Introduction

The multiple regression model as described in the previous chapter assumes that the response variable, y, is continuous and, given the values of the explanatory variables, has a normal distribution with a mean that is a linear function of the explanatory variables and variance, σ^2. But in many studies in medicine, the response variable is binary—for example, improved or not improved, diseased or not diseased, or even dead or alive. Many of the data sets considered in Chapter 4 were of this type. In this chapter, we examine a suitable technique, *logistic regression,* for exploring the effects of explanatory variables on a binary response variable. (Logistic regression can also be applied to categorical responses with more than two categories; see, for example, Hosmer and Lemeshow 2000.)

9.2 Logistic Regression

In any regression problem, the key quantity is the mean or expected value of the response variable, given the values of the explanatory variables. In linear regression, the expected value of a response variable, y, is modelled as a linear function of the explanatory variables $x_1, x_2, \ldots, x_p$, that is,

$$E(y|x_1, \ldots, x_p) = \beta_0 + \beta_1 x_1 \ldots + \beta_p x_p \tag{9.1}$$

For a dichotomous response variable coded 0 and 1, this expected value is simply the probability, π, that the response variable takes the value one. This could be modelled directly as before, but there are two clear problems:

- The predicted value of the probability, π, must satisfy $0 \leq \pi < 1$, whereas a linear predictor can yield values from minus infinity to plus infinity.

- The observed values of y conditional on the values of the explanatory variables will not now follow a normal distribution with mean π, but rather a *Bernoulli distribution*, as we shall explain later.

Having stated the two problems in modelling data where the response is a binary variable, we can now discuss how to solve these problems by developing some of the theory behind logistic regression. Our data now consist of a binary response variable, y, and a set of explanatory variables $x_1, x_2, \ldots, x_p$. The expected value of y is simply $1 \times \Pr(y = 1) + 0 \times \Pr(y = 0) = \Pr(y = 1) = \pi$. (We will assume that the value one is used to code the occurrence of some event of interest and zero is used to code its nonoccurrence). The probability that the event of interest happens, π, should not be modelled directly as a linear function of the explanatory variables since this will not constrain predicted values of π to be in the interval [0,1]. Instead, a suitable transformation of π is modelled. The transformation most often used is the *logit* function of the probability given by $\log \pi/(1 - \pi)$. This leads to the logistic regression model given by

$$\log \mathrm{it}(\pi) = \log \frac{\pi}{1 - \pi} = \beta_0 + \beta_1 x_1 + \cdots \beta_p x_p \tag{9.2}$$

The logit transformation is chosen because, from a mathematical point of view, it is extremely flexible and, from a practical point of view, it leads to meaningful and convenient interpretation, as we explain later. The logit of a probability is nothing more than the log of the odds of the event of interest (see Chapter 4), and since its values can range from $-\infty$ to $+\infty$, the first problem of modelling π directly is overcome. The logistic regression model can be expressed directly in terms of π as

$$\pi = \frac{\exp\left(\beta_0 + \beta_1 x_1 + \cdots \beta_p x_p\right)}{1 + \exp\left(\beta_0 + \beta_1 x_1 + \cdots \beta_p x_p\right)} \tag{9.3}$$

In a logistic regression model, the parameter β_i associated with explanatory variable x_i represents the expected change in the logit when x_i is increased by one unit, conditional on the other explanatory variables remaining the same. Interpretation becomes simpler if we look at $\exp(\beta_i)$, which corresponds to an odds ratio (see Chapter 4). A confidence interval for the latter is obtained by exponentiation of the upper and lower limits of the corresponding confidence interval of the regression coefficient in the logit model. Examples will be given later in the chapter.

In linear regression, the observed value of the outcome variable is expressed as its expected value, given the explanatory variables plus an error term. The error terms are assumed to have a normal distribution with mean zero and a variance that is constant across levels of the explanatory variables. With a binary response, we can express an observed value in the same way as

$$y = \pi + \varepsilon \tag{9.4}$$

However, here the error term, ε, can only assume one of two possible values. If $y = 1$, then $\varepsilon = 1 - \pi$ with probability π; if $y = 0$, then $\varepsilon = -\pi$ with probability $1 - \pi$. Consequently, ε has a distribution with mean zero and variance equal to $\pi(1 - \pi)$. Thus, the conditional distribution of the response variable, y, follows what is known as a *Bernoulli distribution* (which is simply a binomial distribution for a single trial) with probability that it takes the value one given by the mean π, which because it is conditional on the explanatory variables, we shall now denote as $\pi(\mathbf{x})$, where $\mathbf{x}' = [x_1, x_2, \ldots, x_p]$.

In linear regression (both simple and multiple), the method used most often to estimate the unknown parameters is least squares. Under the usual assumptions for the linear regression models (see Chapters 7 and 8), the least squares method yields estimators with a number of desirable statistical properties. Unfortunately, when this method is applied to a model with a dichotomous response, the estimators no longer have these properties. Consequently, the method of *maximum likelihood* is used to estimate the parameters in the logistic regression model. The *log-likelihood function, l,* is given by

$$l(\beta; \mathbf{y}) = \sum_{i=1}^{n} \left\{ y_i \log\left[\pi(\beta' \mathbf{x}_i)\right] + (1 - y_i) \log\left[1 - \pi(\beta' \mathbf{x}_i)\right] \right\} \tag{9.5}$$

where
$\mathbf{x}_i' = [x_{i1}, x_{i2}, \ldots, x_{ip}]$
$\mathbf{y}' = [y_1, y_2, \ldots, y_n]$
$\beta' = [\beta_0, \beta_1, \ldots, \beta_p]$

The estimates of the parameters are found by maximising the log likelihood using an iterative algorithm described in Collett (2003a). Logistic regression can also be used when the response is observed as a proportion rather than directly as a binary variable; an example is the proportion of headache-free days on a number of subjects. The appropriate distribution in this case is the binomial distribution with the correct denominator (in the suggested example, the number of days over which headache status has been recorded).

The lack of fit of a logistic regression model can be measured by a term known as the *deviance*, which is essentially the ratio of the likelihoods of the model of interest to the saturated model that fits the data perfectly (see Collett 2003a for a full explanation). Explicitly, the deviance is defined as

$$D = 2 \sum_{i=1}^{n} \left\{ y_i \log\left(\frac{y_i}{\hat{y}_i}\right) + (n_i - y_i) \log\left(\frac{n_i - y_i}{n_i - \hat{y}_i}\right) \right\} \tag{9.6}$$

where $\hat{y}_i$ is the predicted number of events of interest under the current model—that is, $\hat{y}_i = n_i\hat{\pi}_i$. D compares the observed values y_i with their fitted values, $\hat{y}_i$, under the current model. Differences in deviance can be used to compare alternative *nested* logistic regression models. For example,

$$\text{Model 1 (Deviance } D_1) : \log \text{it}(\pi) = \beta_0 + \beta_1 x_1$$

$$\text{Model 2 (Deviance } D_2) : \log \text{it}(\pi) = \beta_0 + \beta_1 x_1 + \beta_2 x_2 + \beta_3 x_3$$

The difference in deviance $D_1 - D_2$ reflects the combined effect of explanatory variables x_2 and x_3 and under the hypothesis that these variables have no effect (i.e., β_2 and β_3 are both zero). The difference has an approximate chi-squared distribution with degrees of freedom generally equal to the difference in the number of parameters in the two models—in this case, two. The deviance (or likelihood ratio) can be used to test that all regression coefficients in a model are zero.

Two other test statistics are available for the same purpose: the score statistic and Wald's test. Both are described in Collett (2003a). The three tests are asymptotically equivalent but differ in finite samples. The likelihood ratio test is generally considered the most appropriate.

9.3 Two Examples of the Application of Logistic Regression

In this section, we shall look at two examples of the use of logistic regression in medicine beginning with one from psychiatry.

9.3.1 Psychiatric 'Caseness'

Goldberg (1972) describes a psychiatric screening questionnaire, the *General Health Questionnaire* (GHQ), designed to identify people who may be suffering from a psychiatric illness. In Table 9.1 some results from applying this instrument are given; here, what is of interest is how the probability of being classified as a potential psychiatric 'case' by a psychiatrist is related to an individual's score on the GHQ and the individual's gender.

To begin, we can read in the data and plot the estimated probability of being a case against GHQ score, identifying males and females on the plot:

```
data ghq;
  input ghq sex $ cases noncases;
  total=cases+noncases;
  prcase=cases/total;
cards;
```

```
0     F     4     80
1     F     4     29
2     F     8     15


.   .   .


8     M     3     1
9     M     2     0
10    M     2     0
;

proc sgplot data=ghq;
   series y=prcase x=ghq / group=sex;
   scatter y=prcase x=ghq / group=sex;
run;
```

The resulting diagram is shown in Figure 9.1. Clearly, the probability of being considered a case increases with increasing GHQ value, but the relationship is not linear and appears to differ for men and women.

TABLE 9.1

Psychiatric Caseness Data

GHQ score	Sex	Number of Cases	Number of Noncases
0	F	4	80
1	F	4	29
2	F	8	15
3	F	6	3
4	F	4	2
5	F	6	1
6	F	3	1
7	F	2	0
8	F	3	0
9	F	2	0
10	F	1	0
0	M	1	36
1	M	2	25
2	M	2	8
3	M	1	4
4	M	3	1
5	M	3	1
6	M	2	1
7	M	4	2
8	M	3	1
9	M	2	0
10	M	2	0

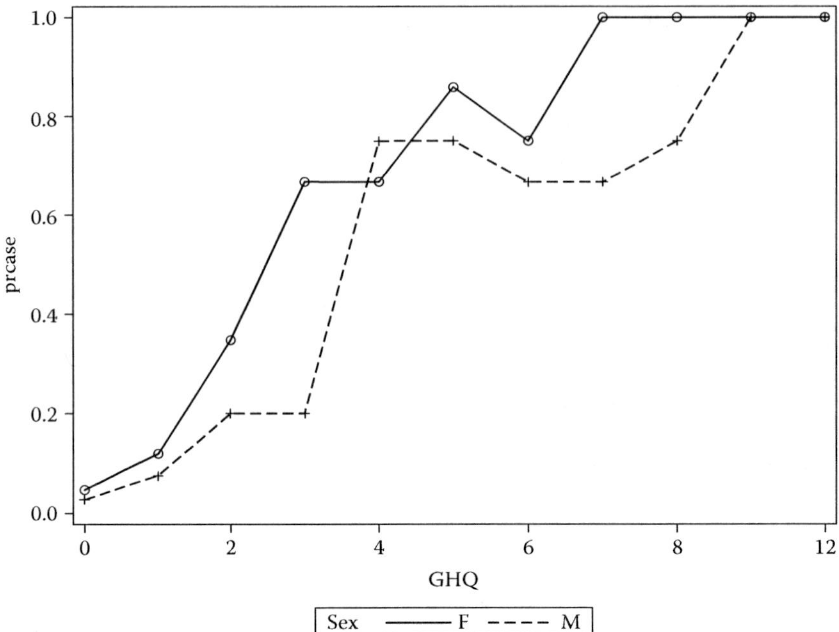

FIGURE 9.1
Plot of probability of being a case against GHQ score identifying males and females.

To begin, we shall ignore gender and compare the fit of both a linear regression and a logistic regression to the probability of being a case with GHQ score as the single explanatory variable; first, linear regression:

```
proc reg data=ghq;
   model prcase=ghq;
   output out=rout p=rpred;
run;
```

The `output` statement creates an output data set that contains all the original variables plus those created by options. The `p=rpred` option specifies that the predicted values are included in a variable named `rpred`. The `out=rout` option specifies the name of the data set to be created.

We then calculate the predicted values from a logistic regression, using `proc logistic`, in the same way:

```
proc logistic data=ghq;
   model cases/total=ghq;
   output out=lout p=lpred;
run;
```

There are two forms of `model` statement within `proc logistic`. This example shows the events/trials syntax, where two variables are specified separated by a slash. The alternative is to specify a single binary response variable before the equal sign.

The two output data sets are combined in a short data step and then plotted together:

```
data lrout;
   set rout;
   set lout;
run;

proc sort data=lrout;
   by ghq;
run;

proc sgplot data=lrout;
   series y=lpred x=ghq / legendlabel='logistic'
   lineatts=(pattern=dash);
   series y=rpred x=ghq / legendlabel='linear';
   scatter y=prcase x=ghq;
run;
```

The resulting diagram is shown in Figure 9.2.

The problems of using the unsuitable linear regression model become apparent on studying Figure 9.2. Using this model, two of the predicted values are greater than one, but the response is a probability constrained to

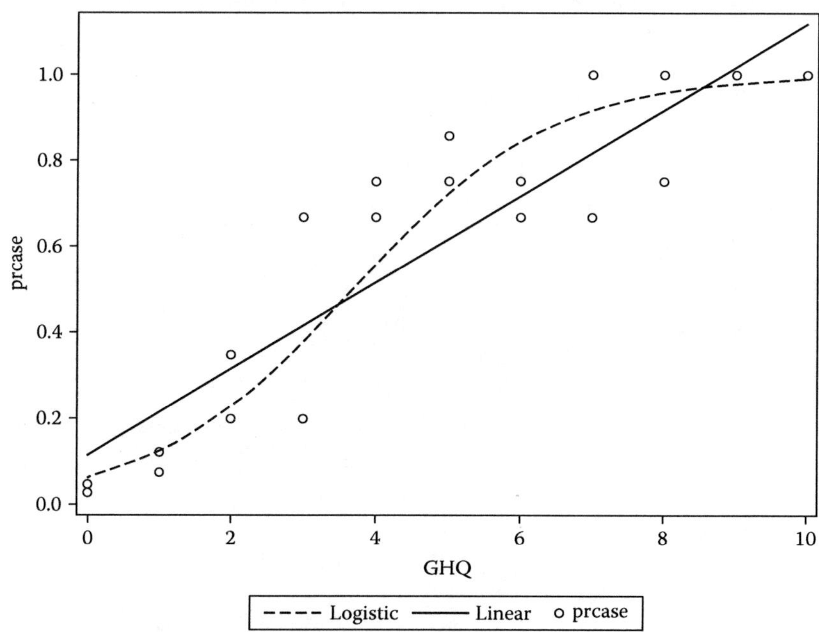

FIGURE 9.2
Probability of caseness versus GHQ score showing the fitted linear and logistic regressions.

be in the interval [0,1]. For an individual with a GHQ score of 10, the linear model predicts that the probability of an individual being judged a case is 1.117. Additionally, the model provides a very poor fit for the observed data. Using the logistic model, on the other hand, leads to predicted values that are satisfactory in that they all lie between 0 and 1, and the model clearly provides a better description of the observed data.

The fitted logistic regression model is

$$\log[\Pr(\text{case})/\Pr(\text{not case})] = -2.71 + 0.74 \times \text{GHQ score}$$

The equation can be rearranged to give the predicted probabilities from the fitted logistic regression model as

$$\Pr(\text{case}) = \exp(-2.71 + 0.74 \times \text{GHQ score})/[1 + \exp(-2.71 + 0.74 \times \text{GHQ score})]$$

For an individual with a GHQ score of 10, this model predicts the probability that the individual is judged a case as 0.99.

The estimated odds ratio for this model is $\exp(0.736) = 2.10$ with 95% confidence interval of $[\exp(0.736 - 1.96 \times 0.0946), \exp(0.736 + 1.96 \times 0.0946)] = [1.734, 2.513]$.

The increase in the odds of being judged a case associated with a one-unit increase in GHQ score is estimated to be between about 73% and 150%.

All three tests of the hypothesis that the regression coefficient of GHQ score is zero given in Table 9.2 have very low associated p-values; clearly, GHQ score is a very strong predictor of the probability of being judged a case.

TABLE 9.2

Results from Fitting a Logistic Regression Model Including Only GHQ to the Psychiatric Caseness Data

Testing Global Null Hypothesis: BETA = 0			
Test	Chi-Square	DF	Pr > ChiSq
Likelihood Ratio	114.0691	1	<.0001
Score	117.1843	1	<.0001
Wald	60.5684	1	<.0001

Analysis of Maximum Likelihood Estimates					
Parameter	DF	Estimate	Standard Error	Wald Chi-Square	Pr > ChiSq
Intercept	1	−2.7107	0.2724	98.9940	<.0001
ghq	1	0.7360	0.0946	60.5684	<.0001

Odds Ratio Estimates		
Effect	Point Estimate	95% Wald Confidence Limits
ghq	2.088	1.734 2.513

Now let us consider a logistic regression model that uses only gender as an explanatory variable:

```
proc logistic data=ghq;
  class sex /param=ref ref=first;
  model cases/total=sex;
run;
```

The `class` statement specifies classification variables, or factors, which may be numeric or character variables. The options, following the slash, allow a choice of coding; `param=ref` specifies reference cell coding, which is equivalent to dummy variable coding and `ref=first` specifies that the first category is the reference category. The results are given in Table 9.3. The estimated regression coefficient is −0.037, but before attempting an interpretation, let us have a look at the 2×2 cross classification that results from collapsing the data over the GHQ score:

```
data ghq2;
  set ghq;
  num=cases; case=1; output;
  num=noncases; case=0; output;
run;

proc freq data=ghq2;
  tables sex*case / relrisk nopercent norow nocol;
  weight num;
run;
```

The resulting table of counts is given in Table 9.4 (associated output has been deleted).

The odds ratio for the data in Table 9.4 calculated as shown in Chapter 4 is $(25 \times 131)/(43 \times 79) = 0.9641$. The estimated variance of the log(odds ratio) is

TABLE 9.3

Results from Fitting a Logistic Model Including Only Sex to the Psychiatric Caseness Data

Analysis of Maximum Likelihood Estimates					
Parameter	**DF**	**Estimate**	**Standard Error**	**Wald Chi-Square**	**Pr > ChiSq**
Intercept	1	−1.1139	0.1758	40.1728	<.0001
Sex M	1	−0.0365	0.2890	0.0159	0.8995

Odds Ratio Estimates			
Effect	**Point Estimate**	**95% Wald Confidence Limits**	
Sex M vs F	0.964	0.547	1.699

TABLE 9.4

Table of Counts after Collapsing the
Psychiatric Caseness Data over GHQ Score

Table of Sex by Case			
sex		**Case**	
Frequency	**0**	**1**	**Total**
F	131	43	174
M	79	25	104
Total	210	68	278

again given in Chapter 4 and is $1/43 + 1/131 + 1/25 + 1/29 = 0.0835$, leading to a 95% confidence interval for the population log(odds ratio) of $[\log(0.964) - 1.96 \times \sqrt{0.084}, \log(0.963) + 1.96 \times \sqrt{0.084}]$—that is, $[-0.603, 0.530]$—so the confidence interval for the population odds ratio itself is $[\exp(-0.603), \exp(0.530)]$, giving $[0.547, 1.699]$. When we compare this with the results from the logistic regression with gender as the single explanatory variable shown in Table 9.3, we find that they are identical.

Now let us consider a logistic regression model that uses GHQ score, gender, and their interaction (GHQ × gender) as explanatory variables:

```
ods graphics on;
proc logistic data=ghq plots=effect(showobs=yes);
  class sex /param=ref ref=first;
  model cases/total=sex ghq sex*ghq / selection=b details;
run;
```

ODS graphics has been enabled and a `plots` option added to the proc statement to generate an effect plot for the model that is a plot of the predicted probabilities. By default, individual observed values are not shown, but are requested here with the `showobs=yes` plot option. The plot could also have been generated with an `effectplot` statement.

The model statement now includes `sex`, `ghq` and their interaction. Within `proc logistic`, effects are specified in the same way as for `proc glm`, so the specification of this model could have been abbreviated to `sex|ghq`. This example illustrates some features of automatic model selection in `proc logistic`, via backward elimination in this case. (The criterion used to judge whether or not to eliminate variables is the change in the likelihoods of the two competing models.) Other possibilities are forward, stepwise, and best subsets—specified with `selection= f, s,` and `score`, respectively. The `details` option provides effect estimates for each step of the model selection process.

The output is shown in Table 9.5. At the first step (step 0), all three effects are entered into the model. From the analysis of effects, neither `sex` nor its interaction with `ghq` would appear to be significant. A naive approach to model selection might drop `sex` from the next step, since it is the least significant

TABLE 9.5

Logistic Regression Results Fitted to Psychiatric Caseness Data with Gender, GHQ Score, and Their Interaction in the Model

Model Information	
Data Set	WORK.GHQ
Response Variable (Events)	Cases
Response Variable (Trials)	Total
Model	binary logit
Optimization Technique	Fisher's scoring

Number of Observations Read	22
Number of Observations Used	22
Sum of Frequencies Read	278
Sum of Frequencies Used	278

Response Profile		
Ordered Value	Binary Outcome	Total Frequency
1	Event	68
2	Nonevent	210

Backward Elimination Procedure

Class Level Information		
Class	Value	Design Variables
sex	F	0
	M	1

Step 0. The following effects were entered: Intercept sex ghq ghq*sex.

Model Convergence Status
Convergence criterion (GCONV=1E-8) satisfied.

Model Fit Statistics		
Criterion	Intercept Only	Intercept and Covariates
AIC	311.319	195.780
SC	314.947	210.291
−2 Log L	309.319	187.780

(Continued)

TABLE 9.5 (*Continued*)

Logistic Regression Results Fitted to Psychiatric Caseness Data with Gender, GHQ Score, and Their Interaction in the Model

Testing Global Null Hypothesis: BETA = 0			
Test	Chi-Square	DF	Pr > ChiSq
Likelihood ratio	121.5390	3	<.0001
Score	121.6891	3	<.0001
Wald	63.3620	3	<.0001

Type 3 Analysis of Effects			
Effect	DF	Wald Chi-Square	Pr > ChiSq
sex	1	0.1367	0.7116
ghq	1	36.0029	<.0001
ghq*sex	1	2.3023	0.1292

Analysis of Maximum Likelihood Estimates						
Parameter		DF	Estimate	Standard Error	Wald Chi-Square	Pr > ChiSq
Intercept		1	−2.7732	0.3586	59.7885	<.0001
sex	M	1	−0.2253	0.6093	0.1367	0.7116
ghq		1	0.9412	0.1569	36.0029	<.0001
ghq*sex	M	1	−0.3020	0.1990	2.3023	0.1292

Association of Predicted Probabilities and Observed Responses			
Percent Concordant	86.4	Somers' D	0.779
Percent Discordant	8.6	Gamma	0.820
Percent Tied	5.0	Tau-a	0.289
Pairs	14280	c	0.889

Analysis of Effects Eligible for Removal			
Effect	DF	Wald Chi-Square	Pr > ChiSq
ghq*sex	1	2.3023	0.1292

Step 1. Effect ghq*sex is removed.

Model Convergence Status
Convergence criterion (GCONV=1E-8) satisfied.

TABLE 9.5 (*Continued*)

Logistic Regression Results Fitted to Psychiatric Caseness Data with Gender, GHQ Score, and Their Interaction in the Model

Model Fit Statistics		
Criterion	**Intercept Only**	**Intercept and Covariates**
AIC	311.319	196.126
SC	314.947	207.009
−2 Log L	309.319	190.126

Testing Global Null Hypothesis: BETA = 0			
Test	**Chi-Square**	**DF**	**Pr > ChiSq**
Likelihood Ratio	119.1929	2	<.0001
Score	120.1327	2	<.0001
Wald	61.9555	2	<.0001

Type 3 Analysis of Effects			
Effect	**DF**	**Wald Chi-Square**	**Pr > ChiSq**
sex	1	4.6446	0.0312
ghq	1	61.8891	<.0001

Analysis of Maximum Likelihood Estimates						
Parameter		**DF**	**Estimate**	**Standard Error**	**Wald Chi-Square**	**Pr > ChiSq**
Intercept		1	−2.4935	0.2816	78.3872	<.0001
sex	M	1	−0.9361	0.4343	4.6446	0.0312
ghq		1	0.7791	0.0990	61.8891	<.0001

Odds Ratio Estimates			
Effect	**Point Estimate**	**95% Wald Confidence Limits**	
sex M vs F	0.392	0.167	0.919
ghq	2.180	1.795	2.646

Association of Predicted Probabilities and Observed Responses			
Percent Concordant	85.8	Somers' D	0.766
Percent Discordant	9.2	Gamma	0.806
Percent Tied	5.0	Tau-a	0.284
Pairs	14280	c	0.883

(*Continued*)

TABLE 9.5 (*Continued*)

Logistic Regression Results Fitted to Psychiatric Caseness Data with Gender, GHQ Score, and Their Interaction in the Model

Residual Chi-Square Test		
Chi-Square	DF	Pr > ChiSq
2.3930	1	0.1219

Analysis of Effects Eligible for Removal			
Effect	DF	Wald Chi-Square	Pr > ChiSq
sex	1	4.6446	0.0312
ghq	1	61.8891	<.0001
Note: No (additional) effects met the 0.05 significance level for removal from the model.			

Summary of Backward Elimination					
Step	Effect Removed	DF	Number In	Wald Chi-Square	Pr > ChiSq
1	ghq*sex	1	2	2.3023	0.1292

effect. However, by default, proc logistic preserves the hierarchy of effects whereby main effects must be included in a model if the interaction between them is included. More generally, higher-order effects will only be retained (or entered) if the lower-order effects which they contain are also present in the model. Hence, in this example, the sex*ghq interaction term is removed from the model in the second step. Fitting the reduced model yields significant main effects for both sex and ghq and the model selection ends there.

The final model is shown graphically in Figure 9.3.

In the model that includes gender and GHQ score, we see that for a given gender the confidence interval of the odds ratio for an increase of one in GHQ score is almost the same as in the model containing only GHQ score. For a given GHQ score, the estimated 95% confidence interval odds ratio for caseness, men against women, is [0.167,0.919]. In the model fitted previously containing only gender, we found that the corresponding confidence interval contained the value one. We might ask, 'Why the difference?' The reason is that the overall odds ratio is dominated by the large number of cases for the lower GHQ scores.

9.3.2 Birth Weight of Babies

For our second example of the application of logistic regression, we will use part of the data set given in Hosmer and Lemeshow (2000) collected during a study to identify risk factors associated with giving birth to a low birth weight baby, defined as weighing less than 2500 g. The risk factors considered

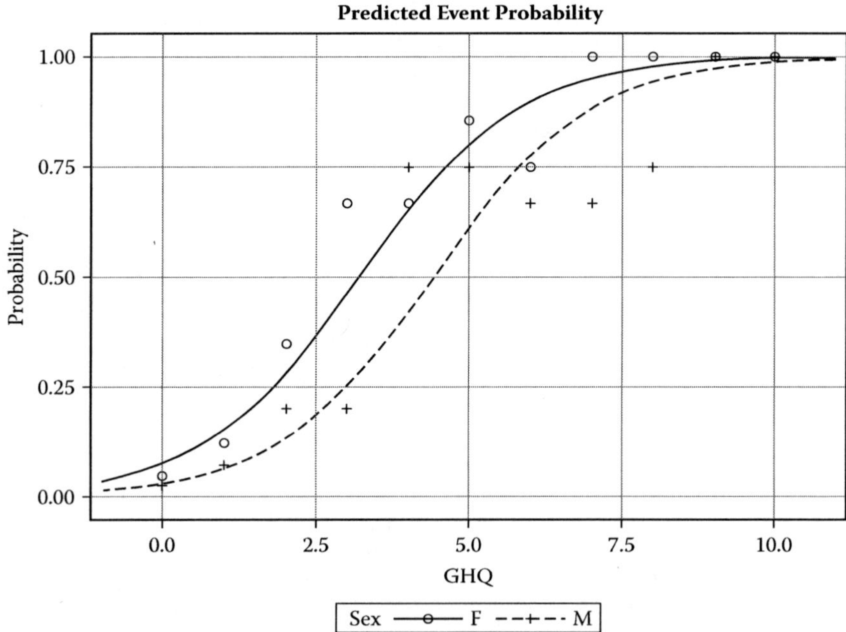

FIGURE 9.3
Plot of predicted probability of caseness from logistic regression model with gender and GHQ score as explanatory variables and observed probabilities labelled by gender.

were age of the mother, weight of the mother at her last menstrual period, race of the mother, and number of physician visits during the first trimester of the pregnancy. Part of the data used is shown in Table 9.6.

The SAS code reading in the data and then fitting the logistic regression model is

```
data lobwgt;
  input id low age lwt race ftv;
cards;
        85    0    19    182    2    0
        86    0    33    155    3    3

. . . .

        82    1    23    94     3    0
        83    1    17    142    2    0
        84    1    21    130    1    3
;

proc logistic data=lobwgt desc;
  class race / param=ref ref=first;
  model low= age lwt race ftv;
run;
```

TABLE 9.6

Data on Infant Low Birth Weight

ID	LOW	AGE	LWT	RACE	FTV
85	0	19	182	2	0
86	0	33	155	3	3
87	0	20	105	1	1
...					
224	0	19	120	1	0
225	0	24	116	1	1
226	0	45	123	1	1
4	1	28	120	3	0
10	1	29	130	1	2
11	1	34	187	2	0
...					
82	1	23	94	3	0
83	1	17	142	2	0
84	1	21	130	1	3

Source:　Hosmer, D. W. and Lemeshow, S. 2002. *Applied Logistic Regression,* 2nd ed. New York: Wiley.

Note:　LOW: 0 = weight of baby > 2500 g; 1 = weight of baby ≤ 2500 g. AGE: age of mother in years. LWT: weight of mother at last menstrual period. RACE: 1 = white; 2 = black; 3 = other. FTV: number of physician visits in the first trimester.

Where a binary response variable is used on the model statement, as opposed to the events/trials used for the GHQ data, SAS models the lower of the two response categories as the 'event'. However, it is common practice for a binary response variable to be coded 0,1, with 1 indicating a response, or event, and 0 indicating no response, or a nonevent. In this case, the seemingly perverse default in SAS will be to model the probability of a nonevent. The `desc` (`descending`) option on the `proc` statement reverses this behaviour.

The specification of explanatory effects on the `model` statement is the same as for `proc glm`, with main effects specified by variable names and interactions by joining variable names with asterisks. The bar operator may also be used as an abbreviated way of entering interactions if these are to be included in the model. The `class` statement specifies reference (dummy variable) coding for `race` with the first category as the reference category. The results are shown in Table 9.7.

Examining first the three tests that all the regression coefficients in the model are zero, we see that both the likelihood ratio and score tests have associated p-values less than 0.05, but that for Wald's test is a little greater than 0.05. Perhaps the most sensible conclusion to draw is that there is *some* evidence that at least one of the regression coefficients differs from zero, but that this evidence is not particularly strong. Looking now at the regression coefficients associated with each of the *five* explanatory variables (remember that race has been recoded

TABLE 9.7

Results from Fitting Logistic Regression Model to Birth Weight Data

Model Information	
Data Set	WORK.LOBWGT
Response Variable	Low
Number of Response Levels	2
Model	binary logit
Optimization Technique	Fisher's scoring

Number of Observations Read	189
Number of Observations Used	189

Response Profile		
Ordered Value	low	Total Frequency
1	1	59
2	0	130

Probability modelled is low = 1.

Class Level Information			
Class	Value	Design Variables	
race	1	0	0
	2	1	0
	3	0	1

Model Convergence Status
Convergence criterion (GCONV=1E-8) satisfied.

Model Fit Statistics		
Criterion	Intercept Only	Intercept and Covariates
AIC	236.672	234.573
SC	239.914	254.023
−2 Log L	234.672	222.573

Testing Global Null Hypothesis: BETA = 0			
Test	Chi-Square	DF	Pr > ChiSq
Likelihood Ratio	12.0991	5	0.0335
Score	11.3876	5	0.0442
Wald	10.6964	5	0.0577

(Continued)

 Applied Medical Statistics Using SAS

TABLE 9.7 (*Continued*)

Results from Fitting Logistic Regression Model to Birth Weight Data

Type 3 Analysis of Effects			
Effect	**DF**	**Wald Chi-Square**	**Pr > ChiSq**
age	1	0.4988	0.4800
lwt	1	4.7428	0.0294
race	2	4.4108	0.1102
ftv	1	0.0869	0.7681

Analysis of Maximum Likelihood Estimates					
Parameter	**DF**	**Estimate**	**Standard Error**	**Wald Chi-Square**	**Pr > ChiSq**
intercept		1	1.2953	1.0714	1.4616	0.2267
age		1	−0.0238	0.0337	0.4988	0.4800
lwt		1	−0.0142	0.00654	4.7428	0.0294
race	2	1	1.0039	0.4979	4.0660	0.0438
race	3	1	0.4331	0.3622	1.4296	0.2318
ftv		1	−0.0493	0.1672	0.0869	0.7681

Odds Ratio Estimates			
Effect	**Point Estimate**	**95% Wald Confidence Limits**	
age	0.976	0.914	1.043
lwt	0.986	0.973	0.999
race 2 vs 1	2.729	1.029	7.240
race 3 vs 1	1.542	0.758	3.136
ftv	0.952	0.686	1.321

Association of Predicted Probabilities and Observed Responses			
Percent Concordant	65.1	Somers' D	0.308
Percent Discordant	34.3	Gamma	0.310
Percent Tied	0.6	Tau-a	0.133
Pairs	7670	c	0.654

in terms of two dummy variables) suggests that weight of mother at her last menstrual period (lwt) and the first of the dummy variables for race may be the most important predictors of low infant birth weight. For lwt the estimated odds ratio is 0.986 with 95% confidence interval [0.973,0.999]; the interval just excludes the value one at its upper end. Thus, we can conclude that the odds of having a low birth weight baby for mothers with weight (lwt + 1) pounds is between about 97.3% and 99.9% of the odds for mothers with weight lwt pounds, conditional on the other variables being unchanged.

Interpretation in terms of a 1-pound weight difference may not be particularly helpful here and it is relatively simple to find the results corresponding to a more meaningful weight difference. Suppose, for example, we want to look at a 10-pound difference. The estimated regression coefficient for such a difference is simply 10 times the original regression coefficient—that is, 10 × (−0.0142), a value of −0.142. The associated standard error of this value is 10 × 0.00654, giving 0.0654. This leads to an estimated value of exp(−0.142) for the odds ratio and a 95% confidence interval for the odds ratio of [exp(−0.142 + 1.96 × 0.0654), exp(−0.142 − 1.96 × 0.0654)]. Therefore, for a 10-pound weight difference, the odds of the heavier mothers giving birth to a low-birth-weight baby are between 76% and 99%; the odds of the lighter mothers are again conditional on the other variables.

For race, the significant dummy variable is that coding the difference between white and black mothers. For the latter, the odds of a low birth weight child are estimated to be 2.729 times the corresponding odds for the former, conditional on the other covariates. But this apparently large effect needs to be considered in terms of the associated 95% confidence interval of [1.029,7.240], which is very wide, with the lower limit being only a little above one.

We can apply backward elimination in an effort to select a more parsimonious model with the following SAS code:

```
proc logistic data=lowbwt desc;
  class race / param=ref ref=first;
  model low=age lwt race ftv / selection=b;
run;
```

The results are shown in Table 9.8. The three explanatory variables, ftv, age, and race, are all eliminated, leaving only lwt. The 95% confidence

TABLE 9.8

Results from Backward Elimination Logistic Regression on the Data on Low Birth Weight

Summary of Backward Elimination					
Step	**Effect Removed**	**DF**	**Number In**	**Wald Chi-Square**	**Pr > ChiSq**
1	Ftv	1	3	0.0869	0.7681
2	Age	1	2	0.5892	0.4427
3	Race	2	1	5.4024	0.0671

Analysis of Maximum Likelihood Estimates					
Parameter	**DF**	**Estimate**	**Standard Error**	**Wald Chi-Square**	**Pr > ChiSq**
Intercept	1	0.9983	0.7853	1.6161	0.2036
lwt	1	−0.0141	0.00617	5.1921	0.0227

Odds Ratio Estimates		
Effect	**Point Estimate**	**95% Wald Confidence Limits**
lwt	0.986	0.974 0.998

interval for lwt is very similar to that when a model with all four explanatory variables is fitted (see Table 9.7).

9.4 Diagnosing a Logistic Regression Model

As with the multiple regression model considered in the previous chapter, fitting a logistic regression model is not complete without checking on model assumptions by examining the properties of some suitably defined 'residuals' or other diagnostics. There are a number of ways in which a fitted logistic model may be inadequate:

- The linear function of the explanatory variables may be inadequate; for example, one or more of the explanatory variables may need to be transformed.
- The logistic transformation of the response probability may not be entirely appropriate—for example, the complementary log–log transformation (see Collett 2003a).
- The data may contain outliers that are not well fitted by the model, or observations with undue impact on the conclusions drawn from the analysis (i.e., influential values).
- The assumption of a binomial distribution may not be correct. For example, with grouped data, the observations y_i can only be assumed to have a binomial distribution when the n_i individual observations on which they are based are independent.

An extremely comprehensive account of residuals and other diagnostics appropriate for checking each of those assumptions is given in Collett (2003a). Here we will describe only the basic residuals and their use. The raw residual for the types of observations modelled by logistic regression is simply $y_i - \hat{y}_i$, where $\hat{y}_i = n_i \pi_i$. But for reasons discussed in Collett, these raw residuals are difficult to interpret. Consequently, the following residuals are more often used:

(1) Pearson residuals:

$$d_i = \frac{y_i - n_i \hat{\pi}_i}{\sqrt{n_i \hat{\pi}_i \left(1 - \hat{\pi}_i\right)}} \tag{9.7}$$

(2) Deviance residuals:

$$d_i = \text{sign}\left(y_i - \hat{y}_i\right)\left[2y_i \log\left(\frac{y_i}{\hat{y}_i}\right) + 2\left(n - y_i\right)\log\left(\frac{n - y_i}{n - \hat{y}_i}\right)\right]^{\frac{1}{2}} \tag{9.8}$$

where sign $(y_i - \hat{y}_i)$ is the function that makes d_i positive when $y_i \geq \hat{y}_i$ and negative when $y_i < \hat{y}_i$. There are various ways of plotting the residuals that give different insights into the possible model inadequacies. Three possibilities are

- An index plot is a plot of residuals against observation number. It is often useful for detecting outliers.

- In a plot of residuals against the linear predictor, the occurrence of a systematic pattern in the plot suggests that the model is incorrect in some way.

- A plot of residuals against explanatory variables may help to identify whether a variable needs to be transformed.

We will illustrate the use of some of the diagnostic plots just described on the logistic regression model arrived at by backward elimination for the birth weight data; the only explanatory variable in this model is lwt. The following code gives plots of deviance residuals plotted against the observation number, the fitted probabilities and the single explanatory variable lwt:

```
proc logistic data=lowbwt desc;
  class race / param=ref ref=first;
  model low=lwt;
  output out=lout p=pred resdev=dres;
run;

proc sgscatter data=lout;
  plot dres*(id pred lwt);
run;
```

The output statement saves the predicted probabilities and deviance residuals in the lout data set. The deviance residuals are then plotted against the predicted probabilities and the three continuous predictors. All the plots are shown in Figure 9.4. The plots of deviance residuals against the linear predictor and each of three of the explanatory variables show no obvious patterns that might suggest the need for, say, a quadratic term in any of the variables to be considered, and there are no obvious outliers in the index plot of the residuals. (The distinct separation of points in these plots is entirely due to the binary nature of the data and does not necessarily reflect any problems with the fitted model, although it does make interpretation more difficult.)

9.5 Logistic Regression for 1:1 Matched Studies

As mentioned in Chapter 4, a frequently used design in medical studies is the matched case-control study in which each patient suffering from a particular

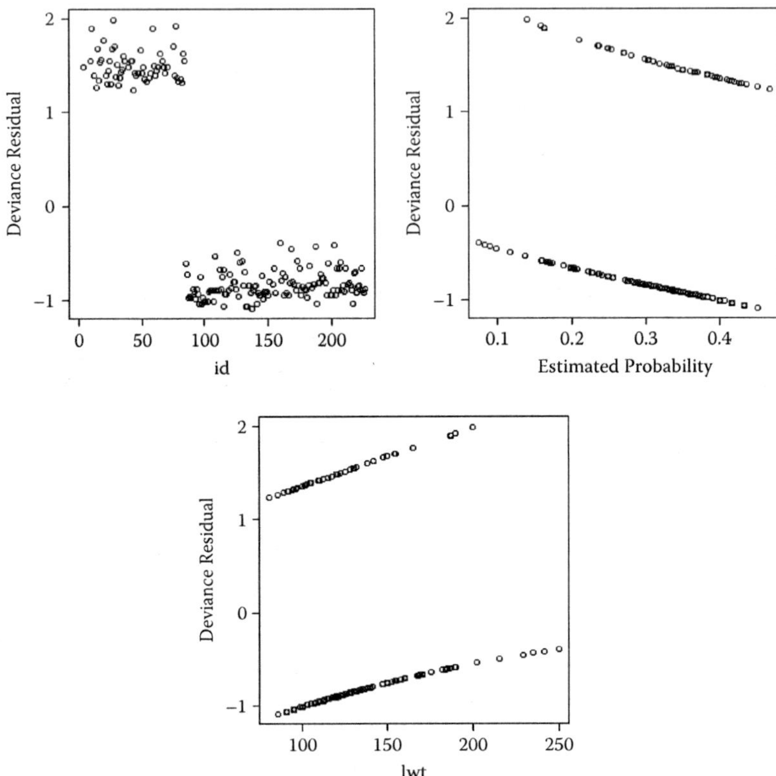

FIGURE 9.4
Diagnostic plots for the logistic regression model fitted to low birth weight data.

condition of interest included in the study is matched to one or more people without the condition. The most commonly used matching variables are age, ethnic group, mental status, etc. A design with m controls per case is known as a 1:m matched study. In many cases, m will be one, and it is the 1:1 matched study that we shall concentrate on here.

Table 9.9 shows the results from a 1:1 matched case-control study. In this study, cases of endometrial cancer were matched on age, race, date of admission, and hospital of admission to a suitable control not suffering from cancer, and past exposure to conjugated estrogens of both case and control was determined.

The form of the logistic model used for these data involves the probability, ϕ, that in matched pair i, for a given value of the explanatory variable x past exposure to conjugated estrogens (yes or no), the member of the pair is a case. Specifically, the model is

$$\log \mathrm{it}(\phi) = \alpha_i + \beta x \tag{9.9}$$

TABLE 9.9

1:1 Matched Case-Control Study

| | Controls | | |
Cases	1	0	Total
1	12	43	55
0	7	121	128
Total	19	164	183

Notes: 1 = exposed; 0 = not exposed.

The odds that a subject with past exposure ($x = 1$) is a cancer case equal $\exp(\beta)$ times the odds that a subject without past exposure ($x = 0$) is a cancer case.

The model generalises to the situation where there are p explanatory variables as

$$\log \mathrm{it}(\phi) = \alpha_i + \beta_1 + x_1 + \cdots \beta_p x_p \tag{9.10}$$

Typically, one x_i is an explanatory variable of real interest, such as past exposure in the preceding example, with the others being used as a form of statistical control in addition to the variables already controlled by virtue of using them to form matched pairs.

The problem with the preceding model is that the number of parameters increases at the same rate as the sample size, with the consequence that maximum likelihood estimation is no longer viable. We can overcome this problem if we regard the parameters α_i as of little interest and thus are willing to forgo their estimation. If we do, we can then create a *conditional likelihood function* that will yield maximum likelihood estimators of the coefficients $\beta_1 \ldots \beta_p$ that are consistent and asymptotically normally distributed. The mathematics behind this are described in Collett (2003a), who shows that this conditional logistic regression model can be applied using standard logistic regression software as follows:

- Set the sample size to the number of matched pairs.
- Use as the explanatory variables the differences between corresponding covariate values for each case and control.
- Set the value of the response variable to one for all observations.
- Exclude the constant term from the model.

To illustrate this approach, we shall apply it to the cancer data in Table 9.8. Exposure to the risk factor, conjugated estrogens, is coded as one and nonexposure by zero. We will first need to set all observed response values to one. Then, corresponding to seven of these observations, the single explanatory variable will take the value –1 (case-control difference in the binary variable denoting exposure); for 43, it will take the value +1; and for (12 + 121), it will take the value 0. The necessary SAS code is

```
data endocal;
   input est num;
   resp=1;
cards;
-1  7
 1 43
 0 133
;

proc logistic data=endocal;
   model resp=est /noint;
   freq num;
run;
```

The `noint` option excludes the intercept term from the model, a feature that is needed for a conditional logistic regression, and the `freq` statement identifies the number of individuals that each observation represents. The results are shown in Table 9.10. The odds that, in a matched pair, past exposure to conjugated estrogens has been suffered by the case are estimated to be between 2.8 and 13.7 times the odds that the control has been exposed. Since there is only one response level, measures of association between the observed and predicted values were not calculated.

The same results can be found directly from Table 9.9 using the information about the estimation of odd ratios for a matched case-control study given in Chapter 4. From this table, the odds ratio is estimated as $43/7 = 6.143$. The variance of ln(odds) is found from $1/7 + 1/43 = 0.166$. Therefore, a 95% confidence interval for the ln(odds ratio) is $[\ln(6.143) - 1.96 \times \sqrt{0.166}, \ln(6.143) + 1.96 \times \sqrt{0.166}]$—that is, $[1.016, 2.614]$, leading to the confidence interval for the odds ratio of $[\exp(1.016), \exp(2.614)]$—that is, $[2.8, 13.7]$.

Now let us look at a more complicated example, again involving the birth weight of babies but now in the context of a matched example. The data arise from looking first at 59 babies who were low weight. The matched data were obtained by randomly selecting, for each woman who gave birth to a low birth weight baby, a mother of the same age who did not give birth to a low birth weight baby. Three of the low birth weight mothers were too young to find a match, so the data consist of 56 matched case-control pairs. The complete data are given in Hosmer and Lemeshow (2000) and data for the first five matched pairs are given here in Table 9.11. Variables selected for investigation were prior preterm delivery (ptd; 1 = yes, 0 = no), smoking status of the mother during pregnancy (smoke; 1 = yes, 0 = no), history of hypertension (ht; 1 = yes, 0 = no), presence of uterine irritability (ui; 1 = yes, 0 = no), and the weight of the mother at the last menstrual period (lwt; pounds).

TABLE 9.10

Results from Fitting a Conditional Logistic Regression Model to the Data in Table 9.9

Model Information	
Data Set	WORK.ENDOCA1
Response Variable	resp
Number of Response Levels	1
Frequency Variable	num
Model	binary logit
Optimisation Technique	Fisher's scoring

Number of Observations Read	3
Number of Observations Used	3
Sum of Frequencies Read	183
Sum of Frequencies Used	183

Response Profile		
Ordered Value	resp	Total Frequency
1	1	183

Probability modelled is resp = 1.

Model Convergence Status
Convergence criterion (GCONV=1E-8) satisfied.

Model Fit Statistics		
Criterion	Without Covariates	With Covariates
AIC	253.692	226.873
SC	253.692	230.083
−2 Log L	253.692	224.873

Testing Global Null Hypothesis: BETA = 0			
Test	Chi-Square	DF	Pr > ChiSq
Likelihood Ratio	28.8184	1	<.0001
Score	25.9200	1	<.0001
Wald	19.8376	1	<.0001

(*Continued*)

TABLE 9.10 (*Continued*)

Results from Fitting a Conditional Logistic Regression Model to the
Data in Table 9.9

Analysis of Maximum Likelihood Estimates					
Parameter	DF	Estimate	Standard Error	Wald Chi-Square	Pr > ChiSq
est	1	1.8153	0.4076	19.8376	<.0001

Odds Ratio Estimates			
Effect	Point Estimate	95% Wald Confidence Limits	
est	6.143	2.763	13.655

TABLE 9.11

Part of the Data from the Matched Case-Control Study of
Babies' Birth Weight

Pair	LoW	Age	LWT	Smoke	PTD	HT	UI
1	0	14	135	0	0	0	0
1	1	14	101	1	1	0	0
2	0	15	98	0	0	0	0
2	1	15	115	0	0	0	1
3	0	16	95	0	0	0	0
3	1	16	130	0	0	0	0
4	0	17	103	0	0	0	0
4	1	17	130	1	1	0	1
5	0	17	122	1	0	0	0
5	1	17	110	1	0	0	0

Notes: LOW: low birth weight; AGE: age of mother; LWT: weight
of mother at last menstrual period; SMOKE: smoking status
during pregnancy; PTD: history of premature labour; HT:
history of hypertension; UI: presence of uterine irritability.

The necessary SAS code to fit the logistic model is

```
data lowbwt11;
  infile 'c:\amsus2\data\lowbwt11.dat';
  input pair LoW Age LWT Smoke PTD HT UI;
run;

proc logistic data=lowbwt11 desc;
  strata pair;
  model low=LWT Smoke PTD HT UI;
run;
```

The `strata` statement is used to specify the variable that identifies the pair to which each observation belongs. Apart from restructuring the data, this is the only change that is needed to perform a conditional analysis of matched pairs. The results are shown in Table 9.12.

The odds ratios in Table 9.12 indicate that smoking during pregnancy, prior preterm deliveries, and presence of hypertension are important risk factors for delivering of a low birth weight baby. The confidence interval estimates in Table 9.10 are very wide for the dichotomous explanatory variables, which is the result of having only relatively few discordant pairs. Hosmer and Lemeshow (2005) point out that the gain in precision obtained from matching and using conditional logistic regression may be offset by a loss owing to a few discordant pairs for dichotomous covariates.

9.6 Propensity Scores

Traditional matching of cases and controls in an observational study is often limited because only a relatively small number of matching factors (or covariates) can be accommodated; consequently, differences that may exist on other covariates not used for matching could lead to biased estimates. One approach to overcoming this potential problem is the use of *propensity scores* where the propensity score of an individual is defined as the conditional probability of being a case, given the individual's values on a (possibly large) number of covariates. In this way, the propensity score provides a scalar summary of *all* the available covariate information and, if we can match cases to controls with similar propensity scores, we can behave as if the subjects had been randomly assigned to the two groups. Alternatively, we use regression to adjust for propensity score. When there are no missing values amongst the set of observed covariates, the required propensity scores can be estimated from logistic regression.

An example of where propensity scores have been used is described in Ye and Kaskutas (2009); in this study, a prospective cohort design was used to investigate the effect of Alcoholics Anonymous (AA) meeting attendance on alcohol abstinence. The relationship between the 'treatment' AA attendance and the outcome abstinence in such an observational study is potentially subject to confounding, in that there may be a number of observable pre-treatment variables—for example, alcohol problem severity, self-motivation, and coercion by others—that affect study participants' decisions to go to AA meetings and independently contribute to their becoming abstinent. Propensity scores were used to adjust the AA effect estimate for selection bias due to observed confounders.

TABLE 9.12

Conditional Logistic Regression Results for the Paired Low Birth Weight Data

Conditional Analysis	
Model Information	
Data Set	WORK.LOWBWT11
Response Variable	LoW
Number of Response Levels	2
Number of Strata	56
Model	binary logit
Optimization Technique	Newton–Raphson ridge

Number of Observations Read	112
Number of Observations Used	112

Response Profile		
Ordered Value	**LoW**	**Total Frequency**
1	0	56
2	1	56
Probability modelled is LoW = 1.		

Strata Summary				
Response Pattern	**LoW** **0**	**1**	**Number of Strata**	**Frequency**
1	1	1	56	112

Newton–Raphson Ridge Optimisation without Parameter Scaling
Convergence criterion (GCONV=1E-8) satisfied.

Model Fit Statistics		
Criterion	**Without Covariates**	**With Covariates**
AIC	77.632	62.474
SC	77.632	76.066
–2 Log L	77.632	52.474

TABLE 9.12 (*Continued*)

Conditional Logistic Regression Results for the Paired
Low Birth Weight Data

Testing Global Null Hypothesis: BETA = 0			
Test	Chi-Square	DF	Pr > ChiSq
Likelihood Ratio	25.1587	5	0.0001
Score	19.7845	5	0.0014
Wald	12.5938	5	0.0275

Analysis of Maximum Likelihood Estimates					
Parameter	DF	Estimate	Standard Error	Wald Chi-Square	Pr > ChiSq
LWT	1	−0.0151	0.00815	3.4281	0.0641
Smoke	1	1.4796	0.5620	6.9305	0.0085
PTD	1	1.6706	0.7468	5.0041	0.0253
HT	1	2.3294	1.0025	5.3984	0.0202
UI	1	1.3449	0.6938	3.7571	0.0526

Odds Ratio Estimates		
Effect	Point Estimate	95% Wald Confidence Limits
LWT	0.985	0.969 1.001
Smoke	4.391	1.459 13.212
PTD	5.315	1.230 22.973
HT	10.271	1.440 73.283
UI	3.838	0.985 14.951

9.7 Summary

The logistic regression model can be used to assess the effects of explanatory variables on a binary response variable. The estimated parameters can
be interpreted in terms of odds and odds ratios. The model can also be used
for the analysis of matched case-control data. As we shall see in the next
chapter, the logistic regression mode—along with multiple linear regression,
analysis of variance, and analysis of covariance—is a member of the family
of *generalised linear models*.

10

Generalised Linear Model

10.1 Introduction

The term 'generalised linear model' (GLM) was first introduced in a landmark paper by Nelder and Wedderburn (1972) in which a wide range of seemingly disparate problems of statistical modelling and inference were set in an elegant unifying framework of great power and flexibility. Generalised linear models include all the modelling techniques described in earlier chapters—that is, analysis of variance, analysis of covariance, multiple linear regression, and logistic regression—and open up the possibility of other models (e.g., *Poisson regression*) that we shall describe in this chapter. A comprehensive account of GLMs is given in McCullagh and Nelder (1989) and a more concise and less technical description in Dobson and Barnett (2008). In the next section, we review the main features of such models.

10.2 Generalised Linear Models

The multiple linear regression model described in Chapter 8 has the following form:

$$y = \beta_0 + \beta_1 x_1 \ldots + \beta_p x_p + \varepsilon \tag{10.1}$$

The error term, ε, is assumed to have a normal distribution with zero mean and variance σ^2. An equivalent way of writing the model is as $y \sim N(\mu,\sigma^2)$, where $\mu = \beta_0 + \beta_1 x_1 + \ldots + \beta_p x_p$. This makes it clear that this model is only suitable for continuous response variables with—conditional on the values of the explanatory variables—a normal distribution with constant variance. The generalisation of such a model made in GLMs consists of allowing each of the following three assumptions associated with the multiple linear regression model to be modified:

- The response variable is normally distributed with a mean determined by the model.
- The mean can be modelled as a linear function of (possibly nonlinear transformations) the explanatory variables (i.e., the effects of the explanatory variables on the mean are additive).
- The variance of the response variable, given the (predicted) mean, is constant.

In a GLM some *transformation* of the mean is modelled by a linear function of the explanatory variables, and the distribution of the response variable around its mean (often referred to as the *error distribution*) is usually generalised in a way that fits naturally with a particular transformation. The result is a very wide class of regression models that includes many other models as special cases, including analysis of variance, multiple linear regression, and logistic regression. The three essential components of a GLM are the following:

(a) A linear predictor, η, formed from the explanatory variables:

$$\eta = \beta_0 + \beta_1 x_1 + \beta_2 x_2 \ldots + \beta_p x_p = \boldsymbol{\beta}'\mathbf{x} \tag{10.2}$$

(b) A transformation of the mean, μ, of the response variable called the *link function*, $g(\mu)$. In a GLM, it is $g(\mu)$ that is modelled by the linear predictor

$$g(\mu) = \eta \tag{10.3}$$

In multiple linear regression and analysis of variance, the link function is the identity function. Other link functions that are used include the log, logit, probit, inverse, and power transformations, although the log and logit are most commonly met in practice. The logit link, for example, is the basis of logistic regression.

(c) The distribution of the response variable, given its mean μ, is assumed to be a distribution from the *exponential family;* this has the form of

$$f(y;\theta,\phi) = \exp\{(y\theta - b(\theta))/a(\phi) + c(y,\phi)\} \tag{10.4}$$

for some specific functions a, b, and c and parameters θ and ϕ. For example, in linear regression, a normal distribution is assumed with mean μ and constant variance σ^2. This can be expressed via the exponential family as follows:

$$f(y;\theta,\phi) = \frac{1}{\sqrt{(2\pi\sigma^2)}} \exp\left\{-(y-\mu)^2 / 2\sigma^2\right\}$$

$$= \exp\left\{(y\mu - \mu^2/2)/\sigma^2 - \frac{1}{2}(y^2/\sigma^2 + \log(2\pi\sigma^2))\right\}$$

(10.5)

so that $\theta = \mu, b(\theta) = \theta^2/2$, $\phi = \sigma^2$ and $a(\phi) = \phi$.

Other distributions in the exponential family include the binomial, Poisson, gamma, inverse Gaussian, and exponential distributions. Particular link functions in GLMs are generally associated with particular error distributions— for example, the identity link with the Gaussian distribution, the logit with the binomial, and the log with the Poisson. The choice of probability distribution determines the relationships between the variance of the response variable (conditional on the explanatory variables) and its mean. This relationship is known as the *variance function*, denoted $V(\mu)$. For the Gaussian distribution, $V(\mu) = \sigma^2$; here, the variance is not a function of the mean and thus can be estimated freely. For the Poisson distribution, however, the variance equals the mean, $V(\mu) = \mu$, so that the variance is constrained and cannot be estimated freely. More will be said about the variance function later in the chapter.

The parameters in GLMs are estimated by maximising the joint likelihood of the observed responses given the parameters of the model and the explanatory variables. This generally requires iterative numerical algorithms; see McCullagh and Nelder (1989) for details.

10.3 Applying the Generalised Linear Model

Multiple linear regression (and analysis of variance and analysis of covariance, which, as mentioned in Chapter 6, are essentially equivalent to multiple regression) can be applied via the GLM approach using an identity link function and a normal error distribution. Logistic regression is applied in the GLM framework by using a logit link function and specifying binomial errors. `Proc genmod` is the main SAS procedure for fitting generalised linear models. Its syntax is broadly similar to that of `proc glm`, with the additional options needed to generalise the linear model. The distribution and the link function are specified on the `model` statement. If the canonical link function is to be used, it is only necessary to specify the distribution. For example, the multiple linear regression of the physical measurements data described in Chapter 8 could be applied using `proc genmod` as follows:

```
proc genmod data=PhysicalMeasures;
  model mass=fore waist height thigh / dist=normal link=id;
run;
```

The results will be the same as those given in Chapter 8. And the logistic regression model for low birth weight babies described in Chapter 9 would be applied with proc genmod as

```
proc genmod data=lowbwt desc;
   class race ;
   model low=race age lwt ftv / dist=b link=logit;
run;
```

In the following two subsections we will look at using GLMs with some less commonly applied link functions and error distributions than those used in the preceding examples. We begin with an account of *Poisson regression*.

10.3.1 Poisson Regression

The Poisson regression model is useful for a response variable, y, that is a count or frequency and for which it is reasonable to assume an underlying Poisson distribution—that is,

$$\Pr(y) = \frac{\mu^y e^{-\mu}}{y!} \quad y = 0, 1, 2 \ldots \tag{10.6}$$

Our first example of the use of Poisson regression involves the data shown in Table 10.1, taken from Seeber (1989). The data arise from 31 male patients treated for superficial bladder cancer and give the number of recurrent tumours during a particular time period after removal of the primary tumour, and the size of the primary tumour (whether smaller or larger than 3 cm).

Before coming to the analysis of the data in Table 10.2, we need to introduce the idea of a *Poisson process*, in which the waiting times between successive events of interest (the tumours in this case) are independent and exponentially distributed with common mean, $1/\lambda$ (say). Then the number of events that occurs up to time t has a Poisson distribution with mean $\mu = \lambda t$. Here the parameter of real interest is the rate at which events occur, λ, and for a single explanatory variable, x, we can adopt a Poisson regression approach using the model

$$\log \lambda = \log \frac{\mu}{t} = \beta_0 + \beta_1 x \tag{10.7}$$

to examine the dependence of λ on x. Rearranging this model, we obtain

$$\log \mu = \beta_0 + \beta_1 x + \log t \tag{10.8}$$

In this form, the model can be fitted within the GLM framework. In this model, $\log t$ is a variable in the model whose regression coefficient is fixed at unity and is usually known as an *offset*.

TABLE 10.1

Bladder Cancer Data

Time	x	n
2	0	1
3	0	1
6	0	1
8	0	1
9	0	1
10	0	1
11	0	1
13	0	1
14	0	1
16	0	1
21	0	1
22	0	1
24	0	1
26	0	1
27	0	1
7	0	2
13	0	2
15	0	2
18	0	2
23	0	2
20	0	3
24	0	4
1	1	1
5	1	1
17	1	1
18	1	1
25	1	1
18	1	2
25	1	2
4	1	3
19	1	4

Source: Seeber, G. U. H. 1989. *Statistics in Medicine* 8:1363–1369. With permission of the publishers, John Wiley & Sons Ltd.

Notes: $x = 0$ tumour < 3 cm; $x = 1$ tumour ≥ 3 cm.

TABLE 10.2

Results from Fitting a Poisson Regression Model to the Data in Table 10.1

Model Information	
Data Set	WORK.BLADDER
Distribution	Poisson
Link Function	Log
Dependent Variable	n
Offset Variable	logtime

Number of Observations Read	31
Number of Observations Used	31

Criteria for Assessing Goodness of Fit			
Criterion	DF	Value	Value/DF
Deviance	29	25.4189	0.8765
Scaled Deviance	29	25.4189	0.8765
Pearson Chi-Square	29	38.5938	1.3308
Scaled Pearson $X2$	29	38.5938	1.3308
Log Likelihood		−33.3234	
Full Log Likelihood		−48.1150	
AIC (smaller is better)		100.2301	
AICC (smaller is better)		100.6586	
BIC (smaller is better)		103.0980	

Algorithm converged.

Analysis of Maximum Likelihood Parameter Estimates							
Parameter	DF	Estimate	Standard Error	Wald 95% Confidence Limits		Wald Chi-Square	Pr > ChiSq
Intercept	1	−2.3394	0.1768	−2.6859	−1.9929	175.13	<.0001
x	1	0.2292	0.3062	−0.3709	0.8293	0.56	0.4541
Scale	0	1.0000	0.0000	1.0000	1.0000		

Note: The scale parameter was held fixed.

To read in the data and apply the Poisson regression model here requires the following SAS code:

```
data bladder;
   input time x n;
   logtime=log(time);
cards;
2      0      1
3      0      1
. . .
25     1      2
4      1      3
19     1      4
;

proc genmod data=bladder;
   model n=x/offset=logtime dist=p;
run;
```

The data step reads in the data and calculates the log of the waiting time to be used as the offset in the analysis. The offset is specified on the `model` statement. The results are shown in Table 10.2.

The estimated model is

$$\log \lambda = -2.339 + 0.229x \tag{10.9}$$

Therefore, for smaller tumours ($x = 0$), the estimated (baseline) rate is exp(–2.339) = 0.096; for larger tumours ($x = 1$), the estimated rate is exp(–2.339 + 0.229) = 0.12. The rate for larger tumours is estimated as 0.12/0.096 = 1.25 times the rate for smaller tumours. In terms of waiting times between recurrences, the means are 1/0.096 = 10.42 months for smaller tumours and 1/0.12 = 8.33 months for larger tumours. But the regression coefficient for the dummy variable coding tumour size is seen from Table 10.2 to be nonsignificant, so the data give no evidence that rates or waiting times for large and small tumours are different. This becomes apparent if we construct a confidence interval for the rate for larger tumours from the confidence limits given in Table 10.2 as [exp(–2.339 – 0.371), exp(–2.339 + 0.829)]—that is, [0.067,0.221]. This interval contains the rate for smaller tumours. There is no evidence that size of primary tumour is associated with number of recurrent tumours.

As a second example of the application of Poisson regression, we shall apply it to the data shown in Table 10.3. These data arise from a prospective study of potential risk factors for coronary heart disease (CHD) (Rosenman et al. 1975). The study looked at 3,154 men aged 40–50 for an average of 8 years and recorded the incidence of cases of CHD. The potential risk factors included smoking, blood pressure, and personality/behaviour type. The data are given in Fitzmaurice, Laird, and Ware (2004) and it is the analysis given in the latter that we follow here.

TABLE 10.3

Data on Incidence of CHD and Associated Risk Factors

Person-Years	Smoking	Blood Pressure	Behaviour	*n* of CHD Cases
5268.2	0	0	0	20
2542.0	10	0	0	16
1140.7	20	0	0	13
614.6	30	0	0	3
4451.1	0	0	1	41
2243.5	10	0	1	24
1153.6	20	0	1	27
925.0	30	0	1	17
1366.8	0	1	0	8
497.0	10	1	0	9
238.1	20	1	0	3
146.3	30	1	0	7
1251.9	0	1	1	29
640.0	10	1	1	21
374.5	20	1	1	7
338.2	30	1	1	12

Notes: Smoking: 0 = nonsmoker; 10 = 1–10 cigarettes a day; 20 = 11–20 cigarettes a day; 30 = 30+ cigarettes a day. Blood pressure: 0 = <140; 1 = ≥140. Behaviour: 0 = type B personality; 1 = type A personality. (Type A is characterised by impatience, competitiveness, aggressiveness, a sense of time urgency, and tenseness. Type B is characterised as easy-going, relaxed about time, not competitive, and not easily angered or agitated.)

Let y_i be the number of cases of CHD and T_i be the person years of follow-up (this is defined as the total duration of observed follow-up, from entry into the study until either disease detection or end of follow-up), where *i* indexes the risk group and takes values 1 to 16. We will begin by looking at a model with a single risk factor—namely, smoking. We shall assume that the values of this variable are quantitative, although this is not strictly the case and an alternative would be to use three dummy variables to code the four categories of smoking. We will use the same model as in the previous example—that is,

$$\log(\mu_i / T_i) = \beta_0 + \beta_1 \text{smoking}_i \tag{10.10}$$

where $\mu_i = E(y_i)$. Remembering that $\log(T_i)$ has to be included as an offset, we can fit this model using the following code:

```
data CHDrisk;
  input pyears smoking BP TypeA Ncases;
  lpyears=log(pyears);
datalines;
5268.2    0    0    0    20
2542.0    10   0    0    16
. . .
```

```
374.5        20     1     1      7
338.2        30     1     1     12
;
```

```
proc genmod data=CHDrisk;
 model ncases=smoking / offset=lpyears dist=p;
run;
```

The results are shown in Table 10.4. The regression coefficient for smoking is highly significant and smoking is clearly an important risk factor for CHD.

Because risk factors for CHD are likely to be correlated (and they clearly are from even a superficial examination of the data in Table 10.3), we next estimate the effect of smoking on CHD rates after adjusting for the potential confounding effects of blood pressure and personality type. The model we need to fit is

$$\log(\mu_i / T_i) = \beta_0 + \beta_1 \text{smoking}_i + \beta_2 \text{BP}_i + \beta_3 \text{Type}_i \qquad (10.11)$$

The required code is

```
proc genmod data=CHDrisk;
   model ncases= smoking BP TypeA/ offset=lpyears dist=p;
run;
```

The results are shown in Table 10.5. Smoking remains a highly significant risk factor even after conditioning on blood pressure and personality type.

As our final example of Poisson regression, we shall apply the method to the data shown in Table 10.6 taken from Piantadosi (1997). The data arise from a study of familial adenomatous polyposis (FAP), an auotsomal dominant genetic defect that predisposes those affected to develop large numbers of polyps in the colon, which, if untreated, may develop into colon cancer. Patients with FAP were randomly assigned to receive an active drug treatment or a placebo. The response variable was the number of colonic polyps at 3 months after starting treatment. Additional covariates of interest were number of polyps before starting treatment, gender, and age.

TABLE 10.4

Results from Fitting a Poisson Regression Model Including Only Smoking to the Data in Table 10.3

Analysis of Maximum Likelihood Parameter Estimates							
Parameter	DF	Estimate	Standard Error	Wald 95% Confidence Limits		Wald Chi-Square	Pr > ChiSq
Intercept	1	–4.7993	0.0885	–4.9728	–4.6258	2939.54	<.0001
smoking	1	0.0318	0.0056	0.0207	0.0428	31.88	<.0001
Scale	0	1.0000	0.0000	1.0000	1.0000		

TABLE 10.5

Results from Fitting a Poisson Regression Model Including Smoking, Blood Pressure, and Personality Type to the Data in Table 10.3

Analysis of Maximum Likelihood Parameter Estimates							
Parameter	DF	Estimate	Standard Error	Wald 95% Confidence Limits		Wald Chi-Square	Pr > ChiSq
Intercept	1	−5.4202	0.1308	−5.6765	−5.1638	1716.79	<.0001
smoking	1	0.0273	0.0056	0.0163	0.0383	23.72	<.0001
BP	1	0.7534	0.1292	0.5001	1.0067	33.98	<.0001
TypeA	1	0.7526	0.1362	0.4856	1.0195	30.53	<.0001
Scale	0	1.0000	0.0000	1.0000	1.0000		

TABLE 10.6

FAP Data

Sex	Treatment	Baseline Count of Polyps	Age	No. of Polyps at 3 Months
0	1	7	17	6
0	0	77	20	67
1	1	7	16	4
0	0	5	18	5
1	1	23	22	16
0	0	35	13	31
0	1	11	23	6
1	0	12	34	20
1	0	7	50	7
1	0	318	19	347
1	1	160	17	142
0	1	8	23	1
1	0	20	22	16
1	0	11	30	20
1	0	24	27	26
1	1	34	23	27
0	0	54	22	45
1	1	16	13	10
1	0	30	34	30
0	1	10	23	6
0	1	20	22	5
1	1	12	42	8

Source: Piatados, S. 1997. *Clinical Trials: A Methodologic Perspective.* New York: Wiley.

Notes: Sex: 0 = female; 1 = male. Treatment: 0 = placebo; 1 = active.

These data can be read in and a Poisson regression model fitted using the following SAS code:

```
data fap;
  input male treat base_n age r_n;
cards;
0        1        7        17        6
0        0        77       20        67
....
0        1        10       23        6
0        1        20       22        5
1        1        12       42        8
;

proc genmod data=fap;
  model r_n=male treat base_n age/dist=p;
run;
```

The results are shown in Table 10.7. The regression coefficients become easier to interpret if they (and the confidence limits) are exponentiated.

TABLE 10.7

Results of Fitting a Poisson Regression Model to the FAP Data in Table 10.6

Model Information	
Data Set	WORK.FAP
Distribution	Poisson
Link Function	Log
Dependent Variable	r_n

Number of Observations Read	22
Number of Observations Used	22

Criteria for Assessing Goodness of Fit			
Criterion	DF	Value	Value/DF
Deviance	17	186.7304	10.9841
Scaled Deviance	17	186.7304	10.9841
Pearson Chi-Square	17	186.0802	10.9459
Scaled Pearson $X2$	17	186.0802	10.9459
Log Likelihood		2946.0059	
Full Log Likelihood		−143.8490	
AIC (smaller is better)		297.6980	
AICC (smaller is better)		301.4480	
BIC (smaller is better)		303.1533	

Algorithm converged.

(Continued)

TABLE 10.7 (*Continued*)

Results of Fitting a Poisson Regression Model to the FAP Data in Table 10.6

Analysis of Maximum Likelihood Parameter Estimates							
Parameter	DF	Estimate	Standard Error	Wald 95% Confidence Limits		Wald Chi-Square	Pr > ChiSq
Intercept	1	3.3610	0.1882	2.9922	3.7298	319.09	<.0001
male	1	0.2814	0.1111	0.0637	0.4991	6.42	0.0113
treat	1	−0.3183	0.0984	−0.5112	−0.1254	10.46	0.0012
base_n	1	0.0089	0.0004	0.0081	0.0097	479.32	<.0001
age	1	−0.0264	0.0073	−0.0408	−0.0120	12.95	0.0003
Scale	0	1.0000	0.0000	1.0000	1.0000		

Note: The scale parameter was held fixed.

For example, the exponentiated confidence interval for the gender regression coefficient is [1.07,1.65]. Men are estimated to have somewhere between 7% and 65% more polyps at 3 months than women, conditional on the other covariates being the same. For treatment, the corresponding interval is [0.60,0.88]. Consequently, patients receiving the active treatment are estimated to have between 60% and 88% the number of polyps at 3 months than those receiving the placebo—again, conditional on the other covariates being equal. One aspect of the fitted model for these data—namely, the value of the deviance divided by degrees of freedom—has implications for the appropriateness of the model, which we shall take up in Section 10.5.

10.3.2 Regression with Gamma Errors

Some of the counts in the polyp data in Table 10.6 are extremely large, indicating that the distribution of counts is very skewed. Consequently, the data might be better modelled by allowing for this with the use of a *gamma distribution* (the distribution is defined in Everitt 2002). Since gamma variables are positive, a log link function will again be used and the SAS code to fit the model is now

```
proc genmod data=fap;
  model r_n=male treat base_n age / dist=g link=log;
run;
```

In this example, we specify both the link function and the error distribution on the model statement, as the log link is not the canonical link for the gamma distribution.

The results are shown in Table 10.8. The gender regression coefficient is now no longer significant at the 5% level, but the *p*-values associated with the other regression coefficients are largely unchanged.

TABLE 10.8

Results from Fitting a Model with Gamma Errors to the FAP Data

Model Information

Data Set	WORK.FAP
Distribution	Gamma
Link Function	Log
Dependent Variable	r_n

Number of Observations Read	22
Number of Observations Used	22

Criteria for Assessing Goodness of Fit

Criterion	DF	Value	Value/DF
Deviance	17	7.5870	0.4463
Scaled Deviance	17	23.1875	1.3640
Pearson Chi-Square	17	5.6485	0.3323
Scaled Pearson $X2$	17	17.2629	1.0155
Log Likelihood		−80.1699	
Full Log Likelihood		−80.1699	
AIC (smaller is better)		172.3398	
AICC (smaller is better)		177.9398	
BIC (smaller is better)		178.8861	

Algorithm converged.

Analysis of Maximum Likelihood Parameter Estimates

Parameter	DF	Estimate	Standard Error	Wald 95% Confidence Limits		Wald Chi-Square	Pr > ChiSq
Intercept	1	3.0155	0.5048	2.0260	4.0049	35.68	<.0001
male	1	0.5093	0.2940	−0.0668	1.0854	3.00	0.0832
treat	1	−0.8358	0.2591	−1.3437	—	10.40	0.0013
base_n	1	0.0132	0.0027	0.0079	0.0186	23.46	<.0001
age	1	−0.0223	0.0186	−0.0588	0.0142	1.44	0.2306
Scale	1	3.0562	0.8759	1.7428	5.3595		

Note: The scale parameter was estimated by maximum likelihood.

10.4 Residuals for GLMs

As with multiple regression and logistic regression, it is important when fitting GLMs to look at suitable residuals to assess assumptions. Two residuals useful in assessing fitted GLMs are described next; in essence, they are equivalent to those described in the previous chapter on logistic regression.

The *deviance residuals* are defined as

$$r_i^D = \text{sign}\left(y_i - \hat{\mu}_i\right)\sqrt{d_i} \tag{10.12}$$

where d_i is the contribution of the ith subject to the deviance, with total deviance given by $D = \sum_i \left(r_i^D\right)^2$.

The *Pearson residuals* are defined as the contribution of the ith subject to the Pearson X^2 statistic

$$r_i^P = \frac{\left(y_i - \hat{\mu}_i\right)}{\sqrt{V\left(\hat{\mu}_i\right)}} \tag{10.13}$$

so that $X^2 = \sum \left(r_y^P\right)^2$.

Both the Pearson and deviance statistics can be used for detecting observations not well fitted by the model. The deviance residuals are more commonly used because their distribution tends to be closer to normal than that of the Pearson residuals.

To illustrate the use of residuals for assessing GLMs, we shall calculate the Pearson residuals for both the Poisson regression model and the gamma errors model fitted to the FAP data. A probability plot will be used in each case to display the residuals. To do this, we rerun the two models, adding an `output` statement to save the Pearson (chi) residuals and then use `proc univariate` for the probability plot, suppressing the printed output with the `noprint` option. The options on the `probplot` statement specify a normal probability plot. Estimating the mean and standard deviation from the data (i.e., the residuals in this case) enables an appropriate reference line to be drawn:

```
proc genmod data=fap;
   model r_n=male treat base_n age/dist=p;
   output out=pout reschi=rs;
run;
```

```
proc univariate data=pout noprint;
  var rs;
  probplot rs/normal(mu=est sigma=est);
run;
proc genmod data=fap;
  model r_n=male treat base_n age/dist=g link=log;
  output out=gout reschi=rs;
run;
proc univariate data=gout noprint;
  var rs;
  probplot rs/normal(mu=est sigma=est);
run;
```

The probability plots are shown in Figures 10.1 and 10.2. The plot associated with the Poisson regression shows a clear departure from linearity, with several very large residuals. The plot associated with the gamma errors model appears to be far more satisfactory. The possible problem with the Poisson model is taken up in the next section.

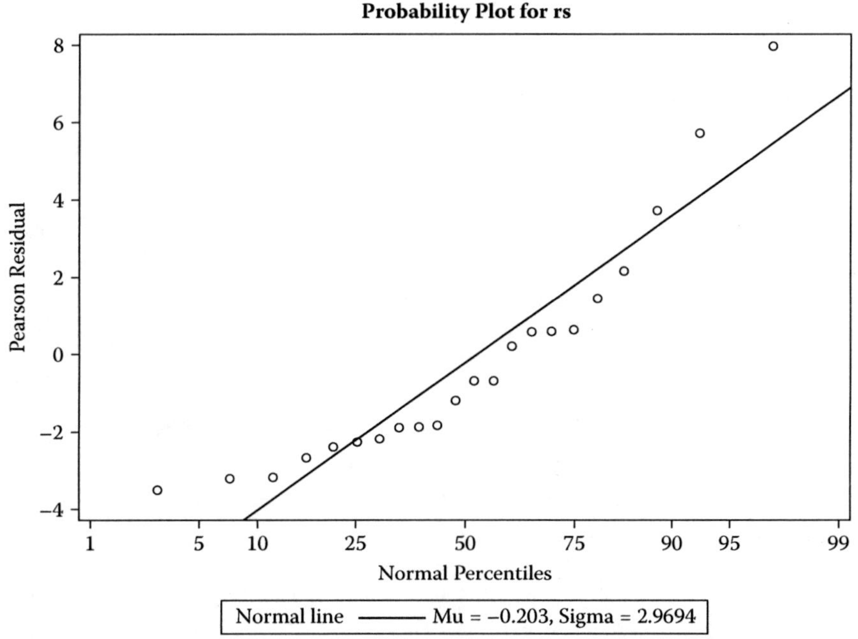

FIGURE 10.1
Normal probability plot of Pearson residuals from the Poisson regression model for the polyp data.

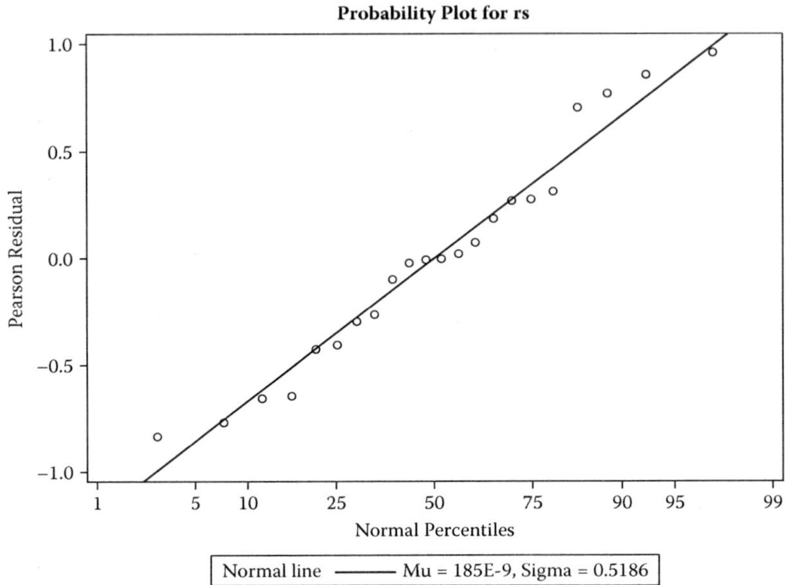

FIGURE 10.2

Normal probability plot of Pearson residuals from the gamma regression model for the polyp data.

10.5 Overdispersion

An important aspect of generalised linear models that thus far we have largely ignored is the variance function, $V(\mu)$, that captures how the variance of a response variable depends upon its mean. The general form of the relationship is var(response) = $\phi V(\mu)$ where ϕ is a constant and $V(\mu)$ specifies how the variance depends on the mean μ. For the error distributions considered previously, this general form becomes

- Normal: $V(\mu) = 1$, $\phi = \sigma^2$; here, the variance does not depend on the mean.

- Binomial: $V(\mu) = \mu(1 - \mu)$, $\phi = 1$.

- Poisson: $V(\mu) = \mu$, $\phi = 1$.

In the case of a Poisson variable, we see that the mean and variance are equal, and in the case of a binomial variable, where the mean is the probability of the occurrence of the event of interest, p, the variance is $p(1 - p)$.

Both the Poisson and binomial distributions have variance functions that are completely determined by the mean. There is no free parameter for the variance since, in applications of the generalised linear model with binomial or Poisson error distributions, the dispersion parameter, ϕ, is defined to be one (see previous results for logistic and Poisson regression). But in some applications, this becomes too restrictive to account fully for the empirical variance in the data; in such cases, it is common to describe the phenomenon as *overdispersion*.

For example, if the response variable is the proportion of family members who have been ill in the past year, observed in a large number of families, then the individual binary observations that make up the observed proportions are likely to be correlated rather than independent. This non-independence can lead to a variance that is greater (less) than that on the assumption of binomial variability. Also, observed counts often exhibit larger variance than would be expected from the Poisson assumption, a fact noted by Greenwood and Yule over 80 years ago (Greenwood and Yule 1920). Greenwood and Yule's suggested solution to the problem was a model in which μ was a random variable with a gamma distribution leading to a *negative binomial distribution* for the count.

There are a number of strategies for accommodating overdispersion, but here we concentrate on a relatively simple approach that retains the use of the binomial or Poisson error distributions as appropriate, but allows estimation of a value of ϕ from the data rather than defining it to be unity for these distributions. The estimate is usually the residual deviance divided by its degrees of freedom—exactly the method used with Gaussian models. Parameter estimates remain the same, but parameter standard errors are increased by multiplying them by the square root of the estimated dispersion parameter. This process can be carried out manually, or almost equivalently the overdispersed model can be formally fitted using a procedure known as *quasilikelihood;* this allows estimation of model parameters without fully knowing the error distribution of the response variable (see McCullagh and Nelder 1989 for full technical details of the approach).

When fitting generalised linear models with binomial or Poisson error distributions, overdispersion can often be spotted by comparing the residual deviance with its degrees of freedom. For a well-fitting model, the two quantities should be approximately equal. If the deviance is far greater than the degrees of freedom, overdispersion may be indicated. In Table 10.7, for example, we see that the ratio of deviance to degrees of freedom is nearly 11, clearly indicating an overdispersion problem. Consequently, we will now refit the Poisson model with the `scale=d` option, which uses the square root of the deviance divided by its degrees of freedom as the scale parameter:

```
proc genmod data=fap;
  model r_n=male treat base_n age/dist=p scale=d;
  output out=pout reschi=rs;
run;
```

TABLE 10.9

Results of Fitting Overdispersed Model Poisson Model to FAP Data

Analysis of Maximum Likelihood Parameter Estimates							
Parameter	DF	Estimate	Standard Error	Wald 95% Confidence Limits		Wald Chi-Square	Pr > ChiSq
Intercept	1	3.3610	0.6236	2.1388	4.5832	29.05	<.0001
Male	1	0.2814	0.3681	−0.4400	1.0028	0.58	0.4445
Treat	1	−0.3183	0.3261	−0.9575	0.3209	0.95	0.3291
base_n	1	0.0089	0.0013	0.0063	0.0115	43.64	<.0001
Age	1	−0.0264	0.0243	−0.0741	0.0213	1.18	0.2776
Scale	0	3.3142	0.0000	3.3142	3.3142		
Note: The scale parameter was estimated by the square root of DEVIANCE/DOF.							

The results are shown in Table 10.9. Comparing these with the results in Table 10.7, we see that the estimated regression coefficients are the same, but their standard errors are now much greater, with the consequence that only the coefficient of baseline polyp count remains significant. Gender, treatment, and age are no longer found to be significant predictors of 3-month polyp count.

10.6 Summary

Generalised linear models provide a very powerful and flexible framework for the application of regression models to medical data. Some familiarity with the basis of such models might allow medical researchers to consider more realistic models for their data rather than to rely solely on linear and logistic regression.

11

Generalised Additive Models

11.1 Introduction

The multiple regression model described in Chapter 8 and the generalised linear model featured in Chapter 10 can accommodate nonlinear functions of the explanatory variables—for example, quadratic or cubic terms—if these are thought to be necessary to provide an adequate fit. In this chapter, however, we consider some alternative and generally more flexible statistical methods for modelling nonlinear relationships between a response variable and one or more explanatory variables. The main component of these methods, known as *generalised additive models* (GAMs), is the fitting of a 'smooth' relationship between the response and each explanatory variable by means of a *scatter plot smoother* (see Chapter 7 and Section 11.2). GAMs are useful when

- The relationship between the variables is expected to be of complex form not easily fitted by standard linear or nonlinear models.
- There is no a priori reason for using a particular model.
- We would like the data themselves to suggest the appropriate functional form for the relationship between an explanatory variable and the response.

Such models should be regarded as philosophically closer to the concepts of exploratory data analysis, in which the form of any functional relationship emerges from a set of data, rather than arising from a theoretical construct. In the health sciences, this can be especially useful because it reflects the uncertainty of knowledge regarding the mechanisms that determine disease and its prognosis.

Since the building blocks of the GAM approach are scatter plot smoothers, these are described in the next section.

11.2 Scatter Plot Smoothers

The scatter plot is an excellent first exploratory graph to study the dependence of two variables. An important second exploratory graph adds a curve to the scatter plot to help us better perceive the pattern of dependence. Most readers will be familiar with adding a parametric curve, such as a simple linear or polynomial regression fit; however, there are nonparametric alternatives that are perhaps less familiar, but can often be more useful, since many bivariate data sets are too complex to be described by a simple parametric family. Perhaps the simplest of these alternatives is a *locally weighted regression* or *loess* fit, first suggested by Cleveland (1979) and introduced in Chapter 7. In essence, this approach assumes that the variables x and y are related by the equation

$$y_i = g(x_i) + \varepsilon_i \tag{11.1}$$

where g is a 'smooth' function and the ε_i are random variables with mean zero and constant scale.

Values $\hat{y}_i$, used to 'estimate' the y_i at each x_i, are found by fitting polynomials using weighted least squares with large weights for points near to x_i and small weights otherwise. Thus, smoothing takes place essentially by local averaging of the y-values of observations having predictor values close to a target value.

Two parameters control the shape of a loess curve; the first is a smoothing parameter, α, with larger values leading to smoother curves (typical values are 0.25 to 1). The second parameter, λ, is the degree of certain polynomials that are fitted by the method; λ can take values 1 or 2. In any specific application, the choice of the two parameters must be based on a combination of judgement and trial and error. Residual plots may be helpful, however, in judging a particular combination of values.

We shall illustrate the use of locally weighted regression on data collected on the oxygen uptake and the expired ventilation of 53 subjects performing a standard exercise task. The data for the first five subjects are given in Table 11.1.

TABLE 11.1

Oxygen Uptake and Expired Ventilation Observations for First 5 of the 53 Subjects in the Data Set

Subject	Oxygen Uptake	Expired Ventilation
1	574	21.9
2	592	18.6
3	664	18.6
4	667	19.1
5	718	19.2

Within SAS, locally weighted regression can be performed with proc loess or proc gam. Although proc loess has more options for choosing the parameters of the locally weighted regression, proc gam fits a wider range of generalised additive models and thus is used here. (The use of proc loess was illustrated in Chapter 7.)

```
data oxygen;
  infile 'c:\amsus\data\oxygen.dat';
  input id o2uptake expired;
run;

proc gam data=oxygen;
  model expired=loess(o2uptake) / method=gcv;
  output out=gamout pred;
run;

proc sgplot data=gamout;
    scatter y=expired x=o2uptake;
    series y=p_expired x=o2uptake;
run;
```

The first point to notice about the syntax of proc gam is that the specification of predictors on the model statement is different from procedures covered in previous chapters. The name of the predictor variable is enclosed in parentheses and prefixed with a keyword indicating the type of smoother to be employed. The keyword param is used for variables that are *not* to be smoothed, but entered as parametric linear predictors; loess is used for a locally weighted regression, spline for a cubic smoothing *spline* (described later in the chapter), and spline2 for a thin plate smoothing spline, which is a multivariate version of the *cubic spline* (again, see later in the chapter).

Parametric effects must be specified before smoothed effects and must be included in the same set of parentheses, where there are more than one. Parametric effects can be categorical but, in that case, must also be named on a class statement. For smoothed effects, the degree of smoothing can be specified for each in terms of its effective number of parameters (analogous to the number of parameters in a parametric fit; see later) or degrees of freedom—for example,

```
model expired = loess(o2uptake,df=6);
```

Alternatively, the method = gcv option on the model statement can be used to select a degree of smoothing using generalised cross validation. The dist= option on the model statement specifies the distribution. Gaussian is the default, and other possibilities are binomial, binary, gamma, igaussian (inverse Gaussian), or poisson.

The output statement creates the gamout data set, which contains the variables used in the model plus predicted values, specified using the

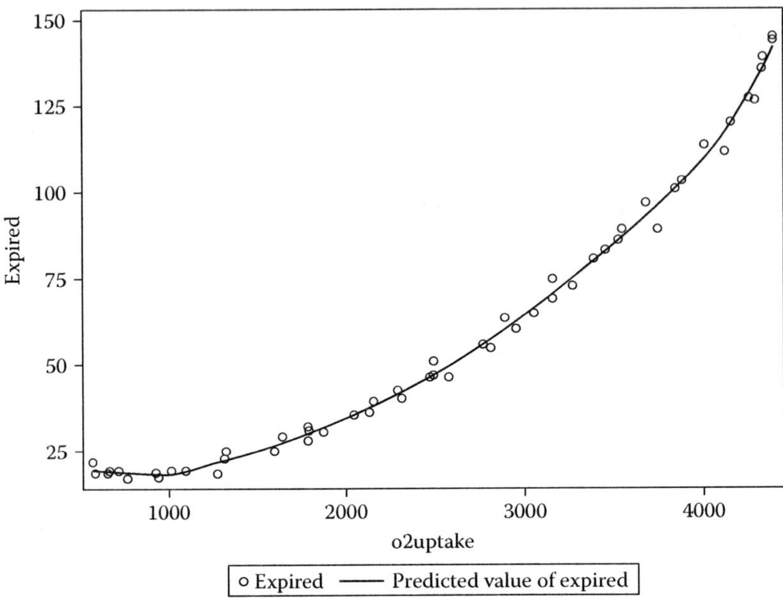

FIGURE 11.1
Plot of oxygen uptake data showing fitted locally weighted regression curve.

keyword `pred`. (The `id` statement can be used to copy additional variables to the output data set.) There are predicted values for each smoothed effect and overall predicted values. These are automatically named by prefixing the original variable name with `p_`, so the `gamout` data set contains both `p_expired` and `p_o2uptake`.

A plot of the data and the overall predicted values is shown in Figure 11.1.

We can compare this result to results from fitting parametric regressions that include various polynomial functions:

```
proc sgplot data=oxygen;
   scatter y=expired x=o2uptake / legendlabel='observed';
   reg y=expired x=o2uptake /degree=2 nomarkers
   lineattrs=(pattern=dot) legendlabel='quadratic';
   reg y=expired x=o2uptake /degree=3 nomarkers
   lineattrs=(pattern=dash) legendlabel='cubic';
   reg y=expired x=o2uptake /degree=4 nomarkers
   lineattrs=(pattern=solid) legendlabel='quartic';
run;
```

Quadratic and cubic functions can be overlaid on a scatter plot using the `reg` plot statement with different `degree` options. To distinguish the curves, we give them different line types and appropriate labels for the legend. The resulting plot is shown in Figure 11.2. Here the locally weighted regression and the polynomial give very similar fits.

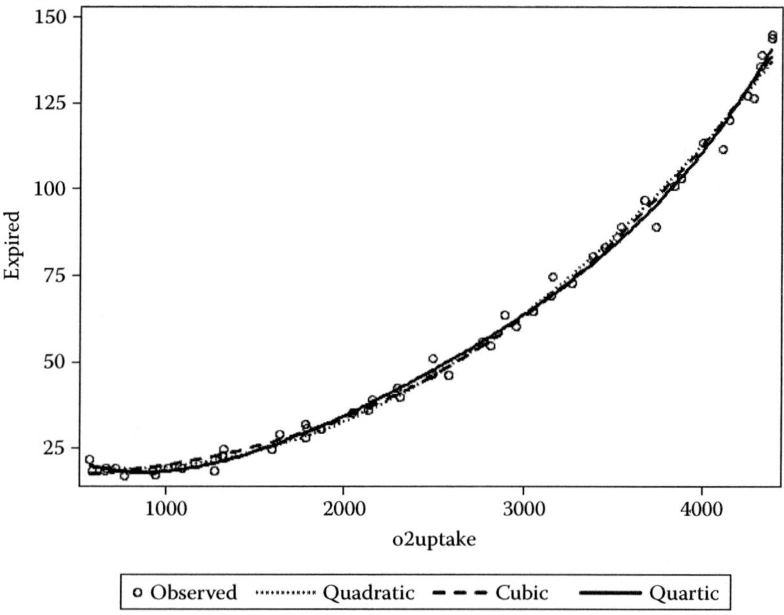

FIGURE 11.2
Plot of oxygen uptake data showing quadratic, cubic, and quartic polynomial fits.

A more difficult challenge for the locally weighted regression approach is provided by the data shown in Table 11.2; these are monthly deaths from bronchitis, emphysema, and asthma in the UK from 1974 to 1979 for both men and women.

First, we read these data in as follows:

```
data respdeaths;
infile cards missover;
 retain obs 0;
 input year @;
 do month=1 to 12;
 input deaths @;
 output;
 obs=obs+1;
 end;
cards;
1974 3035 2552 2704 2554 2014 1655 1721 1524 1596 2074 2199 2512
1975 2933 2889 2938 2497 1870 1726 1607 1545 1396 1787 2076 2837
1976 2787 3891 3179 2011 1636 1580 1489 1300 1356 1653 2013 2823
1977 2996 2523 2540 2520 1994 1964 1691 1479 1596 1877 2032 2484
1978 2899 2990 2890 2379 1933 1734 1617 1495 1440 1777 1970 2745
1979 2841 3535 3010 2091 1667 1589 1518 1348 1392 1619 1954 2633
run;
```

TABLE 11.2

Monthly Deaths from Bronchitis, Emphysema, and Asthma for UK Men and Women, 1974–1979

	Jan	Feb	Mar	Apr	May	Jun	Jul	Aug	Sep	Oct	Nov	Dec
1974	3035	2552	2704	2554	2014	1655	1721	1524	1596	2074	2199	2512
1975	2933	2889	2938	2497	1870	1726	1607	1545	1396	1787	2076	2837
1976	2787	3891	3179	2011	1636	1580	1489	1300	1356	1653	2013	2823
1977	2996	2523	2540	2520	1994	1964	1691	1479	1596	1877	2032	2484
1978	2899	2990	2890	2379	1933	1734	1617	1495	1440	1777	1970	2745
1979	2841	3535	3010	2091	1667	1589	1518	1348	1392	1619	1954	2633

The `retain` statement specifies a variable whose values are to be kept from the previous iteration of the data step and sets its initial value to zero. Then the `year` is read in with the trailing @ holding the line for further data to be read. The `do` loop then reads the number of deaths for each month and writes out an observation. With a single trailing @, the data line is released at the end of the data step iteration.

Now we fit a model using locally weighted regressions with two components—one for year and one for month:

```
proc gam data=respdeaths;
   model deaths=loess(year) loess(month)/method=gcv;
   id obs;
   output out=respout all;
run;


proc sgplot data=respout;
   scatter y=deaths x=obs ;
   series y=p_deaths x=obs;
run;
```

This code is very similar to that given earlier. The `obs` variable is needed for the subsequent plot, so the `id` statement is used to add it to the `respout` data set. The `output` statement also uses the `all` keyword to request all available statistics.

The plot of the observed data and the fitted locally weighted regression are shown in Figure 11.3. The characteristic cyclic nature of the data has been modelled reasonably accurately by the fitted curve.

When the model contains more than one smoothed effect, separate plots of the additive fit of each are useful in assessing their functional form. The plots, referred to in SAS as *component plots,* are produced by default when ODS graphics are on. Here, we explicitly request the plots in order to specify the additional options of confidence limits (`clm`) and common axes for the two plots. The result is shown in Figure 11.4.

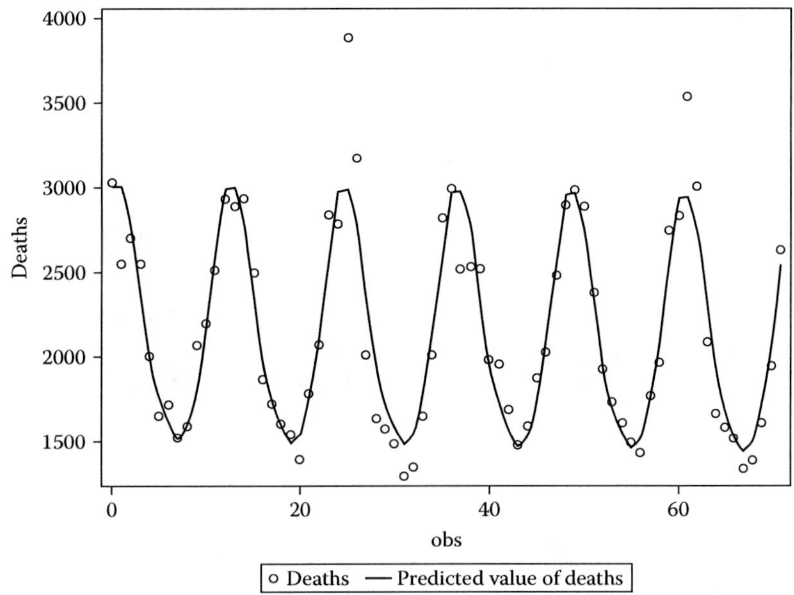

FIGURE 11.3
Plot of monthly deaths from bronchitis showing fitted locally weighted regression.

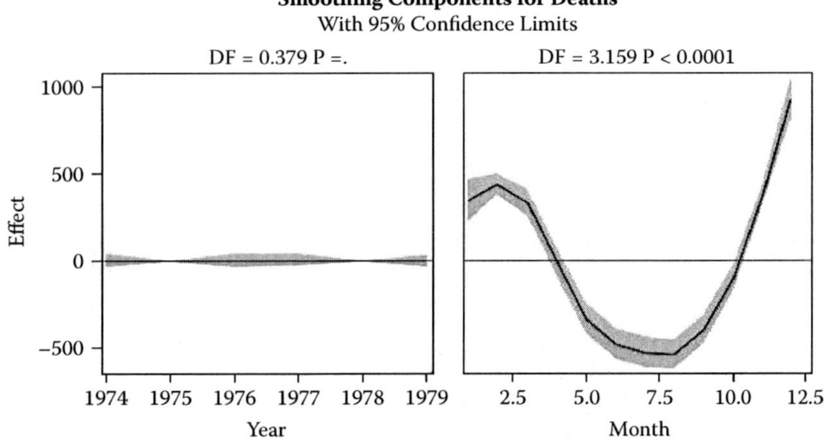

FIGURE 11.4
Component plots for the locally weighted regression model for the bronchitis data.

```
ods graphics on;
proc gam data=respdeaths plots=components(clm commonaxes);
  model deaths=loess(year) loess(month)/ method=gcv;
run;
```

In the right-hand panel, we see more clearly the pattern of winter excess of respiratory deaths, whereas there is little evidence of a year-to-year change. In fact, a formal test of the two components shows that the effect of year is nonsignificant. (Such tests will be described later in the chapter.)

An alternative smoother that can often usefully be applied to bivariate data is some form of *spline function*. (A spline is a term for a flexible strip of metal or rubber used by a draftsman to draw curves.) Spline functions are polynomials within intervals of the x-variable that are connected across different values of x. Figure 11.5, for example, shows a linear spline function (i.e., a piecewise linear function) of the form

$$f(x) = \beta_0 + \beta_1 X + \beta_2 (X-a)_+ + \beta_3 (X-b)_+ + \beta_4 (X-c)_+ \qquad (11.2)$$

where $(u)_+ = u \quad u > 0$

$$ = 0 \quad u \le 0$$

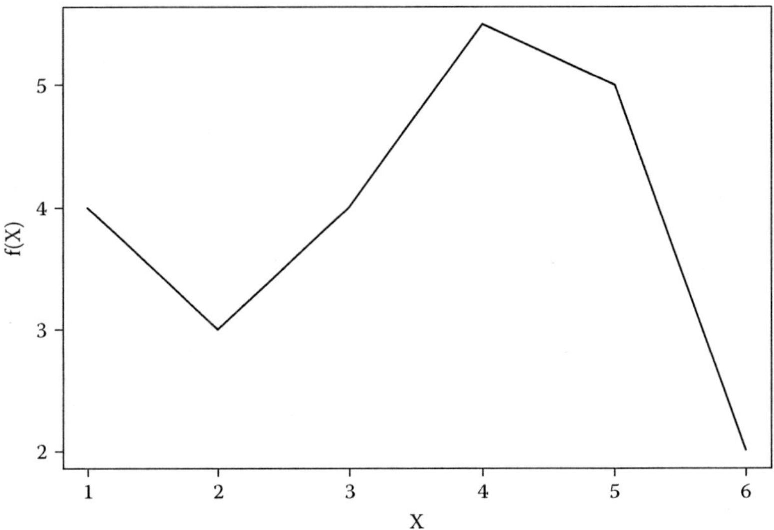

FIGURE 11.5

A linear spline function with knots at $a = 1$, $b = 3$, $c = 5$. (Taken from Harrell, F. E. 2001. *Regression Modeling Strategies*. With permission of New York: Springer.)

The interval endpoints, *a, b,* and *c* are called *knots.* The number of knots can vary according to the amount of data available for fitting the function.

The linear spline is simple and can approximate some relationships, but it is not smooth, so it will not fit highly curved functions well. The problem is overcome by using piecewise polynomials—in particular, cubics, which have been found to have nice properties with good ability to fit a variety of complex relationships. The result is a cubic spline, which is a smooth curve $f(x)$ that summarises the dependence of a response variable, y, on an explanatory variable, x, and fitted by minimising

$$\sum_{i=1}^{n}\left[y_i - f(x_i)\right]^2 + \lambda \int f''(x)^2\, dx \tag{11.3}$$

where $f''(x)$ is the second derivative of $f(x)$ with respect to x. The first term represents the sum of squares criterion used in least squares. The integral in the second term, $\int f''(x)^2\, dx$, measures the departure from linearity of f (for linear f, the term is zero) and λ is a nonnegative smoothing parameter. It governs the trade-off between the goodness of fit to the data and the degree of smoothness of f. Larger values of λ force f to be smoother.

For any value of λ, the solution to (11.3) is a cubic spline—a piecewise cubic polynomial with pieces joined at the unique observed values x_i of the explanatory variable. The 'effective number of parameters' (analogous to the number of parameters in a parametric fit) or degrees of freedom of a cubic spline smoother is generally used to specify its smoothness rather than λ directly. A numerical search is then used to determine the value of λ corresponding to the required degrees of freedom. Roughly, the complexity of a cubic spline is about the same as a polynomial of degree one less than the degrees of freedom. But the cubic spline smoother 'spreads out' its parameters in a more even way and, hence, is much more flexible than is polynomial regression. (The preceding account follows that given in Hastie and Tibshirani 1990.)

As mentioned earlier, `proc gam` can also fit spline smoothers and very similar results to those shown above for the two-component locally weighted regression fit for the bronchitis data can be obtained by changing the `model` statement to

```
model deaths=spline(year) spline(month)/ method=gcv;
```

For exploratory analysis of bivariate data, spline and loess smoothers are also available as plot types within proc sgplot (see Figure 11.6):

```
proc sgplot data=respdeaths;
  pbspline y=deaths x=obs;
  loess y=deaths x=obs;
run;
```

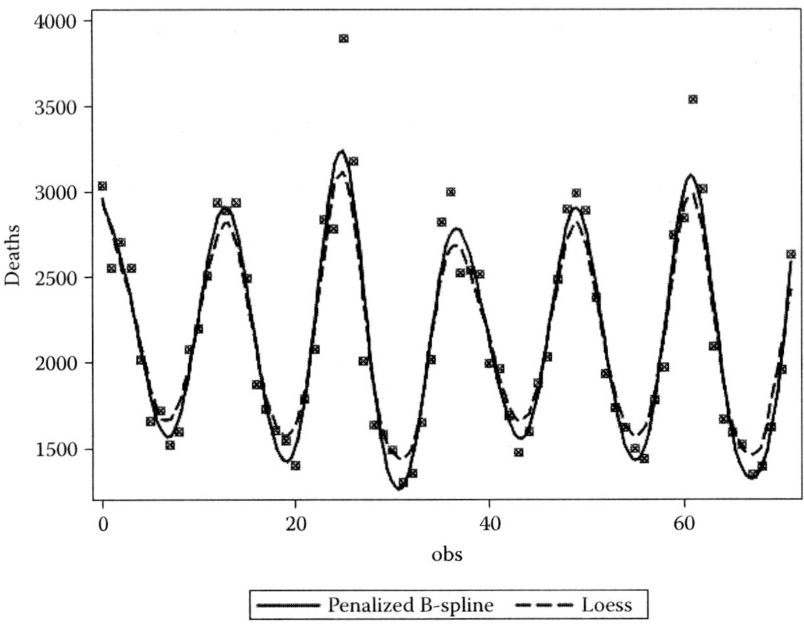

FIGURE 11.6
Spline and loess smoothers fitted to the bronchitis data.

11.3 Additive and Generalised Additive Models

In a linear regression model, there is a dependent variable, y, and a set of explanatory variables, $x_1, \ldots, x_p$; the model assumed is

$$y = \beta_0 + \sum_{j=1}^{p} \beta_j x_j + \varepsilon \tag{11.4}$$

Additive models replace the linear function $\beta_j x_j$ by a smooth nonparametric function to give

$$y = \beta_0 + \sum_{j=1}^{p} g_j(x_j) + \varepsilon \tag{11.5}$$

where g_i can be one of the scatter plot smoothers described in the previous section or, if the investigator chooses, a linear function for particular x_j.

Models can therefore include a mixture of linear and smooth functions if necessary.

A generalised additive model arises from Equation (11.5) in the same way as a generalised linear model arises from a multiple regression model—namely, that some function of the expectation of the response variable is now modelled by a sum of nonparametric functions. For example, the logistic additive model is

$$\operatorname{logit}\left[\Pr(y=1)\right]=\beta_0+\sum_{j=1}^{p}g_j(x_j) \tag{11.6}$$

Fitting a generalised additive model involves what is known as a *back-fitting algorithm*. The smooth functions g_i are fitted one at a time by taking the residual

$$y-\sum_{k\neq j}g_k(x_k) \tag{11.7}$$

Then they are fitted against x_j using one of the scatter plot smoothers described in Section 11.2. The process is repeated until it converges. Linear terms in the model are fitted by least squares. Full details are given in Chambers and Hastie (1993).

Various tests are available to assess the nonlinear contributions of the fitted smoothers, and generalised additive models can be compared with, say, linear models fitted to the same data by means of likelihood ratio tests often set out in an analysis of deviance table (see Chapter 10). In this process, the fitted smooth curve is assigned an estimated equivalent number of degrees of freedom. For full details, again, see Chambers and Hastie (1993).

11.4 Examples of the Application of GAMs

Our first example will involve applying a generalised additive model to data given in Hastie and Tibshirani (1990) that come from a study of the factors affecting patterns of insulin-dependent diabetes mellitus in children (Socket et al. 1987). The objective was to investigate the dependence of the level of serum C-peptide on various other factors in order to understand the patterns of residual insulin secretion. The response measure to be used is the logarithm of C-peptide concentration at diagnosis, and the two explanatory variables are age and base deficit, a measure of acidity. The data set contains observations on 43 children; Table 11.3 shows the observations for the first 5 children.

TABLE 11.3

Insulin-Dependent Diabetes in Five Children

Subject	Age	Base Deficit	Peptide
1	5.2	−8.1	4.8
2	8.8	−16.1	4.1
3	10.5	−0.9	5.2
4	10.6	−7.8	5.5
5	10.4	−29.0	5.0

Source: Hastie, T. J. and Tibshirani, R. J. 1990. *Generalized Additive Models*, London: CRC/ Chapman and Hall.

We begin by reading in the data and examining scatter plots of log (peptide) against age and against base:

```
data diabetes;
  infile 'c:\amsus\data\diabetes.dat';
  input id age base peptide;
  logpeptide=log10(peptide);
run;

proc sgscatter data=diabetes;
   plot logpeptide*(age base)/reg pbspline;
run;
```

We use $\log_{10}$ of the peptide value following Hastie and Tibshirani (1990). Log peptide is then plotted against age and base, superimposing on each the associated linear regression and a spline smooth. The results are shown in Figure 11.7. In both plots, there appears to be at least some evidence of a departure from linearity, although this is stronger for age than base deficit.

To begin, we fit a generalised additive model to these data, using locally weighted regression fits for both age and base:

```
ods graphics on;
proc gam data=diabetes plots(clm commonaxes);
  model logpeptide=loess(age) loess(base) / method=gcv;
run;
```

In this example, we use ods graphics to generate the component plots. The plots are automatically generated when ODS graphics are on, but the plots option on the proc statement is used to specify confidence bands and common vertical axes for the plots. The plots are shown in Figure 11.8 and the procedure output in Table 11.4.

The results shown in Table 11.4 confirm the need for a nonlinear function for age, but it appears there is not a strong case for fitting a nonlinear term for base. The plot of the fitted functions in Figure 11.8 shows the wide standard error limits for the base curve.

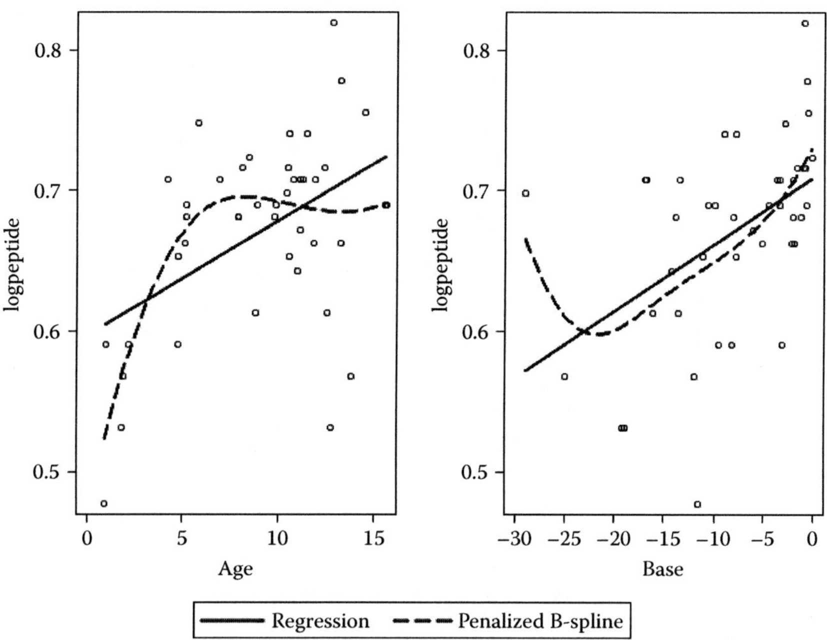

FIGURE 11.7
Plots of log peptide against base and age for insulin dependence data, showing linear and spline fits.

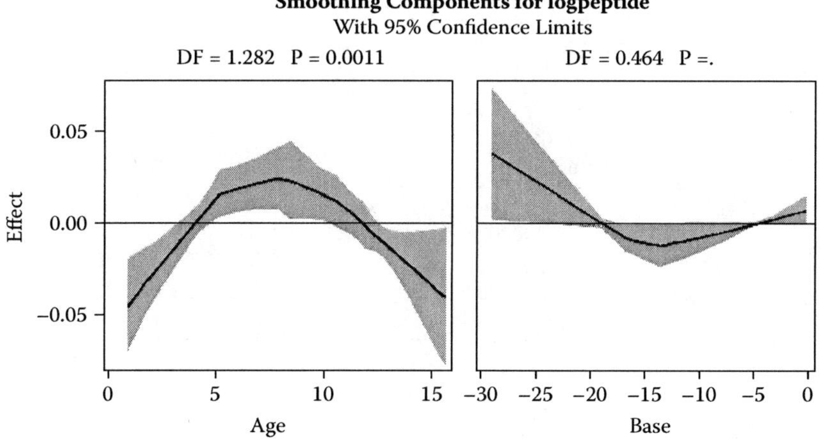

FIGURE 11.8
Fitted functions for age and base deficit.

TABLE 11.4

Results from Fitting a GAM with Spline Functions for Both Age
and Base to the Insulin Dependence Data in Table 11.3

Dependent Variable: Logpeptide	
Smoothing Model Component(s): Loess(age) Loess(base)	
Summary of Input Data Set	
Number of Observations	43
Number of Missing Observations	0
Distribution	Gaussian
Link Function	Identity

Iteration Summary and Fit Statistics	
Final Number of Backfitting Iterations	4
Final Backfitting Criterion	2.3603574E-9
Deviance of the Final Estimate	0.0912805666

The backfitting algorithm converged.

Regression Model Analysis Parameter Estimates				
Parameter	**Parameter Estimate**	**Standard Error**	**t Value**	**Pr > |t|**
Intercept	0.64112	0.02255	28.43	<.0001
Linear(age)	0.00658	0.00193	3.41	0.0015
Linear(base)	0.00360	0.00109	3.31	0.0020

Smoothing Model Analysis: Fit Summary for Smoothing Components				
Component	**Smoothing Parameter**	**DF**	**GCV**	**Num Unique Obs**
Loess(age)	0.686047	1.282008	0.000059665	43
Loess(base)	1.000000	0.464229	0.000056241	43

Smoothing Model Analysis: Analysis of Deviance				
Source	**DF**	**Sum of Squares**	**Chi-Square**	**Pr > ChiSq**
Loess(age)	1.28201	0.027463	11.5091	0.0011
Loess(base)	0.46423	0.008214	3.4424	.

We now fit a model which includes a locally weighted regression fit for age but a linear term for base; the results are given in Table 11.5. A comparison of this model with the one described before shows that allowing for possible nonlinearity of base contributes very little to the model.

Finally, we can compare the fit of the model with a locally weighted regression term for age and a linear term for base, with a multiple regression model which includes linear effects for both explanatory variables only. This leads to the results for the comparison in the following:

	Terms	Resid. DF	RSS	Test	DF	SS	F	Pr(F)
Model 1	Age + base	40	0.1261					
Model 2	Lo(age) + base	39.14	0.1016	1v2	0.86	0.0245	10.97	0.003

Allowing for nonlinearity in age contributes significantly to the model. We could, of course, allow for this nonlinearity in the classical way (by including, say, a quadratic term for age), but it is the fitting of the GAM models that has identified the need for such a term.

The next data set we shall consider relates to air pollution in 41 US cities. For each city, a binary variable is recorded to indicate whether the annual mean concentration of sulphur dioxide is below 30 µg per cubic metre or equal to or above this value. Also recorded are six other variables, two of which relate to human ecology and four to climate. (The data are taken from Sokal and Rohlf 1981.) The observations for the first five cities are given in Table 11.6.

We will use this example to illustrate how GAM models may uncover a relationship that could easily be overlooked, if the data were analysed using logistic regression. A naïve approach using logistic regression might conclude that none of the six predictor variables is related to sulphur dioxide concentration. However, some exploratory plots suggest the possibility of nonlinear relationships. We concentrate on two of the six variables: population size and average rainfall.

```
data usair;
   infile 'c:\amsus\data\usair.dat';
   input city $16. hiso2 temperature factories population
windspeed rain rainydays;
run;
```

We begin with some box plots with the `datalabel` option to identify any outliers by name:

```
proc sgplot data=usair;
   vbox population / category=hiso2 datalabel=city;
run;
proc sgplot data=usair;
   vbox rain / category=hiso2 datalabel=city;
run;
```

TABLE 11.5

Results from Fitting a GAM with Spline Function for Age and a Linear
Term for Base to the Insulin Dependence Data in Table 11.3

Dependent Variable: Logpeptide
Regression Model Component(s): Base
Smoothing Model Component(s): Loess(age)

Summary of Input Data Set	
Number of Observations	43
Number of Missing Observations	0
Distribution	Gaussian
Link Function	Identity

Iteration Summary and Fit Statistics	
Final Number of Backfitting Iterations	4
Final Backfitting Criterion	2.919605E-11
Deviance of the Final Estimate	0.1016127205

The backfitting algorithm converged.

Regression Model Analysis Parameter Estimates				
Parameter	Parameter Estimate	Standard Error	t Value	Pr > |t|
Intercept	0.64090	0.02353	27.24	<.0001
base	0.00363	0.00113	3.20	0.0027
Linear(age)	0.00663	0.00201	3.30	0.0021

Smoothing Model Analysis Fit Summary for Smoothing Components				
Component	Smoothing Parameter	DF	GCV	Num Unique Obs
Loess(age)	0.779070	0.857962	0.000064786	43

Smoothing Model Analysis Analysis of Deviance				
Source	DF	Sum of Squares	Chi-Square	Pr > ChiSq
Loess(age)	0.85796	0.024478	9.4292	0.0016

TABLE 11.6

Air Pollution Data for First 5 of 41 Cities

City	Hiso2	Temperature	Factories	Population	Wind Speed	Rain	Rainy Days
Phoenix	0	70.3	213	582	6.0	7.05	36
Little Rock	0	61.0	91	132	8.2	48.52	100
San Francisco	0	56.7	453	716	8.7	20.66	67
Denver	0	51.9	454	515	9.0	12.95	86
Hartford	1	49.1	412	158	9.0	43.37	127

Source: Sokal, R. R., and Rohlf, R. J. 1981. *Biometry*, 2nd ed. San Francisco: W. H. Freeman.

The results shown in Figure 11.9 show that Chicago is an outlier in population size, so it is dropped from the analysis:

```
data usair;
  set usair;
  if city=:'Chicago' then delete;
run;
```

The spline smoothing plot introduced earlier can also be useful with binary data:

```
proc sgscatter data=usair;
  plot hiso2*(population rain)/pbspline;
run;
```

Figure 11.10 shows the resulting plots, both of which suggest nonlinear relationships. We now fit a logistic model with a spline smooth of average rainfall:

```
ods graphics on;
proc gam data=usair;
 model hiso2=spline(rain,df=2)/dist=binary;
 output out=gamout p;
run;
ods graphics off;
```

The `dist` = option on the `model` statement specifies that the outcome is binary. The degree of smoothing for spline smooth of rain is set to two degrees of freedom. In the case of a spline smooth, one of these degrees of freedom is allocated to the linear component. ODS graphics are used to generate the component plot, which is shown in Figure 11.11. The `output` statement with the p option saves the predicted values in the `gamout` data set. The output is shown in Table 11.7. There we see that the linear component is not significant but that the nonlinear smooth is. The predicted values (p_hiso2) in the

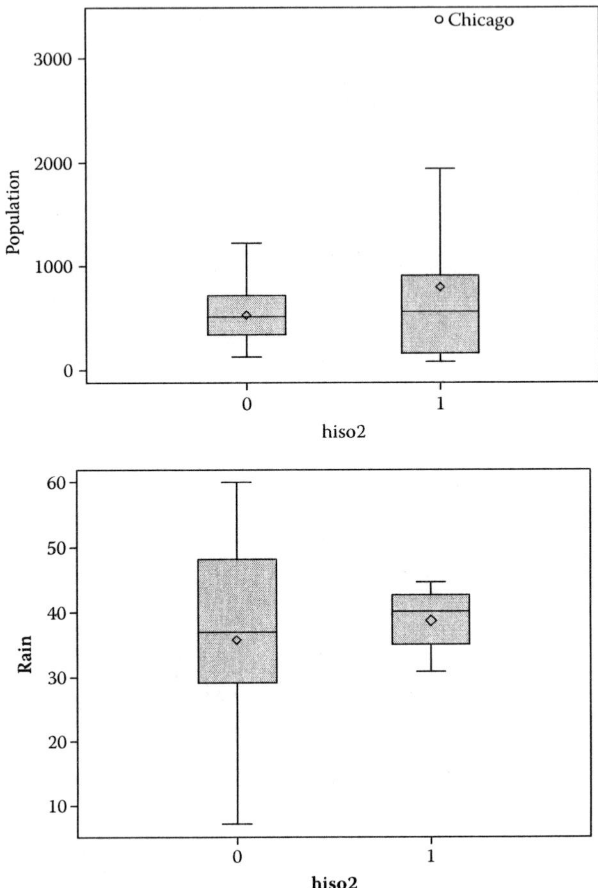

FIGURE 11.9
Box plots for average rainfall and population size for the air pollution data.

output data set are the log odds of a high SO_2 value. The predicted probabilities can be calculated and plotted as follows:

```
data gamout;
  set gamout;
  odds=exp(P_hiso2);
  pred=odds/(1+odds);
run;

proc sort data=gamout; by rain; run;
proc sgplot data=gamout;
  series y=pred x=rain;
run;
```

The resulting plot is shown in Figure 11.12.

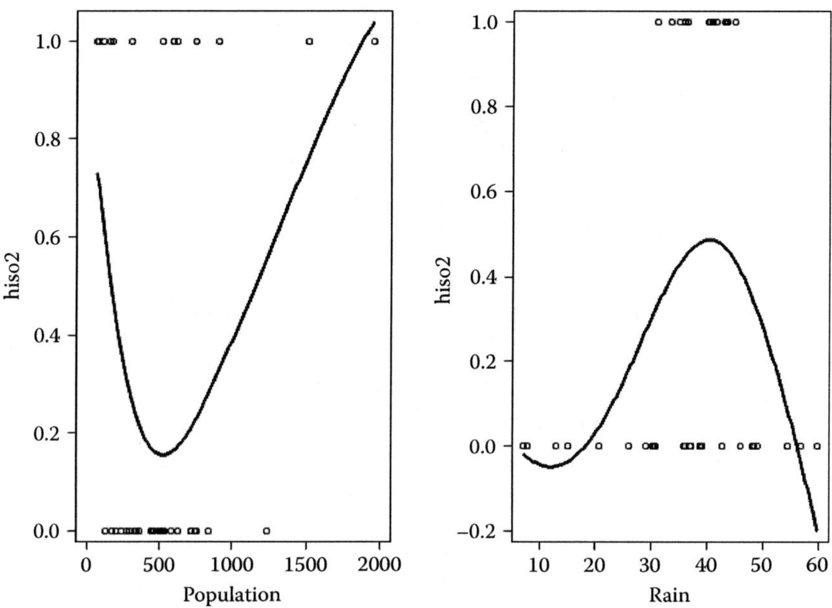

FIGURE 11.10
Plots of average rainfall and population size against high SO_2 for the US air pollution data.

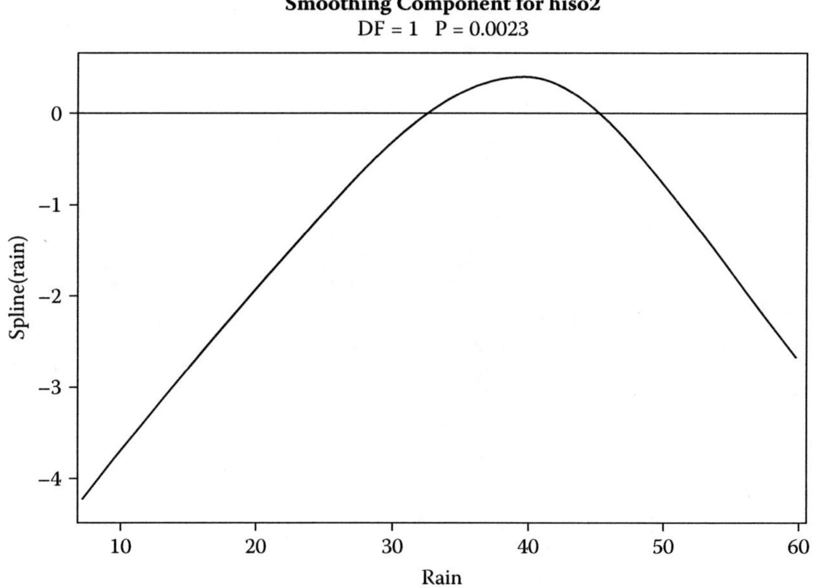

FIGURE 11.11
Fitted function for average rainfall for the air pollution data.

TABLE 11.7

Results from Fitting a GAM to the Air Pollution Data in Table 11.6

| *Dependent Variable: Hiso2* |
| *Smoothing Model Component(s): Spline(rain)* |

Summary of Input Data Set	
Number of Observations	40
Number of Missing Observations	0
Distribution	Binomial
Link Function	Logit

Response profile		
Ordered Value	hiso2	Total Frequency
1	0	27
2	1	13

Note: PROC GAM is modelling the probability that hiso2 = 1. One way to change this in order to model the probability that hiso2 = 0 is to specify the response variable option EVENT='0'.

Iteration Summary and Fit Statistics	
Number of Local Scoring Iterations	17
Local Scoring Convergence Criterion	8.619436E-10
Final Number of Backfitting Iterations	1
Final Backfitting Criterion	6.0285409E-9
Deviance of the Final Estimate	40.425572908

The local scoring algorithm converged.

Regression Model Analysis Parameter Estimates				
Parameter	Parameter Estimate	Standard Error	t Value	Pr > |t|
Intercept	−0.85734	2.05467	−0.42	0.6789
Linear(rain)	0.00886	0.05190	0.17	0.8654

TABLE 11.7 (*Continued*)

Results from Fitting a GAM to the Air Pollution Data in Table 11.6

Smoothing Model Analysis Fit Summary for Smoothing Components				
Component	Smoothing Parameter	DF	GCV	Num Unique Obs
Spline(rain)	0.999899	1.000000	29.622066	40

Smoothing Model Analysis Analysis of Deviance				
Source	DF	Sum of Squares	Chi-Square	Pr > ChiSq
Spline(rain)	1.00000	9.312978	9.3130	0.0023

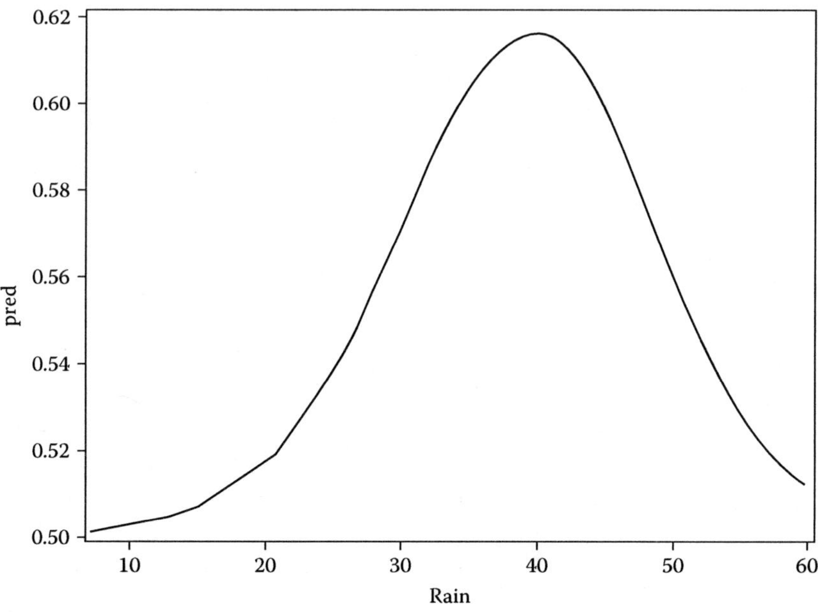

FIGURE 11.12

Predicted values for average rainfall for the US air pollution data.

11.5 Summary

Generalised additive models provide a useful addition to the tools available for exploring the relationship between a response variable and a set of explanatory variables. Such models allow possible nonlinear terms in the latter to be uncovered and, perhaps, then to be modelled in terms of more familiar low-degree polynomials. The GAM model can deal with nonlinearity in covariates that are not the main interest in a study and 'adjust' for those effects appropriately.

12

Analysis of Longitudinal Data I

12.1 Introduction

Longitudinal data arise when participants in a study are measured on the same variable (or variables) on several different occasions. Such data arise frequently in medical investigations, particularly from clinical trials. An example (taken from Davis 2002) is shown in Table 12.1. Here, 40 male subjects were randomly assigned to one of two treatment groups; each patient had been rated on the brief psychiatric rating scale (BPRS) measured before treatment (week 0) and at weekly intervals for 8 weeks. The BPRS assesses the level of 18 symptom constructs such as hostility, suspiciousness, hallucination, and grandiosity; each is rated from 1 (not present) to 7 (extremely severe). The scale is used to evaluate patients suspected of having schizophrenia. Longitudinal data can be analysed in a variety of ways ranging from the simple to the relatively complex. In this chapter, we concentrate on the former, leaving the latter until Chapters 13 and 14.

12.2 Graphical Displays of Longitudinal Data

Graphical displays of data are almost always useful for exposing patterns in the data, particularly when these are unexpected; this might be of great help in suggesting which class of models might be most sensibly applied in the later, more formal analysis. According to Diggle, Liang, and Zeger (2002), there is no single prescription for making effective graphical displays of longitudinal data, although they do offer the following simple guidelines:

- Show as much of the relevant raw data as possible rather than only data summaries.
- Highlight aggregate patterns of potential scientific interest.
- Identify both cross-sectional and longitudinal patterns.

TABLE 12.1

BPRS Measurements from 40 Subjects

		Week								
	Subject	**0**	**1**	**2**	**3**	**4**	**5**	**6**	**7**	**8**
Treatment 1	1	42	36	36	43	41	40	38	47	51
	2	58	68	61	55	43	34	28	28	28
	3	54	55	41	38	43	28	29	25	24
	4	55	77	49	54	56	50	47	42	46
	5	72	75	72	65	50	39	32	38	32
	6	48	43	41	38	36	29	33	27	25
	7	71	61	47	30	27	40	30	31	31
	8	30	36	38	38	31	26	26	25	24
	9	41	43	39	35	28	22	20	23	21
	10	57	51	51	55	53	43	43	39	32
	11	30	34	34	41	36	36	38	36	36
	12	55	52	49	54	48	43	37	36	31
	13	36	32	36	31	25	25	21	19	22
	14	38	35	36	34	25	27	25	26	26
	15	66	68	65	49	36	32	27	30	37
	16	41	35	45	42	31	31	29	26	30
	17	45	38	46	38	40	33	27	31	27
	18	39	35	27	25	29	28	21	25	20
	19	24	28	31	28	29	21	22	23	22
	20	38	34	27	25	25	27	21	19	21
Treatment 2	1	52	73	42	41	39	38	43	62	50
	2	30	23	32	24	20	20	19	18	20
	3	65	31	33	28	22	25	24	31	32
	4	37	31	27	31	31	26	24	26	23
	5	59	67	58	61	49	38	37	36	35
	6	30	33	37	33	28	26	27	23	21
	7	69	52	41	33	34	37	37	38	35
	8	62	54	49	39	55	51	55	59	66
	9	38	40	38	27	31	24	22	21	21
	10	65	44	31	34	39	34	41	42	39
	11	78	95	75	76	66	64	64	60	75
	12	38	41	36	27	29	27	21	22	23
	13	63	65	60	53	52	32	37	52	28
	14	40	37	31	38	35	30	33	30	27
	15	40	36	55	55	42	30	26	30	37
	16	54	45	35	27	25	22	22	22	22
	17	33	41	30	32	46	43	43	43	43
	18	28	30	29	33	30	26	36	33	30

TABLE 12.1 (*Continued*)

BPRS Measurements from 40 Subjects

					Week				
Subject	**0**	**1**	**2**	**3**	**4**	**5**	**6**	**7**	**8**
19	52	43	26	27	24	32	21	21	21
20	47	36	32	29	25	23	23	23	23

Source: Davis, C. S. 2002. *Statistical Methods for the Analysis of Repeated Measurements.* New York: Springer.

- Try to make the identification of unusual individuals or unusual observations simple.

A number of graphical displays which can be useful in the preliminary assessment of longitudinal data from clinical trials will now be illustrated using the data shown in Table 12.1. But before this, we need a small digression to explain how data sets for longitudinal and repeated-measures data can be structured in two ways. In the first form, there is one observation per subject (typically per person) and the repeated measurements are held in separate variables. We shall refer to this form as the 'wide' form. Alternatively, there may be a separate observation for each measurement occasion, with variables indicating which subject and occasion it belongs to. This is the 'long' form of the data set. Usually, both forms will be needed. The wide form is useful for calculating summary measures, whereas the long form is needed for plots and the types of analyses covered in the next chapter.

Returning to the example involving the BPRS scores, we begin by reading in the data in the 'wide' format:

```
data bprs;
   input id x0-x8;
   group=1;
   if _n_>20 then group=2;
   id=100*group+id;
cards;
       1       42      36      36      43      41      40      38      47      51
       2       58      68      61      55      43      34      28      28      28
...
      20       38      34      27      25      25      27      21      19      21
       1       52      73      42      41      39      38      43      62      50
       2       30      23      32      24      20      20      19      18      20
...
      20       47      36      32      29      25      23      23      23      23
;
```

The subjects are numbered consecutively within treatment groups. The SAS automatic variable `_n_` is used to assign them to groups and a unique `id` variable is calculated. We then reformat the data set to the long form:

```
data bprsl;
  set bprs;
  array xs {*} x0-x8;
  do week=0 to 8;
   bprs=xs{week+1};
   output;
  end;
  keep id group week weekgroup bprs;
run;
proc print data=bprsl(obs=45) noobs;
run;
```

The key elements of the data step needed to do this are the `array` statement, the iterative do group, and the `output` statement. These were introduced in Chapter 2, in which we dealt with the equivalent situation where each line of raw data contained values for several subjects. To recap briefly, the `array` statement declares a shorthand alias, `xs`, for the variables `x0` to `x8`. The iterative do statement repeats the following statements, up to the corresponding end statement, a number of times with the index variable changing at each repetition. In this instance, there are nine repetitions with the index variable—week—taking values 0, 1, 2, ..., 8. The elements of an array are always numbered from 1, so we need to add one to week. The `output` statement writes out an observation to the data set being created with the current values of all variables. As this is between the do statement and the end statement, nine observations are created for every one read in.

The resulting long form of the data for the first five subjects in Table 12.1 is given in Table 12.2.

Having reformatted the data, we can plot the BPRS values for all 40 men, differentiating between the treatment groups into which the men have been randomised:

```
proc sgpanel data=bprsl;
  panelby group / spacing=10;
  series y=bprs x=week /group=id;
run;
```

The resulting diagram is shown in Figure 12.1. This simple graph makes a number of features of the data readily apparent. First, the BPRS factor of almost all the men is decreasing over the 8 weeks of the study. Second, the men who have higher BPRS values at the beginning tend to have higher values throughout the study. This phenomenon is generally referred to as *tracking*. Third, there are substantial individual differences and variability appears to decrease with time.

The tracking phenomenon can be seen more clearly in a plot of the standardised values of each observation—that is, the values obtained by subtracting the relevant occasion mean from the original observation and then dividing by the corresponding visit standard deviation. The following code produces Figure 12.2:

TABLE 12.2

Long Form of the Data for the First Five
Subjects in Table 12.1

Id	Group	Week	bprs
101	1	0	42
101	1	1	36
101	1	2	36
101	1	3	43
101	1	4	41
101	1	5	40
101	1	6	38
101	1	7	47
101	1	8	51
102	1	0	58
102	1	1	68
102	1	2	61
102	1	3	55
102	1	4	43
102	1	5	34
102	1	6	28
102	1	7	28
102	1	8	28
103	1	0	54
103	1	1	55
103	1	2	41
103	1	3	38
103	1	4	43
103	1	5	28
103	1	6	29
103	1	7	25
103	1	8	24
104	1	0	55
104	1	1	77
104	1	2	49
104	1	3	54
104	1	4	56
104	1	5	50
104	1	6	47
104	1	7	42
104	1	8	46
105	1	0	72
105	1	1	75
105	1	2	72
105	1	3	65

(Continued)

TABLE 12.2 (*Continued*)

Long Form of the Data for the First Five
Subjects in Table 12.1

Id	Group	Week	bprs
105	1	4	50
105	1	5	39
105	1	6	32
105	1	7	38
105	1	8	32

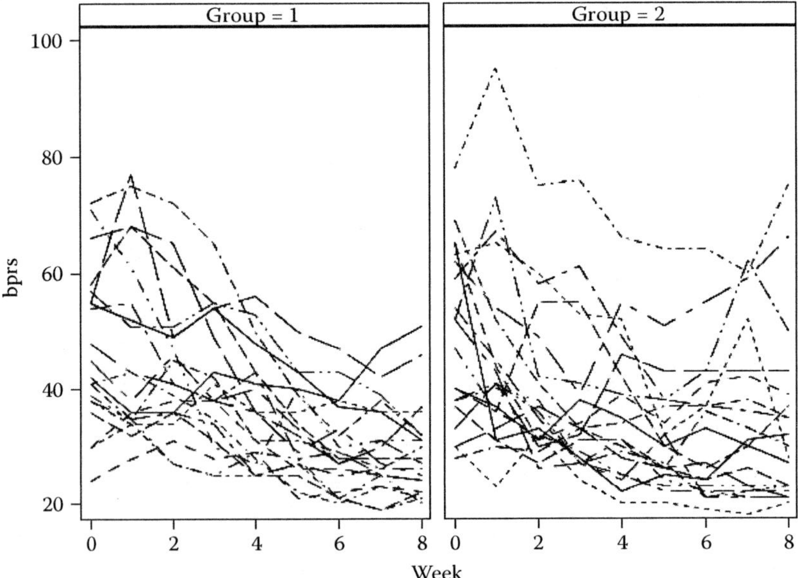

FIGURE 12.1
Individual response profiles by treatment group for the BPRS data.

```
proc sort data=bprsl;
 by week;
run;
proc stdize data=bprsl out=bprslz method=std;
  var bprs;
  by week;
run;
proc sgpanel data=bprslz;
  panelby group / spacing=10;
  series y=bprs x=week /group=id;
run;
```

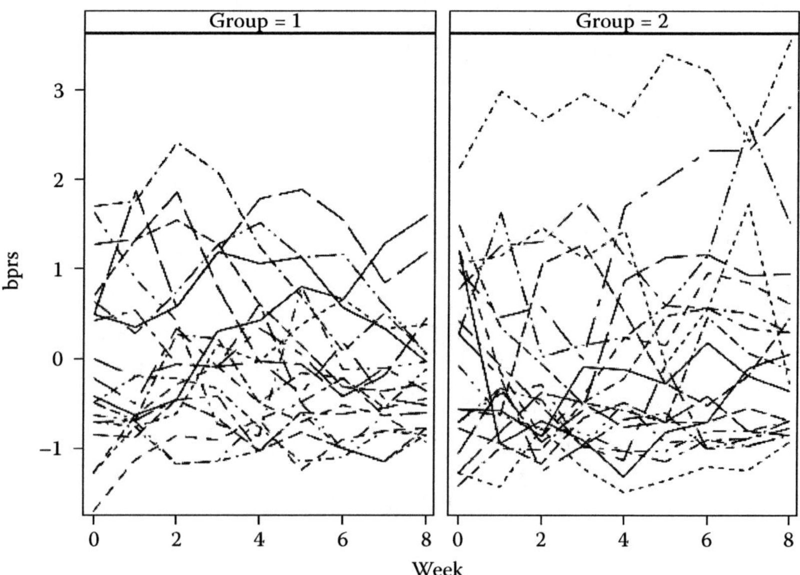

FIGURE 12.2
Individual response profiles for BPRS data after standardization.

The data are first sorted by week. `Proc stdize`, with the `method=std` option and the `by week` statement, then standardises within each measurement occasion. The `var bprs` statement specifies the variable to be standardised; the default is for all numeric variables to be. The standardised values are saved in the data set `bprslz`.

With large numbers of observations, graphical displays of individual response profiles are of little use and investigators then commonly produce graphs showing average profiles for each treatment group along with some indication of the variation of the observations at each time point. Such a graph can be constructed by using a `vline` plot within `proc sgplot`:

```
proc sgplot data=bprsl;
  vline week/response=bprs stat=mean group=group
  limitstat=stderr;
run;
```

The result is shown in Figure 12.3. There is considerable overlap in the mean profiles of the two treatment groups, suggesting perhaps that there is little difference between the two groups with respect to the mean BPRS values.

A possible alternative to plotting the mean profiles as in Figure 12.3 is to graph side-by-side box plots of the observations at each time point:

```
proc sgplot data=bprsl;
  vbox bprs/category=week group=group nomean nocaps;
run;
```

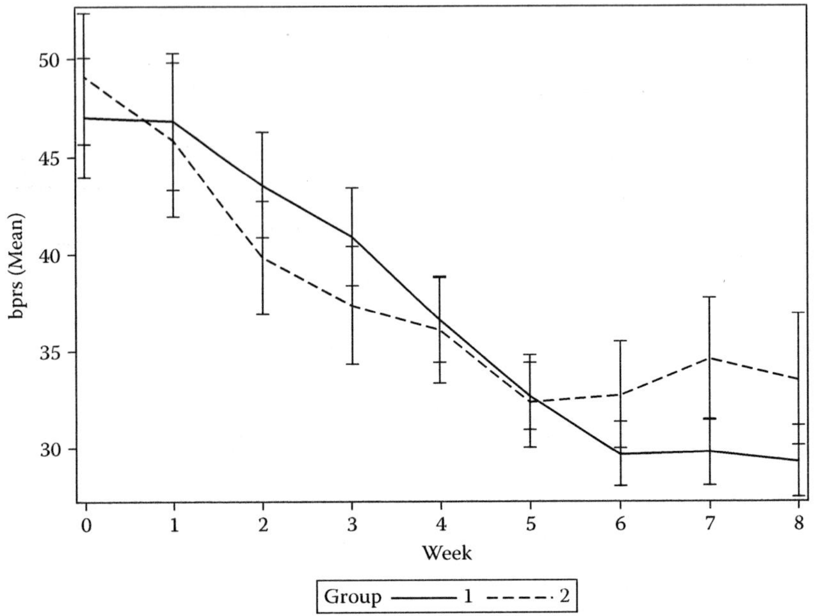

FIGURE 12.3
Mean response profiles for the two treatment groups in the BPRS data.

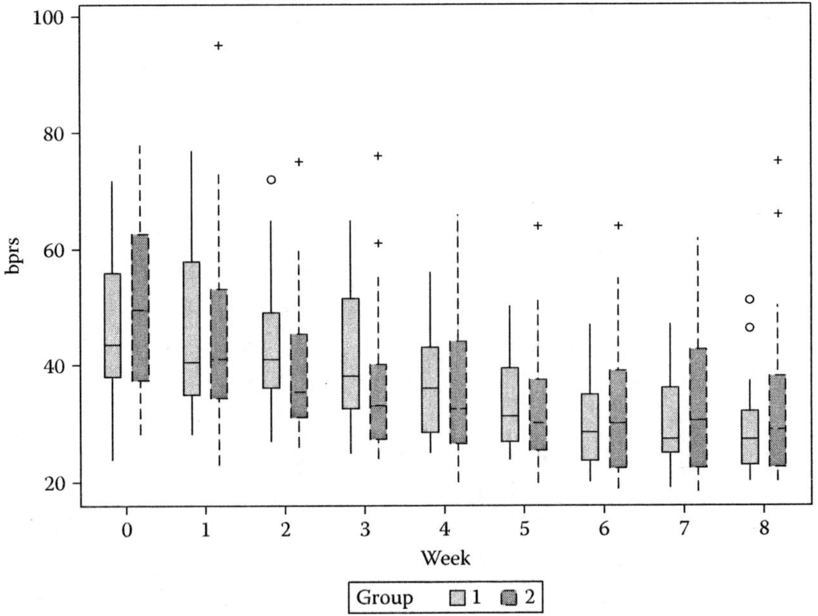

FIGURE 12.4
Box plots for the BPRS data.

The resulting plot is shown in Figure 12.4. The plot suggests the presence of some possible 'outliers' at a number of time points and indicates again the general decline in BPRS values over the 8 weeks of the study in both treatment groups.

Another graphic for longitudinal data that is often helpful in making informed decisions about models that might be appropriate for the data is the scatter plot matrix (see Chapter 8). But we shall leave consideration of this type of plot until the next chapter, when we begin to discuss possible models for longitudinal data.

12.3 Summary Measure Analysis of Longitudinal Data

According to Matthews (2005), 'the use of summary measures is one of the most important and straightforward methods for the analysis of longitudinal data'. The approach is certainly straightforward, but as to 'most important'—we think not. The models to be described in the next two chapters are of far greater importance for dealing appropriately with longitudinal data. Nevertheless, we will describe the summary measure method (often also called the *response feature method*) here because it may be helpful in some cases for a 'quick-and-dirty' assessment of longitudinal data.

The summary measure method operates by transforming the T repeated measurements made on the ith individual in the study, $\mathbf{x}'_i = [x_{i1} \ldots x_{iT}]$, into a single value that captures some essential feature of the patient's response over time (see later discussion). Analysis then proceeds by applying standard univariate methods to the summary measures from the sample of patients (see later examples). The approach has been in use for many years and is described in Oldham (1962), Yates (1982), and Matthews et al. (1990).

12.3.1 Choosing Summary Measures

The key step to a successful summary measure analysis of longitudinal data is the choice of a relevant summary measure. The chosen measure needs to be relevant to the particular questions of interest in the study and in the broader scientific context in which the study takes place. In some longitudinal studies, more than a single summary measure might be deemed relevant or necessary, in which case the problem of combined inference may need to be addressed. More often in practice, however, it is likely that the different measures will deal with substantially different questions so that each will have a notional interpretation in its own right. In most investigations, the decision over what summary measure to use needs to be made before the data are collected.

A wide range of possible summary measures have been proposed. Those given in Table 12.3, for example, were suggested by Matthews et al. (1990).

TABLE 12.3

Possible Summary Measures

Type of Data	Question of Interest	Summary Measure
Peaked	Is overall value of outcome variable the same in different groups?	Overall mean (equal time intervals) or area under curve (unequal intervals)
Peaked	Is maximum (minimum) response different between groups?	Maximum (minimum) value
Peaked	Is time to maximum (minimum) response different between groups?	Time to maximum (minimum) response
Growth	Is rate of change of outcome different between groups?	Regression coefficient
Growth	Is eventual value of outcome different between groups?	Final value of outcome or difference between last and first values or percentage change between first and last values
Growth	Is response in one group delayed relative to the other?	Time to reach a particular value (e.g., a fixed percentage of baseline)

Frison and Pocock (1992) argue that the average response to treatment over time is often likely to be the most relevant summary statistic in treatment trials. In some cases, the response on a particular visit may be chosen as the summary statistic of most interest, but this must be distinguished from the generally flawed approach, which separately analyses the observations at each and every time point.

12.3.2 Applying the Summary Measure Approach

As our first example of the summary measure approach, it will be applied to the post-treatment values of the BPRS in Table 12.1. The mean of weeks 1 to 8 will be the chosen summary measure. We first calculate this measure and then look at box plots of the measure for each treatment group:

```
data bprs;
 set bprs;
 mnbprs=mean(of x1-x8);
run;
proc sgplot data=bprs;
   vbox mnbprs / category=group;
run;
```

When a variable list is to be used with the mean function it must be preceded by of.

The resulting plot is shown in Figure 12.5. The diagram indicates that the mean summary measure is more variable in the second treatment group and

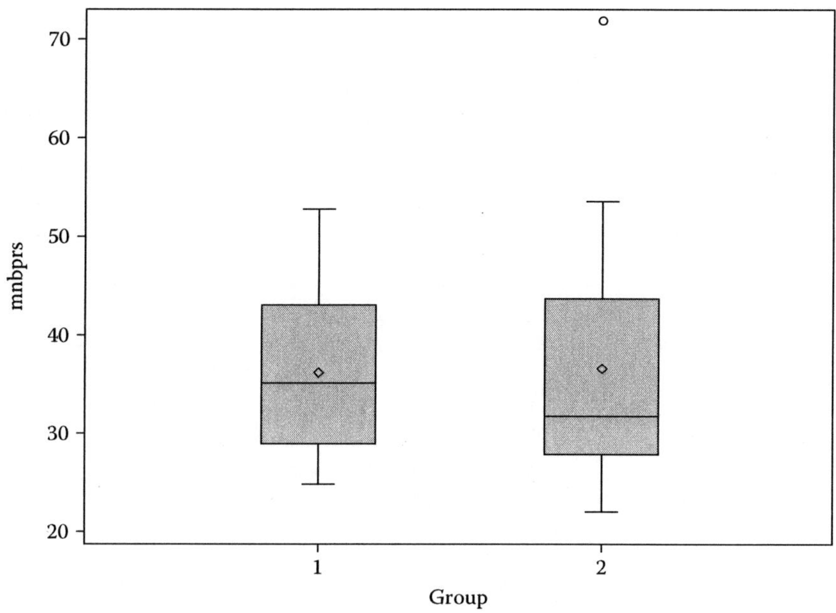

FIGURE 12.5
Box plots of mean summary measures for the two treatment groups in the BPRS data.

its distribution in this group is somewhat skewed. There is little evidence of a difference in location of the summary measure distributions in each group.

Although all the informal graphical material presented up to now has indicated a lack of difference in the two treatment groups, most investigators would still require a formal test for a difference. Consequently, we shall now apply a *t*-test to assess any difference between the treatment groups and also calculate a confidence interval for this difference:

```
proc ttest data=bprs;
   class group;
   var mnbprs;
run;
```

The results are shown in Table 12.4. The *t*-test confirms the lack of any evidence for a group difference.

12.3.3 Incorporating Pretreatment Outcome Values into the Summary Measure Approach

Baseline measurements of the outcome variable in a longitudinal study are often correlated with the chosen summary measure, and using such

TABLE 12.4

Results from an Independent Sample *t*-Test on the Mean Summary Measure
for the BPRS Data in Table 12.1

			Variable: mnbprs			
group	N	Mean	Std Dev	Std Err	Minimum	Maximum
1	20	36.1688	8.3691	1.8714	24.8750	52.6250
2	20	36.5625	12.2090	2.7300	22.0000	71.8750
Diff (1–2)		–0.3937	10.4667	3.3098		

group	Method	Mean	95% CL Mean		Std Dev	95% CL Std Dev	
1		36.1688	32.2519	40.0856	8.3691	6.3646	12.2236
2		36.5625	30.8485	42.2765	12.2090	9.2848	17.8321
Diff (1–2)	Pooled	–0.3937	–7.0942	6.3067	10.4667	8.5538	13.4892
Diff (1–2)	Satterthwaite	–0.3937	–7.1229	6.3354			

Method	Variances	DF	t Value	Pr > |t|
Pooled	Equal	38	–0.12	0.9059
Satterthwaite	Unequal	33.626	–0.12	0.9060

	Equality of Variances			
Method	Num DF	Den DF	F Value	Pr > F
Folded F	19	19	2.13	0.1083

measures in the analysis can often lead to substantial gains in precision when
used appropriately as a covariate in an analysis of covariance (see Everitt and
Pickles 2004). We can illustrate the analysis on the data in Table 12.1 using the
BPRS value corresponding to time zero taken prior to the start of treatment
as the baseline covariate. The SAS code needed for the analysis of covariance
of the mean summary measure with treatment group and week 0 value as
covariates is

```
proc glm data=bprs;
  class group;
  model mnbprs=x0 group;
run;
```

The results are shown in Table 12.5. We see that the baseline BPRS is strongly
related to the BPRS values taken after treatment has begun, but there is
still no evidence of a treatment difference even after conditioning on the
baseline value.

TABLE 12.5

Results from an Analysis of Covariance of the BPRS Data with Baseline BPRS and Group as Covariates

Class–Level Information		
Class	**Levels**	**Values**
group	2	1 2

Number of Observations Read	40
Number of Observations Used	40

Dependent Variable: mnbprs					
Source	**DF**	**Sum of Squares**	**Mean Square**	**F Value**	**Pr > F**
Model	2	1871.515626	935.757813	15.10	<.0001
Error	37	2292.965234	61.972033		
Corrected Total	39	4164.480859			

R-Square	**Coeff Var**	**Root MSE**	**mnbprs Mean**
0.449400	21.64745	7.872232	36.36563

Source	**DF**	**Type I SS**	**Mean Square**	**F Value**	**Pr > F**
x0	1	1868.066649	1868.066649	30.14	<.0001
group	1	3.448977	3.448977	0.06	0.8148

Source	**DF**	**Type III SS**	**Mean Square**	**F Value**	**Pr > F**
x0	1	1869.965235	1869.965235	30.17	<.0001
group	1	3.448977	3.448977	0.06	0.8148

12.3.4 Dealing with Missing Values When Using the Summary Measure Approach

One of the problems that often occurs in the collection of longitudinal data is that a patient may not have values of the outcome measure recorded on all the occasions intended. This problem will be considered in detail in the next chapter, but as an example of where it has arisen, we can examine the data shown in Table 12.6 (taken from Davis 2002). The data come from a clinical trial comparing two treatments for maternal pain relief during labour. In this study, 83 women in labour were randomised to receive an experimental pain

TABLE 12.6

Pain Scores from 83 Women in Labour: First 20 Subjects in Each Group

	Patient	**Self-Reported Pain Scores at 30-Minute Intervals**						
		0	**30**	**60**	**90**	**120**	**150**	**180**
Group 1	1	0.0	0.0	0.0	0.0			
	2	0.0	0.0	0.0	0.0	2.5	2.3	14.0
	3	38.0	5.0	1.0	1.0	0.0	5.0	
	4	6.0	48.0	85.0	0.0	0.0		
	5	19.0	5.0					
	6	7.0	0.0	0.0	0.0			
	7	44.0	42.0	42.0	45.0			
	8	1.0	0.0	0.0	0.0	0.0	6.0	24.0
	9	24.5	35.0	13.0				
	10	1.0	30.5	81.5	67.5	98.5	97.0	
	11	35.5	44.5	55.0	69.0	72.5	39.5	26.0
	12	0.0	0.0	0.0	0.0	0.0	0.0	0.0
	13	8.0	30.5	26.0	24.0	29.0	45.0	91.0
	14	7.0	6.5	7.0	4.0	10.0		
	15	6.0	8.5	19.5	16.5	42.5	45.5	48.5
	16	32.5	9.5	7.5	5.5	4.5	0.0	7.0
	17	10.5	10.0	18.0	32.5	0.0	0.0	0.0
	18	11.5	20.5	32.5	37.0	39.0		
	19	72.0	91.5	4.5	32.0	10.5	10.5	10.5
	20	0.0	0.0	0.0	0.0	13.54	7.0	
Group 2	1	4.0	9.0	30.0	75.0	49.0	97.0	
	2	0.0	0.0	1.0	27.5	95.0	100.0	
	3	9.0	6.0	25.0				
	4	52.5	18.0	12.5				
	5	90.5	99.0	100.0	100.0	100.0	100.0	100.0
	6	74.0	70.0	81.5	94.5	97.0		
	7	0.0	0.0	0.0	1.5	0.0	18.0	71.0
	8	0.0	51.5	56.0				
	9	6.5	7.0	7.0	9.0	25.0	36.0	20.0
	10	19.0	31.0	41.0	58.0			
	11	6.0	23.0	45.0	67.0	90.5		
	12	42.0	64.0	6.0				
	13	86.5	53.0	88.0	100.0	100.0		
	14	50.0	100.0	100.0	100.0	100.0		
	15	27.5	36.5	74.0	97.0	100.0	100.0	95.0
	16	0.0	0.0	6.0	6.0			
	17	62.0	79.0	80.5	85.0	90.0	97.5	97.0
	18	17.5	27.5	21.0	60.0	80.0	97.0	
	19	6.5	5.5	18.5	20.0	36.5	63.5	81.5
	20	8.0	9.0	35.5	39.0	70.0	92.0	98.0

medication (43 subjects) or placebo (40 subjects). Treatment was initiated when the cervical dilation was 8 cm. At 30-minute intervals, the amount of pain was self-reported by placing a mark on a 100 mm line ($0 =$ no pain, $100 =$ very much pain). Table 12.6 gives the data for the first 20 subjects in each group.

If we use the mean as a summary measure for these data, we can deal with the missing values simply by calculating, for each subject, the mean of her *available* values. For example, for subject 1, this would be the mean of four values and, for subject 2, the mean of three values. This is clearly very straightforward, but Matthews (1993) points out a number of possible problems:

- If the summary measures are based on observations that have widely differing structures, then, even within apparently homogeneous groups, they will not share a common distribution, contrary to the assumptions of most of the methods of analysis that are likely to be applied.

- The reason that observations are missing needs to be considered. (This problem is discussed in the next chapter.)

Here, we shall ignore these possible difficulties and carry out the summary measure analysis using the following SAS code:

```
data labour;
   infile cards missover;
   input id x0-x6;
   group=1;
   if _n_ >20 then group=2;
   mnpain=mean(of x0-x6);
cards;
       1      0.0     0.0     0.0     0.0
       2      0.0     0.0     0.0     0.0     2.5     2.3    14.0
       3     38.0     5.0     1.0     1.0     0.0     5.0
....
      19      6.5     5.5    18.5    20.0    36.5    63.5    81.5
      20      8.0     9.0    35.5    39.0    70.0    92.0    98.0
;

proc ttest data=labour;
   class group;
   var mnpain;
run;
```

The `infile` statement is not usually needed when the data are instream— that is, included at the end of the data step after a `cards` or `datalines` statement. Including it allows options to be used to modify the way the data are read. In this case, the `missover` option prevents SAS from going to a new line when there are fewer data values than variables. Instead, the remaining variables are set to missing values. The results are shown in Table 12.7.

TABLE 12.7

Results from an Independent Sample *t*-Test for the Mean Summary Measure Used on the Data in Table 12.6

Variable: mnpain						
group	N	Mean	Std Dev	Std Err	Minimum	Maximum
1	20	19.5002	18.2679	4.0848	0	62.6667
2	20	48.1040	28.7643	6.4319	3.0000	98.5000
Diff (1–2)		−28.6038	24.0946	7.6194		

group	Method	Mean	95% CL Mean		Std Dev	95% CL Std Dev	
1		19.5002	10.9506	28.0499	18.2679	13.8926	26.6816
2		48.1040	34.6420	61.5661	28.7643	21.8749	42.0123
Diff (1–2)	Pooled	−28.6038	−44.0285	−13.1792	24.0946	19.6912	31.0526
Diff (1–2)	Satterthwaite	−28.6038	−44.1206	−13.0871			

Method	Variances	DF	t Value	Pr > |t|
Pooled	Equal	38	−3.75	0.0006
Satterthwaite	Unequal	32.182	−3.75	0.0007

Equality of Variances				
Method	Num DF	Den DF	F Value	Pr > F
Folded F	19	19	2.48	0.0547

There is strong evidence of a treatment difference for these data. The 95% confidence interval for the difference is [−44.03,−13.18]. The experimental treatment appears to have lowered the average pain score by between 13 and 44 points on the visual analogue scale.

12.4 Summary Measure Approach for Binary Responses

Table 12.8 shows part of the data collected in a clinical trial comparing two treatments for a respiratory illness (Davis 1991). In each of the two centres, eligible patients were randomly assigned to active treatment or placebo. During treatment, the respiratory status (categorised as 0 = poor, 1 = good) was determined at four visits. There were 111 patients (54 active, 57 placebo) with no missing data for responses or covariates. Data for the first five patients are shown in Table 12.8.

TABLE 12.8

Respiratory Disorder Data for First 5 of 111 Patients

Patient	Centre	Treatment	Sex	Age	BL	V1	V2	V3	V4
1	1	1	1	46	0	0	0	0	0
2	1	1	1	28	0	0	0	0	0
3	1	2	1	23	1	1	1	1	1
4	1	1	1	44	1	1	1	1	0
5	1	1	2	13	1	1	1	1	1

Notes: Treatment: 1 = placebo; 2 = active. Sex: 1 = male; 2 = female.

Here we shall consider how the response feature approach can be applied to this binary response, with the initial analysis ignoring all covariates except treatment group. We might, of course, simply ignore the binary nature of the response variable and compare the 'mean' responses over time in the two treatment groups by a *t*-test. Since the mean in this case is the proportion (p) of visits at which a patient's respiratory status was good, we could consider performing the test after taking some appropriate transformation, for example, arcsin (p) or arcsin ($\sqrt{p}$):

```
data resptrial;
  input id centre treat sex age bl v1-v4;
  ngood=sum(of v1-v4);
  visits=4;
  mnstatus=mean(of v1-v4);
  arcsin=arsin(mnstatus);
  arcroot=arsin(sqrt(mnstatus));
cards;
1    1    1    1    46    0    0    0    0    0
2    1    1    1    28    0    0    0    0    0
3    1    2    1    23    1    1    1    1    1
....
110  2    2    2    63    1    1    1    1    1
111  2    2    1    31    1    1    1    1    1
;

proc ttest data=resptrial;
  class treat;
  var mnstatus arcsin arcroot;
run;
```

The results are shown in Table 12.9. There is clear evidence of a treatment difference, whether the untransformed or transformed summary measure is analysed. On average, there is a higher proportion of 'good' responses in the active treatment group.

TABLE 12.9

Results from Summary Measure Analysis Applied to the Respiratory Data in Table 12.8

			Variable: mnstatus			
treat	N	Mean	Std Dev	Std Err	Minimum	Maximum
1	57	0.4430	0.3981	0.0527	0	1.0000
2	54	0.6852	0.3704	0.0504	0	1.0000
Diff (1–2)		−0.2422	0.3849	0.0731		

treat	Method	Mean	95% CL Mean		Std Dev	95% CL Std Dev	
1		0.4430	0.3373	0.5486	0.3981	0.3361	0.4884
2		0.6852	0.5841	0.7863	0.3704	0.3114	0.4573
Diff (1–2)	Pooled	−0.2422	−0.3871	−0.0973	0.3849	0.3399	0.4438
Diff (1–2)	Satterthwaite	−0.2422	−0.3868	−0.0976			

Method	Variances	DF	t Value	Pr > |t|
Pooled	Equal	109	−3.31	0.0013
Satterthwaite	Unequal	108.97	−3.32	0.0012

Equality of Variances				
Method	Num DF	Den DF	F Value	Pr > F
Folded F	56	53	1.16	0.5984

			Variable: arcsin			
treat	N	Mean	Std dev	Std Err	Minimum	Maximum
1	57	0.5907	0.6082	0.0806	0	1.5708
2	54	0.9715	0.6169	0.0840	0	1.5708
Diff (1–2)		−0.3809	0.6124	0.1163		

treat	Method	Mean	95% CL Mean		Std Dev	95% CL Std Dev	
1		0.5907	0.4293	0.7520	0.6082	0.5134	0.7460
2		0.9715	0.8031	1.1399	0.6169	0.5186	0.7616
Diff (1–2)	Pooled	−0.3809	−0.6114	−0.1503	0.6124	0.5408	0.7061
Diff (1–2)	Satterthwaite	−0.3809	−0.6115	−0.1502			

Method	Variances	DF	t Value	Pr > |t|
Pooled	Equal	109	−3.27	0.0014
Satterthwaite	Unequal	108.48	−3.27	0.0014

TABLE 12.9 (*Continued*)

Results from Summary Measure Analysis Applied to the Respiratory Data in Table 12.8

Equality of Variances				
Method	**Num DF**	**Den DF**	**F Value**	**Pr > F**
Folded F	53	56	1.03	0.9141

Variable: arcroot						
treat	**N**	**Mean**	**Std Dev**	**Std Err**	**Minimum**	**Maximum**
1	57	0.6981	0.6046	0.0801	0	1.5708
2	54	1.0666	0.5614	0.0764	0	1.5708
Diff (1–2)		−0.3685	0.5840	0.1109		

treat	**Method**	**Mean**	**95% CL Mean**		**Std Dev**	**95% CL Std Dev**	
1		0.6981	0.5377	0.8586	0.6046	0.5104	0.7417
2		1.0666	0.9134	1.2198	0.5614	0.4719	0.6930
Diff (1–2)	Pooled	−0.3685	−0.5883	−0.1487	0.5840	0.5157	0.6733
Diff (1–2)	Satterthwaite	−0.3685	−0.5878	−0.1491			

Method	**Variances**	**DF**	**t Value**	**Pr > |t|**
Pooled	Equal	109	−3.32	0.0012
Satterthwaite	Unequal	108.96	−3.33	0.0012

Equality of Variances				
Method	**Num DF**	**Den DF**	**F Value**	**Pr > F**
Folded F	56	53	1.16	0.5881

A linear regression of the arcsin-transformed proportion of positive responses over the four postbaseline measurement occasions might be used to assess the effects of the baseline measurement, age, sex, and centre:

```
proc glm data=resptrial;
  class centre treat sex;
  model arcroot=centre age sex bl treat;
run;
```

The results are shown in Table 12.10. Here, we should use the type III sums of squares because these give a test of each covariate *conditional* on all the other covariates in the model. The regression coefficient for centre is marginally

TABLE 12.10

Results from the Linear Regression on the Arcsin-Transformed Proportion of Positive Responses for the Respiratory Data in Table 12.8

Class–Level Information		
Class	**Levels**	**Values**
centre	2	1 2
treat	2	1 2
sex	2	1 2

Number of Observations Read	111
Number of Observations Used	111

Dependent Variable: arcroot

Source	DF	Sum of Squares	Mean Square	F Value	Pr > F
Model	5	16.51257785	3.30251557	14.20	<.0001
Error	105	24.42553350	0.23262413		
Corrected Total	110	40.93811135			

R-Square	Coeff Var	Root MSE	arcroot Mean
0.403355	54.97165	0.482311	0.877382

Source	DF	Type I SS	Mean Square	F Value	Pr > F
centre	1	3.14379291	3.14379291	13.51	0.0004
age	1	1.00083354	1.00083354	4.30	0.0405
sex	1	0.40002818	0.40002818	1.72	0.1926
bl	1	8.27903368	8.27903368	35.59	<.0001
treat	1	3.68888954	3.68888954	15.86	0.0001

Source	DF	Type III SS	Mean Square	F Value	Pr > F
centre	1	0.97656959	0.97656959	4.20	0.0430
age	1	0.43858914	0.43858914	1.89	0.1726
sex	1	0.01684248	0.01684248	0.07	0.7884
bl	1	8.74201567	8.74201567	37.58	<.0001
treat	1	3.68888954	3.68888954	15.86	0.0001

TABLE 12.11

Results from an Overdispersed Logistic Model Fitted to the Proportion of Positive Responses in the Respiratory Data in Table 12.8

Response Profile		
Ordered Value	Binary Outcome	Total Frequency
1	Event	249
2	Nonevent	195

Class–Level Information		
Class	Value	Design Variables
centre	1	0
	2	1
treat	1	0
	2	1
sex	1	0
	2	1

Model Convergence Status
Convergence criterion (GCONV=1E-8) satisfied.

Deviance and Pearson Goodness-of-Fit Statistics				
Criterion	Value	DF	Value/DF	Pr > ChiSq
Deviance	259.2222	105	2.4688	<.0001
Pearson	222.9025	105	2.1229	<.0001

Number of events/trials observations: 111
Note: The covariance matrix has been multiplied by the heterogeneity factor (deviance/DF) 2.46878.

Model Fit Statistics		
Criterion	Intercept Only	Intercept and Covariates
AIC	248.652	207.731
SC	252.748	232.306
−2 Log L	246.652	195.731

(Continued)

TABLE 12.11 (*Continued*)

Results from an Overdispersed Logistic Model Fitted to the Proportion of Positive Responses in the Respiratory Data in Table 12.8

Testing Global Null Hypothesis: BETA = 0			
Test	Chi-Square	DF	Pr > ChiSq
Likelihood Ratio	50.9209	5	<.0001
Score	46.0339	5	<.0001
Wald	37.0374	5	<.0001

Type 3 Analysis of Effects			
Effect	DF	Wald Chi-Square	Pr > ChiSq
centre	1	3.1834	0.0744
age	1	1.7011	0.1921
sex	1	0.0663	0.7968
bl	1	24.6428	<.0001
treat	1	12.1889	0.0005

Analysis of Maximum Likelihood Estimates						
Parameter		DF	Estimate	Standard Error	Wald Chi-Square	Pr > ChiSq
Intercept		1	−0.9002	0.5305	2.8789	0.0897
centre	2	1	0.6716	0.3764	3.1834	0.0744
age		1	−0.0182	0.0139	1.7011	0.1921
sex	2	1	0.1192	0.4630	0.0663	0.7968
bl		1	1.8820	0.3791	24.6428	<.0001
treat	2	1	1.2992	0.3721	12.1889	0.0005

Odds Ratio Estimates			
Effect	Point Estimate	95% Wald Confidence Limits	
centre 2 vs 1	1.957	0.936	4.093
age	0.982	0.956	1.009
sex 2 vs 1	1.127	0.455	2.792
bl	6.567	3.124	13.806
treat 2 vs 1	3.666	1.768	7.603

significant at the 5% level, but both the baseline response and treatment group are highly significant.

A more satisfactory analysis of the respiratory data can be achieved by using the generalised linear modelling approach described in Chapter 10. A standard logistic regression model might be applied, but since the number of occasions on which infection was present out of the four visits made by each participant is unlikely to be binomially distributed (the observations are likely to be correlated rather than independent), we need to allow for possible overdispersion. Fitting a model with logistic link and with treatment, sex, age, and baseline respiratory status as the main effects gives

```
proc logistic data=resptrial;
   class centre treat sex /param=ref ref=first;
   model ngood/visits=centre age sex bl treat /scale=d;
run;
```

The events/trials syntax is used on the `model` statement and `scale=d` sets the dispersion parameter to be the deviance divided by its degrees of freedom. The results are shown in Table 12.11. The estimated value of the scale parameter, 2.47, is substantially above 1, confirming the presence of overdispersion. The estimated odds ratio for the effect of treatment is 3.67 with a 95% confidence interval of [1.77, 7.60]. The active treatment considerably increases the odds of a 'good' respiratory status. The *p*-values from the linear regression in Table 12.10 and the logistic regression in Table 12.11 are comparable, but the estimates from the logit model are on a more natural scale. There is no relatively straightforward interpretation of the estimates from the model fitted to the arcsin-transformed responses, although calculation of an odds ratio at the mean value of the sample covariates could be attempted.

12.5 Summary

The methods described in this chapter are most (only) suitable for an initial exploration and analysis of longitudinal data (often collected in the course of a clinical trial). The graphical methods can provide insights into both potentially interesting patterns of response over time and the structure of any treatment differences. In addition, they can indicate possible outlying observations that may need special attention. The response feature approach to analysis has the distinct advantage that it is straightforward, can be tailored to consider aspects of the data thought to be particularly relevant, and produces results which are relatively simple to understand. Depending on the chosen summary measure, the approach can often accommodate data containing missing values without difficulty, although it might be misleading if the observations are anything other than missing completely at random (see Chapter 13).

But, although simple to apply, the summary measure approach has a number of distinct drawbacks; one is that it forces the investigator to focus on only a single aspect of the repeated measurements over time. It seems intuitively clear that when *T* repeated measures are replaced by a single number summary, there must necessarily be some loss of information. And it is possible for individuals with quite different response profiles to have the same or similar values for the chosen summary measure. Finally, the simplicity of the summary measure method is lost when there are missing data or the repeated measures are irregularly spaced, as is the methods efficiency; the methods to be described in the next two chapters are more efficient than a summary measure analysis and can also handle missing data with minimal difficulty.

13

Analysis of Longitudinal Data II: Linear Mixed-Effects Models for Normal Response Variables

13.1 Introduction

The summary measure approach to the analysis of longitudinal data described in the previous chapter sometimes provides a useful first step in making inferences about the data, but it is really only ever a first step; a more complete and a more appropriate analysis will involve fitting a suitable model to the data and estimating parameters that link the explanatory variables of interest to the repeated measures of the response variable. The main objective in longitudinal studies is to characterise change in the repeated values of the response variable and to determine the explanatory variables most associated with any change.

But because several observations of the response variable are made on the same individual, it is likely that the measurements will be correlated rather than independent, even after conditioning on the explanatory variables. A consequence of this is that suitable models for longitudinal data need to include parameters analogous to the regression coefficients in the usual multiple regression model (see Chapter 8) that relate the explanatory variables to the repeated measurements, *and*, in addition, parameters that account adequately for the correlational structure of the repeated measurements of the response variable.

It is the regression coefficients that are generally of most interest, with the correlational structure parameters often being regarded as *nuisance parameters*. But providing an adequate model for the correlational structure of the repeated measures *is* necessary to avoid misleading inferences about those parameters that are of most importance to the researcher, as is made clear in Fitzmaurice, Laird, and Ware (2004). These authors emphasise that, although the estimation of the correlational structure of the repeated measurements is usually regarded as a secondary aspect of any analysis (relative to the mean response over time), the estimated correlational structure must describe the actual correlational structure present in the data relatively accurately to avoid making misleading inferences on the substantive parameters.

Over the last decade, methodology for the analysis of repeated measures data has been the subject of much research and development and there are now a variety of powerful techniques available. A comprehensive account of these methods is given in Diggle, Liang, and Zeger (2002) and Davis (2002). In this chapter, we will concentrate on a single class of methods, *linear mixed-effects models,* suitable for responses that can be assumed to be approximately normally distributed after conditioning on the explanatory variables. Non-normal responses will be the subject of Chapter 14.

13.2 Linear Mixed-Effects Models for Repeated Measures Data

Linear mixed-effects models for repeated measures data formalise the sensible idea that an individual's pattern of responses is likely to depend on many characteristics of that individual, including some that are unobserved. These unobserved variables are then included in the model as random variables—that is, *random effects.* The essential feature of the model is that the (usually positive) correlation amongst the repeated measurements on the same individual arises from shared, unobserved variables. Fitzmaurice et al. (2004) suggest several possible sources of correlation in longitudinal data, including:

- Between-individual heterogeneity reflecting natural variation in individuals' propensity to respond: some consistently respond higher than the average and others consistently lower. The result is a positive correlation between the repeated measurements of the response.

- Within-individual biological variation: the notion here is that some underlying biological process or processes that change through time in a relatively smooth and continuous fashion lead to random deviations from an individual's underlying response trajectory and are more similar when measurements are obtained very closely together in time. Consequently, measurements taken closely together will typically be more highly correlated than measurements that are further separated in time.

Conditional on the values of the random effects, the repeated measurements are assumed to be independent—the so-called *local independence assumption.*

Two examples of linear mixed-effects models—namely, the *random intercept model* and the *random intercept and slope model*—are introduced and described in the next subsection.

13.2.1 Random Intercept and Random Intercept and Slope Models

Consider a simple set of longitudinal data in which a number of individuals have values of a response variable of interest recorded at times $t_1, t_2, \ldots, t_r$. (In this account of the models, we assume the same set of time points for each individual but this is for convenience only; data sets where individuals are measured at different time points can also be easily dealt with.) Let y_{ij} represent the value of the response for individual i at time t_j. A possible model for the y_{ij} might be

$$y_{ij} = \beta_0 + \beta_1 t_j + u_i + \varepsilon_{ij} \tag{13.1}$$

Here, the total residual that would be present in the usual linear regression model has been partitioned into a subject-specific random component u_i, which is constant over time plus a residual ε_{ij}, which varies randomly over time. The u_i terms are assumed to be normally distributed with zero mean and variance σ_u^2. Similarly, the residual (or error) terms, ε_{ij}, are assumed normally distributed with zero mean and variance σ^2. The u_i effects and the ε_{ij} effects are assumed to be independent of each other and of the t_j.

The model in (13.1) is known as a *random intercept model*, the u_i being the random intercepts. The repeated measurements for an individual vary about that individual's own regression line, which can differ in intercept but not in slope from the regression lines of other individuals. The random-effects model possible heterogeneity in the intercepts of the individuals. In the model in Equation (13.1), time has a *fixed effect*.

The random intercept model implies that the total variance of each repeated measurement is given by

$$\operatorname{Var}\left(u_i + \varepsilon_{ij}\right) = \sigma_u^2 + \sigma^2 \tag{13.2}$$

Due to this decomposition of the total residual variance into a between-subject component, σ_u^2, and a within-subject component, σ^2, the model is sometimes referred to as a *variance component model*.

The covariance between the total residuals at two time points t_j and $t_{j'}$ in the same individual i is

$$\operatorname{Cov}\left(u_i + \varepsilon_{ij}, u_i + \varepsilon_{ij'}\right) = \sigma_u^2 \tag{13.3}$$

Note that these covariances are induced by the shared random intercept. For individuals with $u_i > 0$, the total residuals will tend to be greater than the mean; for individuals with $u_i < 0$, they will tend to be less than the mean. It follows from Equations (13.2) and (13.3) that the residual correlations are given by

$$\operatorname{Cor}\left(u_i + \varepsilon_{ij}, u_i + \varepsilon_{ij'}\right) = \frac{\sigma_u^2}{\sigma_u^2 + \sigma^2} \tag{13.4}$$

This is an *intraclass correlation* (see Chapter 2) interpreted as the proportion of the total residual variance that is due to residual variability between subjects. A random intercept model constrains the variance of each repeated measure to be the same and the covariance between any pair of measurements to be equal. This is usually called the *compound symmetry* structure. These constraints are often not realistic for longitudinal data, where it is commonly the case that measurements taken more closely to each other in time will be more highly correlated than those taken further apart. In addition, the variances of the later repeated measures are often greater than those taken earlier. Consequently, for many such data sets, the random intercept model will not do justice to the observed pattern of covariances between the repeated measures.

A model that allows a more realistic structure for the covariances is one that allows heterogeneity in both slopes and intercepts: the *random slope and intercept model*. In this model, there are two types of random effects—the first modelling heterogeneity in intercepts, u_{i_1}, and the second modelling heterogeneity in slopes, u_{i_2}. Explicitly, the model is

$$y_{ij} = \beta_0 + \beta_1 t_j + u_{i_1} + u_{i_2} t_j + \varepsilon_{ij} \tag{13.5}$$

where the parameters are not, of course, the same as in Equation (13.1).

Now the two random effects, u_{i_1} and u_{i_2}, are assumed to have a *bivariate* normal distribution with zero means for both variables, variances $\sigma_{u_1}^2, \sigma_{u_2}^2$, and covariance $\sigma_{u_1 u_2}$. With this model, the total residual is $u_{i_1} + u_{i_2} t_j + \varepsilon_{ij}$ with variance

$$\mathrm{Var}\left(u_{i_1} + u_{i_2} x_j + \varepsilon_{ij}\right) = \sigma_{u_1}^2 + 2\sigma_{u_1 u_2} t_j + \sigma_{u_2}^2 x_j^2 + \sigma^2 \tag{13.6}$$

which is no longer constant for different values of t_j. Similarly, the covariance between two total residuals of the same individual

$$\mathrm{Cov}\left(u_{i_1} + u_{i_2} t_j + \varepsilon_{ij}, u_{i_1} + u_{i_2} t_{j'} + \varepsilon_{ij'}\right) = \sigma_{u_1}^2 + \sigma_{u_1 u_2}\left(t_j + t_{j'}\right) + \sigma_{u_2}^2 t_j t_{j'} \tag{13.7}$$

is not constrained to be the same for all pairs j and j'.

Linear mixed-effects models can be estimated by maximum likelihood; details are given in Fitzmaurice et al. (2004). However, maximum likelihood tends to produce biased estimates of the variance components; consequently, a modified version of maximum likelihood, known as *restricted maximum likelihood* (REML), is often recommended. This method provides consistent estimates of the variance components. Details are given in Diggle et al. (2003) and Fitzmaurice et al. (2004). Often, the two estimation methods will give very similar results.

Competing linear mixed-effects models can be compared using a likelihood ratio test. If, however, the models have been estimated by restricted maximum likelihood, this test can be used only if both models have the same set of fixed effects (see Longford 1993). (It should also be noted that reestimating the model after adding or subtracting a constant from each t_j—for example, the mean of the time values—will lead to different estimates of the variances and covariances of the random effects, but will not affect fixed effects. Centring time in this way is often helpful when the times of recording the response variable do not include zero to avoid the intercept representing measurement at time zero.)

13.2.2 Applying the Random Intercept and Random Intercept and Slope Models

We will use the data in Table 13.1, reported in Zerbe (1979) and also given in Davis (2003), to illustrate the application of linear mixed-effects models, in particular the two models described in Section 13.2.1. These data consist of plasma inorganic phosphate measurements obtained from 13 control and 20 obese patients 0, 0.5, 1, 1.5, 2, and 3 hours after an oral glucose challenge. The data are read in as follows:

```
data pip;
  infile 'c:\amsus\data\pip.dat';
  input id x1-x8;
  if id>13 then group=2;
  else group=1;
run;

data pipl;
  set pip;
  array xs {*} x1-x8;
  array t{8} t1-t8 (0 .5 1 1.5 2 3 4 5);
  do i=1 to 8;
    time=t{i};
    pip=xs{i};
    output;
  end;
  label time='hours after glucose';
  keep id time group pip;
run;

proc format;
  value group 1='Control' 2='Obese';
run;

proc print data=pipl;
  where id in(1 13 14 33);
run;
```

Both wide and long forms of the data set are created as described in the previous chapter. One difference in this example arises because the measurement times are not evenly spaced, so the index to the array cannot be used as the 'time' variable. Instead, a separate array of measurement times is set up. We also create a format for later labelling of the two groups. The fact

TABLE 13.1

Plasma Inorganic Phosphate Levels from 33 Subjects

		Hours after Glucose Challenge							
Group	ID	0	0.5	1	1.5	2	3	4	5
Control	1	4.3	3.3	3.0	2.6	2.2	2.5	3.4	4.4
	2	3.7	2.6	2.6	1.9	2.9	3.2	3.1	3.9
	3	4.0	4.1	3.1	2.3	2.9	3.1	3.9	4.0
	4	3.6	3.0	2.2	2.8	2.9	3.9	3.8	4.0
	5	4.1	3.8	2.1	3.0	3.6	3.4	3.6	3.7
	6	3.8	2.2	2.0	2.6	3.8	3.6	3.0	3.5
	7	3.8	3.0	2.4	2.5	3.1	3.4	3.5	3.7
	8	4.4	3.9	2.8	2.1	3.6	3.8	4.0	3.9
	9	5.0	4.0	3.4	3.4	3.3	3.6	4.0	4.3
	10	3.7	3.1	2.9	2.2	1.5	2.3	2.7	2.8
	11	3.7	2.6	2.6	2.3	2.9	2.2	3.1	3.9
	12	4.4	3.7	3.1	3.2	3.7	4.3	3.9	4.8
	13	4.7	3.1	3.2	3.3	3.2	4.2	3.7	4.3
Obese	14	4.3	3.3	3.0	2.6	2.2	2.5	2.4	3.4
	15	5.0	4.9	4.1	3.7	3.7	4.1	4.7	4.9
	16	4.6	4.4	3.9	3.9	3.7	4.2	4.8	5.0
	17	4.3	3.9	3.1	3.1	3.1	3.1	3.6	4.0
	18	3.1	3.1	3.3	2.6	2.6	1.9	2.3	2.7
	19	4.8	5.0	2.9	2.8	2.2	3.1	3.5	3.6
	20	3.7	3.1	3.3	2.8	2.9	3.6	4.3	4.4
	21	5.4	4.7	3.9	4.1	2.8	3.7	3.5	3.7
	22	3.0	2.5	2.3	2.2	2.1	2.6	3.2	3.5
	23	4.9	5.0	4.1	3.7	3.7	4.1	4.7	4.9
	24	4.8	4.3	4.7	4.6	4.7	3.7	3.6	3.9
	25	4.4	4.2	4.2	3.4	3.5	3.4	3.8	4.0
	26	4.9	4.3	4.0	4.0	3.3	4.1	4.2	4.3
	27	5.1	4.1	4.6	4.1	3.4	4.2	4.4	4.9
	28	4.8	4.6	4.6	4.4	4.1	4.0	3.8	3.8
	29	4.2	3.5	3.8	3.6	3.3	3.1	3.5	3.9
	30	6.6	6.1	5.2	4.1	4.3	3.8	4.2	4.8
	31	3.6	3.4	3.1	2.8	2.1	2.4	2.5	3.5
	32	4.5	4.0	3.7	3.3	2.4	2.3	3.1	3.3
	33	4.6	4.4	3.8	3.8	3.8	3.6	3.8	3.8

Source: Zerbe, G. O. 1979. *Journal of the American Statistical Association*, 74:215–221.

that the format bears the same name, group, as the variable to which it is to be applied is not a problem. Indeed, it can be useful when formats are defined for a large number of variables. Selected cases are then printed from the long version of the data set to check that the reorganisation is correct. The results are shown in Table 13.2.

TABLE 13.2

Part of Glucose Challenge Data in 'Long' Form

Obs	id	group	time	pip
1	1	Control	0.0	4.3
2	1	Control	0.5	3.3
3	1	Control	1.0	3.0
4	1	Control	1.5	2.6
5	1	Control	2.0	2.2
6	1	Control	3.0	2.5
7	1	Control	4.0	3.4
8	1	Control	5.0	4.4
97	13	Control	0.0	4.7
98	13	Control	0.5	3.1
99	13	Control	1.0	3.2
100	13	Control	1.5	3.3
101	13	Control	2.0	3.2
102	13	Control	3.0	4.2
103	13	Control	4.0	3.7
104	13	Control	5.0	4.3
105	14	Obese	0.0	4.3
106	14	Obese	0.5	3.3
107	14	Obese	1.0	3.0
108	14	Obese	1.5	2.6
109	14	Obese	2.0	2.2
110	14	Obese	3.0	2.5
111	14	Obese	4.0	2.4
112	14	Obese	5.0	3.4
257	33	Obese	0.0	4.6
258	33	Obese	0.5	4.4
259	33	Obese	1.0	3.8
260	33	Obese	1.5	3.8
261	33	Obese	2.0	3.8
262	33	Obese	3.0	3.6
263	33	Obese	4.0	3.8
264	33	Obese	5.0	3.8

Here we will begin by plotting the data to gain some idea of what form of linear mixed-effects model might be appropriate. First, we plot the raw data separately for the control and the obese groups:

```
proc sgpanel data=pipl noautolegend;
   panelby group/columns=2 spacing=10 novarname;
   series y=pip x=time/group=id;
   format group group.;
run;
```

To do this, we use `proc sgpanel` with the long format of the data set. This allows us to produce separate line plots for each person using the `group` option on the `series` statement with the person identifier, `id`. The `panelby` statement specifies separate plots for each group. Adding 10 pixels of spacing between plots and removing the variable name from the heading enhance the appearance of the plots, especially when used with a format. The resulting plot is shown in Figure 13.1.

The profiles in both groups show some curvature, suggesting that a quadratic effect of time may be needed in any model. There also appears to be some suspicion of a difference in the shape of the curves in the two groups, suggesting perhaps the need to consider a group × time interaction.

Next, we plot the scatter plot matrices of the repeated measurements for the two groups using the following:

```
proc sgscatter data=pip;
  matrix x1-x8;
  by group notsorted;
  format group group.;
run;
```

The wide version of the data set is used with `proc sgscatter` and the `matrix` statement. The `by` statement can be used to produce separate plots even though the data set has not been sorted (with `proc sort`), provided

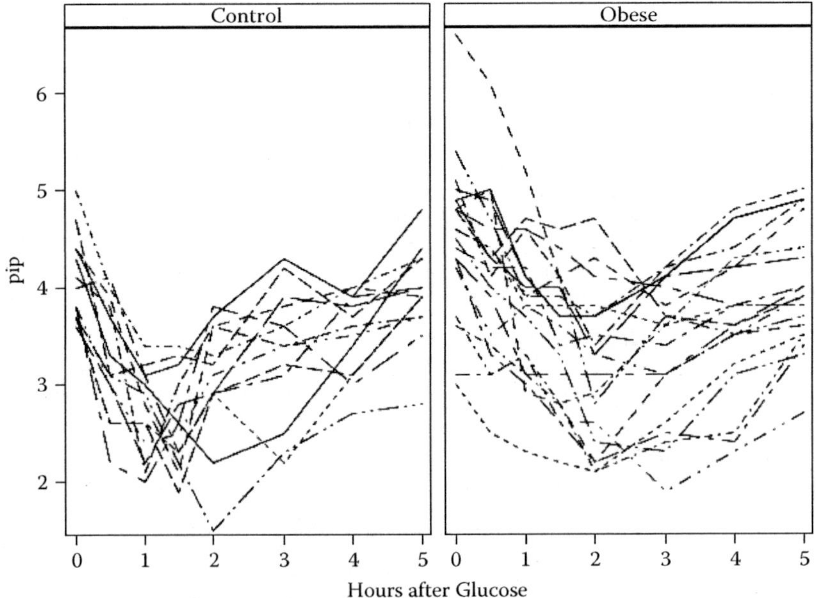

FIGURE 13.1
Glucose challenge data for control and obese groups.

that `notsorted` is specified. The plots are shown in Figures 13.2 and 13.3. Both plots indicate that the correlations of pairs of measurements made at different times differ, so the compound symmetry structure for these correlations (see Section 13.2.1) is unlikely to be appropriate.

On the basis of the plots in Figure 13.1 to 13.3, it is clear that a suitable model for the glucose challenge data will need to include a quadratic effect for time and allow the correlations structure to depart from the compound symmetry assumption outlined in Section 13.2.1. We will begin by fitting the following random intercept and slope model, in which group is a dummy variable identifying the two groups of patients and linear time has a random effect with quadratic time having a fixed effect:

$$y_{ij} = \beta_0 + \beta_1 \text{group} + \beta_2 \text{time} + \beta_3 \text{time}^2 + u_{i1} + u_{i2}\text{time} + \varepsilon_{ij} \tag{13.8}$$

We can fit this model using `proc mixed` as follows (note that time is centred by subtracting mean time from each recording time):

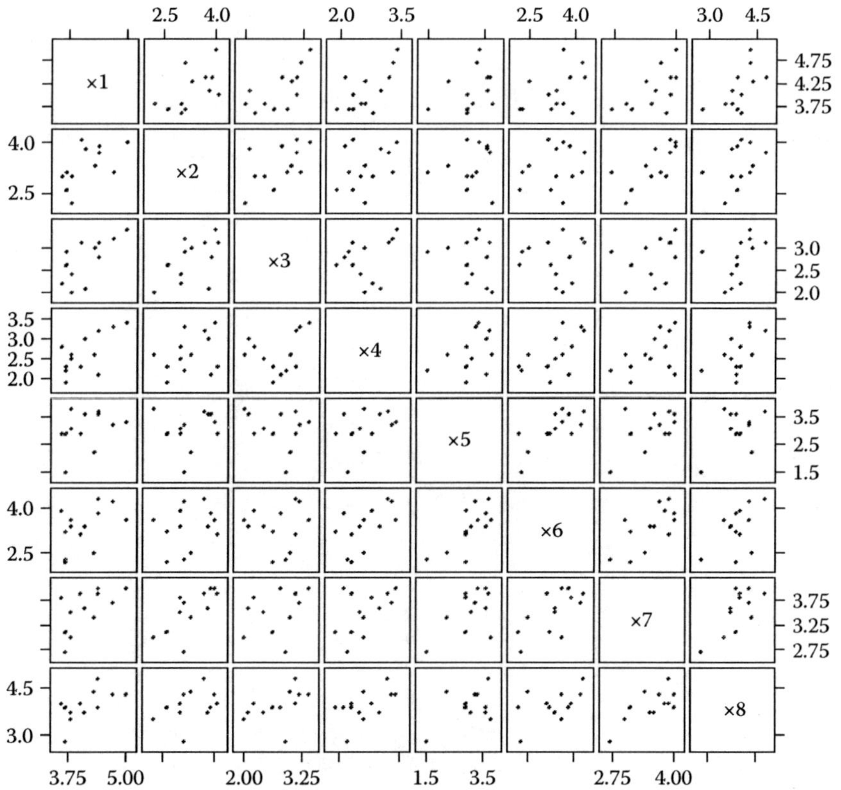

FIGURE 13.2
Scatter plot matrix for control group in Table 13.1.

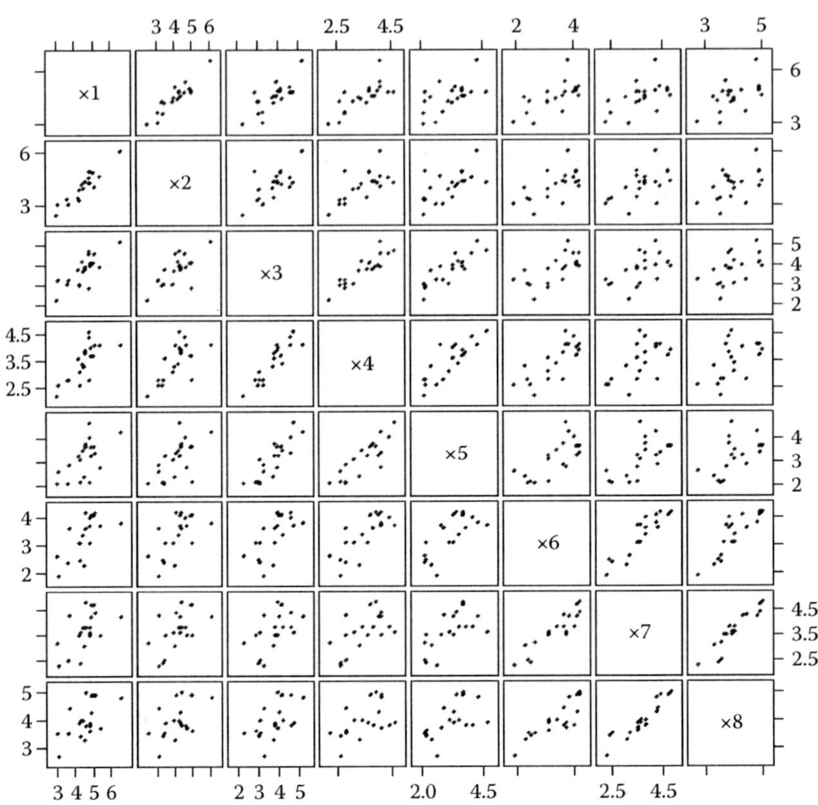

FIGURE 13.3
Scatter plot matrix for obese group in Table 13.1.

```
proc stdize data=pipl out=pipl method=mean;
   var time;
run;

proc sort data=pipl; by id time; run;

proc mixed data=pipl covtest noclprint;
   class group id;
   model pip=group time|time /s ddfm=bw;
   random int time /subject=id type=un;
run;
```

Proc mixed is the SAS procedure for linear mixed models with normal
responses. Its syntax is similar to that of proc glm with additional statements and options to deal with the random effects. The first point to note
is that it takes as input the long form of the data set. With large data sets,
it is advisable to sort the data by subject and measurement occasion within

subject. The `class` statement performs its usual function of identifying categorical variables. If the subject identifier is not a numeric variable or the data have not been sorted, it should be included on the `class` statement. The `noclprint` option on the `proc` statement stops the levels of the categorical variables being listed in the output, which is useful when the data contain observations on a large number of subjects. In that case, `noclprint=n` could be used to suppress the class level listing for variables with more than n levels.

The `model` statement specifies the fixed effects in the model in the same way as for `proc glm`. Here we use the bar operator (|) as the shorthand for time `time*time` and, as this implies, interactions and polynomial terms can be specified with the asterisk. The `s` (solution) option requests that the fixed-effects parameter estimates are included in the output. In mixed models, the denominator degrees of freedom for the F- and t-tests of the fixed effects need to be estimated from the data. `Proc mixed` offers five methods of estimation. In general, these will lead to different results, but for longitudinal analyses with reasonably sized samples, any method is likely to yield degrees of freedom large enough to lead to very similar p-values. We have selected the bw (`betweenwithin`) method as suitable for longitudinal analysis, although the Satterthwaite or Kenward–Roger methods could also have been chosen.

The `random` statement specifies the random effects and their related options. A random intercept is not included in the model by default and needs to be specified as `int` or `intercept` on the `random` statement. Including `time` as a random effect specifies random slopes in `time` (i.e., the u_{i2} time term in the model). The `subject=` option specifies the subject identifier. The `type=` option specifies the covariance structure of the random effects. In the terminology adopted by SAS, the random parameters are referred to as 'covariance parameters' and are represented in the model as a covariance matrix, which has a structure specified by the `type` option. `Type=vc` (variance components) is the default and estimates the variance for each random effect whilst constraining any covariance between them to zero. `Type=un` (unstructured) allows the random intercepts and slopes to covary and estimates the covariance between them. The `covtest` option on the `proc mixed` statement produces asymptotic standard errors and Wald tests for the covariance parameters.

The results are shown in Table 13.3. The regression coefficients for linear and quadratic time are both highly significant. The group effect just fails to reach significance at the 5% level. When an unstructured covariance matrix is specified for the random effects, their estimates are labelled in the output with the row and column number of the matrix. UN(1,1) is the variance of the random intercept term u_{i1} and is estimated to be 0.28. UN(2,2) is the variance of the random slopes in time, u_{i2}, estimated as 0.016, and UN(2,1) is the intercept-slope covariance term estimated as −0.01.

Here, to demonstrate what happens if we make a very misleading assumption about the correlational structure of the repeated measurements, we will compare the results in Table 13.3 with those obtained if we assume that the repeated measurements are independent and fit the corresponding

TABLE 13.3

Results from Random Slope and Intercept Model with Fixed Quadratic
Time Effect Fitted to the Glucose Challenge Data

Model Information	
Data Set	WORK.PIPL
Dependent Variable	Pip
Covariance Structure	Unstructured
Subject Effect	Id
Estimation Method	REML
Residual Variance Method	Profile
Fixed Effects SE Method	Model-Based
Degrees of Freedom Method	Between-Within

Class–Level Information		
Class	Levels	Values
group	2	1 2
id	33	Not printed

Dimensions	
Covariance Parameters	4
Columns in X	5
Columns in Z Per Subject	2
Subjects	33
Max Obs Per Subject	8

Number of Observations	
Number of Observations Read	264
Number of Observations Used	264
Number of Observations Not Used	0

Iteration History			
Iteration	Evaluations	−2 Res Log Like	Criterion
0	1	570.33709221	
1	2	424.01656924	0.00000368
2	1	424.01647003	0.00000000

Convergence criteria met.

TABLE 13.3 (*Continued*)

Results from Random Slope and Intercept Model with Fixed Quadratic Time Effect Fitted to the Glucose Challenge Data

		Covariance Parameter Estimates			
Cov Parm	Subject	Estimate	Standard Error	Z Value	Pr Z
UN(1,1)	id	0.2760	0.07612	3.63	0.0001
UN(2,1)	id	−0.01093	0.01768	−0.62	0.5366
UN(2,2)	id	0.01592	0.006092	2.61	0.0045
Residual		0.1757	0.01770	9.92	<.0001

Fit Statistics	
−2 Res Log Likelihood	424.0
AIC (smaller is better)	432.0
AICC (smaller is better)	432.2
BIC (smaller is better)	438.0

Null Model Likelihood Ratio Test		
DF	Chi-Square	Pr > ChiSq
3	146.32	<.0001

		Solution for Fixed Effects				
Effect	group	Estimate	Standard Error	DF	t Value	Pr > |t|
Intercept		3.3098	0.1253	31	26.41	<.0001
group	1	−0.3826	0.1928	31	−1.98	0.0562
group	2	0				
time		−0.1358	0.02825	229	−4.81	<.0001
time*time		0.1636	0.01125	229	14.55	<.0001

Type 3 Tests of Fixed Effects				
Effect	Num DF	Den DF	F Value	Pr > F
group	1	31	3.94	0.0562
time	1	229	23.11	<.0001
time*time	1	229	211.56	<.0001

model to that in Equation (13.8), but without the random effects (i.e., the model):

$$y_{ij} = \beta_0 + \beta_1\text{group} + \beta_2\text{time} + \beta_3\text{time}^2 + \varepsilon_{ij} \qquad (13.9)$$

We have used the same terms to refer to the various regression coefficients in the preceding model as in the model defined by Equation (13.7), but remember that this is for convenience—the terms are, of course, not the same in the two models.

The independence model can be fitted in the usual way using `proc glm` as follows:

```
proc glm data=pipl;
  class group;
  model pip=group time|time /solution;
run;
```

The results are shown in Table 13.4. We see that, under the independence assumption, the standard error for the group effect is about one-half of that given in Table 13.3 and, if it were used, would lead to the claim of strong evidence of a difference between control and obese patients. For between-subject effects (here, group), the independence model estimated standard error will almost always be lower than for a nonindependence model unless, of course, the repeated measurements are actually independent of one another. For the time regression coefficient, however, the estimated standard errors for the two models are very similar; Pickles (2005) makes the point that, for within-subject effects (here, the time trend), the independence model may lead to standard error estimates that are too large.

To assess informally how well the fitted linear mixed-effects model defined in Equation (13.8) describes the glucose challenge data, we will now plot the predicted values from the model separately for each group. To do this, we use the same `proc mixed` step as before, changing the model statement to

```
model pip=group time|time/s ddfm=bw outp=mixout;
```

The `outp=mixout` option saves the predicted values to the `mixout` data set. `Proc mixed` has two types of predicted values and residuals, referred to

TABLE 13.4

Results from Independence Model Fitted to Glucose Challenge Data

Parameter	Estimate		Standard Error	t Value	Pr > |t|
Intercept	3.339104980	B	0.07391650	45.17	<.0001
group 1	−0.457019231	B	0.08723374	−5.24	<.0001
group 2	0.000000000	B			
time	−0.135803943		0.02934081	−4.63	<.0001
time*time	0.163609832		0.01858531	8.80	<.0001

as 'marginal' and 'conditional'. Marginal values do not include the random effects in the predicted values, whereas conditional predicted values do. The marginal predicted values are saved with the outpm= option. Here, the conditional predicted values are saved and then plotted in the same way as the observed values were for Figure 13.1. The result is shown in Figure 13.4. We can see that the model has captured the profiles of the control group relatively well but not, perhaps, those of the obese group. We need to consider a further model that contains a group × time interaction by amending the model statement to

```
model pip=group time|time group*time/s ddfm=bw outp=mixout;
```

The results for this model are given in Table 13.5. The interaction effect is highly significant. The fitted values from this model are plotted in Figure 13.5 (the code is very similar to that given for producing Figure 13.4). The plot shows that the new model has produced predicted values that more accurately reflect the raw data plotted in Figure 13.1. The predicted profiles for the obese group are 'flatter', as required.

The random effects are not estimated as part of the model. However, having estimated the model, we can *predict* the values of the random effects. In general, the problem of predicting a random variable can be shown to be

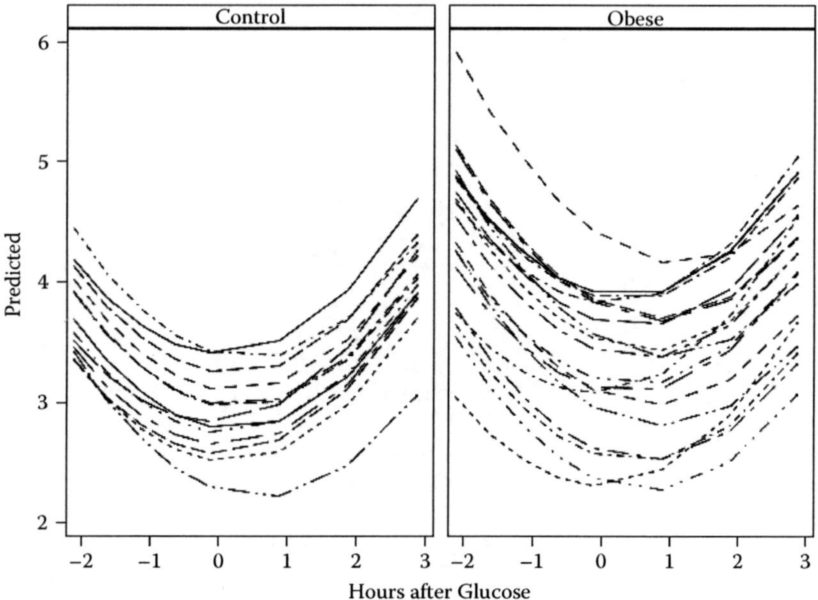

FIGURE 13.4
Fitted values from random intercept and slope model with fixed quadratic effect for glucose challenge data.

TABLE 13.5

Results from Random Intercept and Slope Model with Fixed Quadratic
Time Effect and Group × Time Interaction Fitted to the Glucose
Challenge Data

Model Information	
Data Set	WORK.PIPL
Dependent Variable	Pip
Covariance Structure	Unstructured
Subject Effect	id
Estimation Method	REML
Residual Variance Method	Profile
Fixed Effects SE Method	Model-Based
Degrees of Freedom Method	Between-Within

Dimensions	
Covariance Parameters	4
Columns in X	7
Columns in Z Per Subject	2
Subjects	33
Max Obs Per Subject	8

Number of Observations	
Number of Observations Read	264
Number of Observations Used	264
Number of Observations Not Used	0

Iteration History			
Iteration	Evaluations	−2 Res Log Like	Criterion
0	1	564.72900461	
1	1	417.95581545	0.00000000

Convergence criteria met.

Covariance Parameter Estimates					
Cov Parm	Subject	Estimate	Standard Error	Z Value	Pr Z
UN(1,1)	id	0.2774	0.07539	3.64	0.0001
UN(2,1)	id	−0.00817	0.01323	−0.62	0.5367
UN(2,2)	id	0.009834	0.004660	2.11	0.0174
Residual		0.1757	0.01770	9.92	<.0001

TABLE 13.5 (*Continued*)

Results from Random Intercept and Slope Model with Fixed Quadratic Time Effect and Group × Time Interaction Fitted to the Glucose Challenge Data

Fit Statistics	
−2 Res Log Likelihood	418.0
AIC (smaller is better)	426.0
AICC (smaller is better)	426.1
BIC (smaller is better)	431.9

Null Model Likelihood Ratio Test		
DF	Chi-Square	Pr > ChiSq
3	146.77	<.0001

			Solution for Fixed Effects			
Effect	group	Estimate	Standard Error	DF	t Value	Pr > |t|
Intercept		3.3391	0.1255	31	26.62	<.0001
group	1	−0.4570	0.1941	31	−2.36	0.0250
group	2	0				
time		−0.2006	0.03113	228	−6.44	<.0001
time*time		0.1636	0.01125	228	14.55	<.0001
time*group	1	0.1644	0.04787	228	3.43	0.0007
time*group	2	0				

	Type 3 Tests of Fixed Effects			
Effect	Num DF	Den DF	F Value	Pr > F
group	1	31	5.55	0.0250
time	1	228	21.92	<.0001
time*time	1	228	211.56	<.0001
time*group	1	228	11.79	<.0007

that of predicting its conditional mean, given the available data. Thus, the best predictor of a random effect is its conditional mean, given the vector of responses and the estimated regression coefficients in the model. Having a prediction of the random effects allows prediction of a subject's response profile. Full details of predicting random effect in linear mixed models are given in Fitzmaurice et al. (2004).

Using the estimated random effects, we now check the assumptions of the final model fitted to the glucose challenge data (i.e., that the

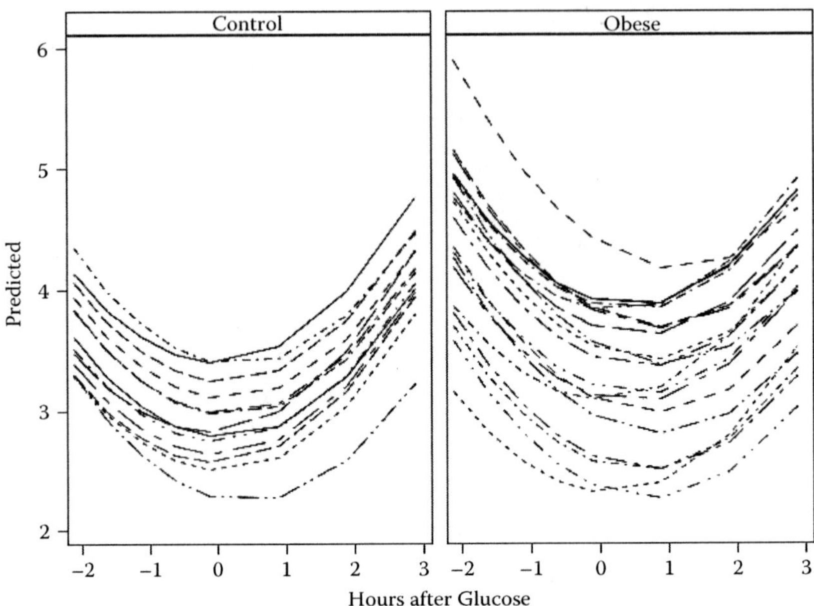

FIGURE 13.5
Fitted values from random intercept and slope model with fixed quadratic effect and group ×
time interaction for glucose challenge data.

random-effect terms and residuals are normally distributed). The residuals are in the same data set as the predicted values, created with the `outp` option on the `model` statement shown earlier. They are produced and saved as follows:

```
proc mixed data=pip1 covtest noclprint;
  class group id;
  model pip=group time|time group*time/s ddfm=bw outp=mixout;
  random int time /subject=id type=un s;
  ods output solutionr=reffs;
  ods listing exclude solutionr;
run;
```

Three elements have been added to the `proc mixed` step. The `s` (solution) option has been added to the `random` statement. This requests that the random effects be calculated and, by default, they are printed in the output. The `ods output` statement is used to store them in a data set. `Solutionr` is the ODS table name and `reffs` is the name we have chosen for the data set being created. Finally, the `ods listing` statement excludes the random-effects table from the output listing. With a large number of subjects, the random-effects table will run to several pages of output, so it is useful to be able to suppress it when it is not required.

`Proc univariate` is used to produce normal probability plots:

```
proc sort data=reffs; by effect; run;
proc univariate data=reffs noprint;
  var estimate;
  probplot estimate /normal(mu=est sigma=est);
  by effect;
run;
proc univariate data=mixout noprint;
  var resid;
  probplot resid /normal(mu=est sigma=est);
run;
```

The resulting plots are shown in Figures 13.6 through 13.8. The plots of the residuals are each essentially linear as required, although there is some slight deviation from linearity for each of the predicted random effects. A further plot that can be helpful is a scatter plot of the residuals against predicted values. In a correctly specified model, the scatter plot should not display any systematic pattern; the fitting of a loess curve (see Chapter 7) can often help in assessing the scatter plot. Similarly, scatter plots of the residuals against selected covariates from the model for the mean response can be examined for systematic trends, which, if present, may indicate the

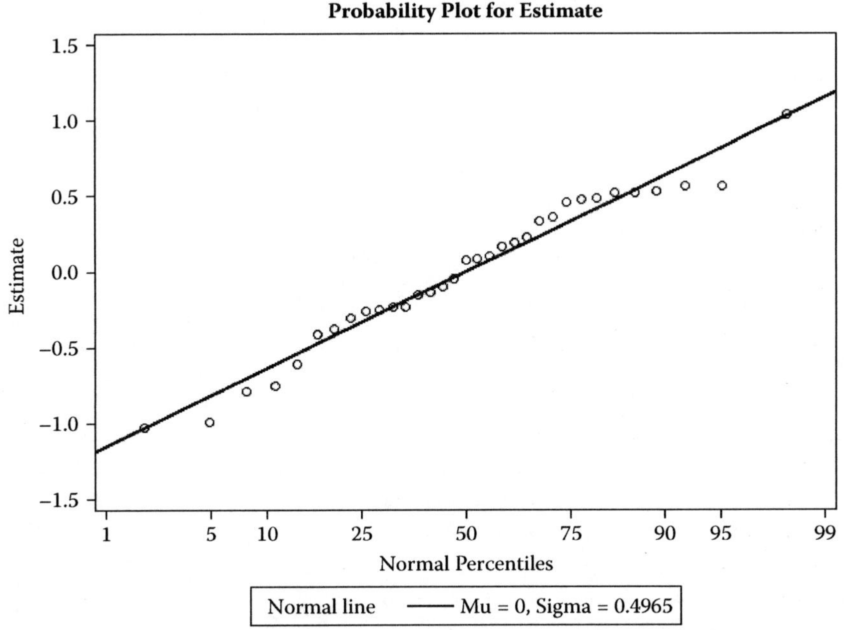

FIGURE 13.6
Probability plot for random intercepts.

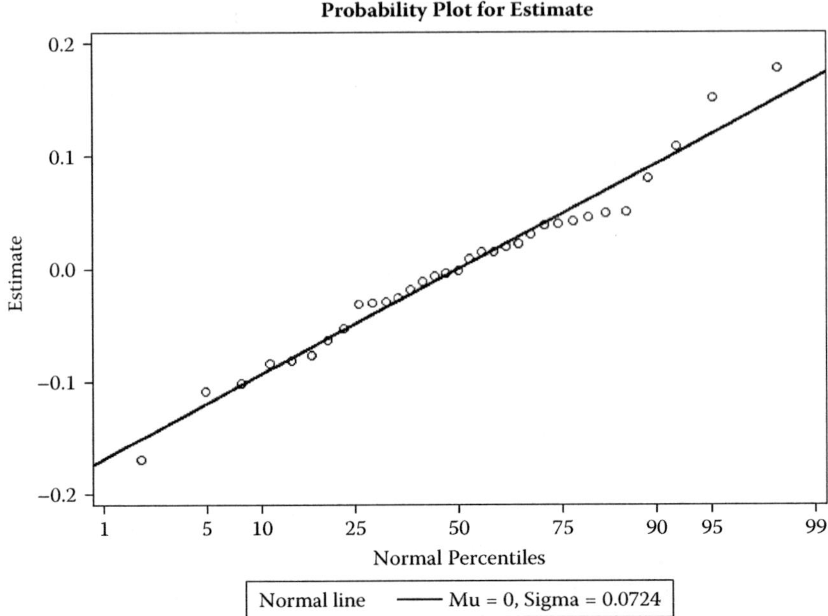

FIGURE 13.7
Probability plot for random slopes.

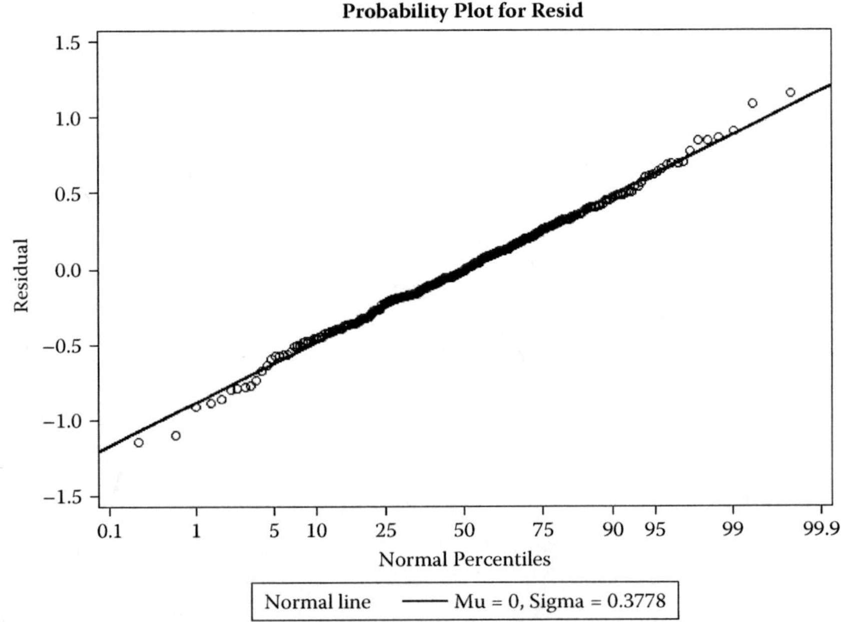

FIGURE 13.8
Probability plot for residuals.

omission of a quadratic term or the need for transformation of a covariate. We can construct the residual against predicted and residual against time scatter plots for the final model fitted to the glucose challenge data using the code

```
proc sgscatter data=mixout;
   plot resid *(pred time)/group=group loess=(clm);
run;
```

The plots are shown in Figure 13.9. There are no clear patterns in either plot that may cause concern about the validity of the fitted model.

For interest, the corresponding plots for a model that includes the group × time interaction, but only a linear effect for time, are shown in Figure 13.10 (the code is very similar to that used directly before). Here, the plot of residuals against time shows a clear pattern indicating that a quadratic effect is needed in the model.

There are some problems with using the raw residuals because they are correlated and do not necessarily have constant variance; Fitzmaurice et al. (2004) show how to produce transformed residuals, which may, in some cases, give a clearer indication of departures from the assumptions of the modelling process.

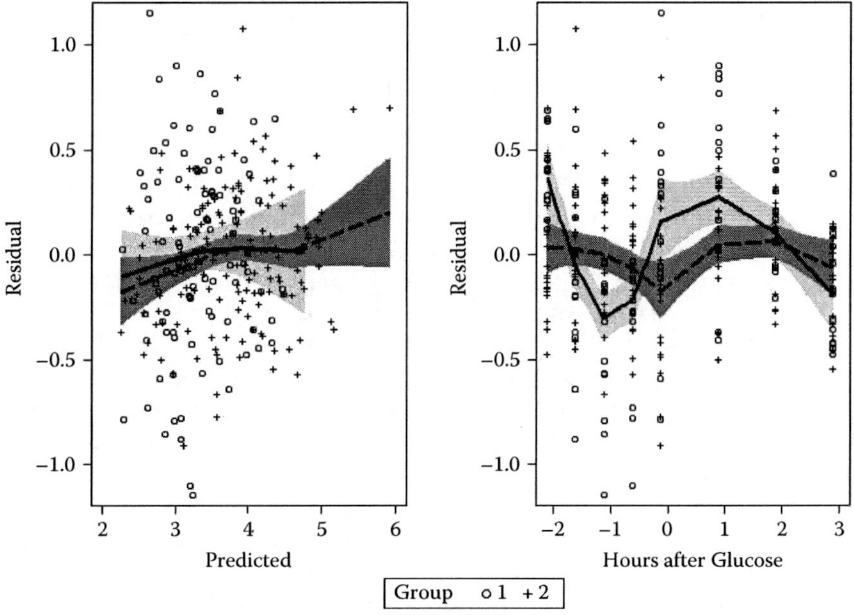

FIGURE 13.9

Plots of residuals against predicted value and residuals against time for the random intercept and slope model with quadratic time and group × time interaction fitted to the glucose challenge data.

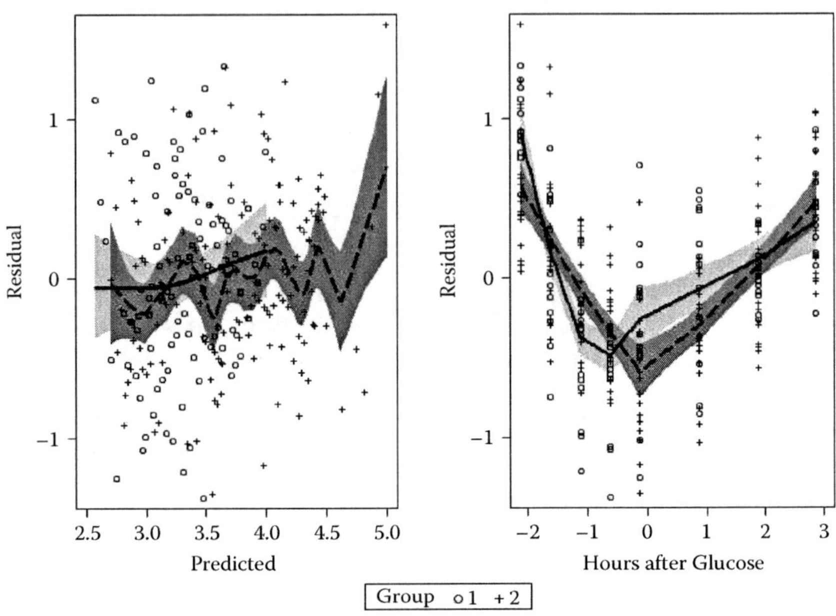

FIGURE 13.10
Plots of residuals against predicted value and residuals against time for the random intercept and slope model with only linear time and group × time interaction fitted to the glucose challenge data.

13.3 Dropouts in Longitudinal Data

A problem that frequently occurs when collecting longitudinal data is that some of the intended measurements are, for one reason or another, not made. In clinical trials, for example, some patients may miss one or more protocol scheduled visits after treatment has begun and thus fail to have the required outcome measure taken. There will be other patients who do not complete the intended follow-up for some reason and drop out of the study before the end date specified in the protocol. Both situations result in missing values of the outcome measure; in the first case, these are intermittent, but dropping out of the study implies that, once an observation at a particular time point is missing, so are all the remaining planned observations. Many studies will contain missing values of both types, although in practice it is dropouts that cause most problems when turning to analysing the resulting data set.

An example of a set of longitudinal data in which a number of patients have dropped out is given in Table 13.6; data for only five patients are given in the table but the data to be analysed here have 100 patients and are a subset of the data collected in a clinical trial that is described in detail in Proudfoot et al. (2003). The trial was designed to assess the effectiveness of an interactive

TABLE 13.6

Data for Five Patients from the Original BtB Clinical Trial

Sub	DRUG	Duration	Treatment	BDIpre	BDI2m	BDI3m	BDI5m	BDI8m
1	N	>6 m	TAU	29	2	2	NA	NA
2	Y	>6 m	BtB	32	16	24	17	20
3	Y	<6 m	TAU	25	20	NA	NA	NA
4	N	>6 m	BtB	21	17	16	10	9
5	Y	>6 m	BtB	26	23	NA	NA	NA

program using multimedia techniques for the delivery of cognitive behavioural therapy for depressed patients and is known as Beating the Blues (BtB). In a randomised controlled trial of the program, patients with depression recruited in primary care were randomised either to the BtB program or to treatment as usual (TAU). The outcome measure used in the trial was the Beck Depression Inventory II (Beck, Steer, and Brown 1996), with higher values indicating more depression.

Measurements of this variable were made on five occasions, one prior to the start of treatment and at two monthly intervals after treatment began. In addition, whether or not a participant in the trial was already taking antidepressant medication was noted along with the length of time he or she had been depressed, divided into greater than 6 months or less than or equal to 6 months; 'NA' denotes 'not available' (i.e., a missing value).

We can read the data in creating both the wide and long formats in the same data step:

```
data btb (keep=sub--treatment BDIpre--BDI8m)
     btbl (keep=sub--treatment bdi time);
infile 'c:\amsus\data\btb.dat' missover;
 array bdis {*} BDIpre BDI2m BDI3m BDI5m BDI8m;
 array t {*} t1-t5 (0 2 3 5 8);
 input sub drug$ Duration$ Treatment$ @;
 do i=1 to 5;
   input bdi @;
   bdis{i}=bdi;
   time=t{i};
   output btbl;
 end;
 output btb;
run;
```

We have already seen how to use the `array`, iterative `do`, and `output` statements to restructure a data set. This example shows the use of two `output` statements, each naming the data set that the observation is to be written to. The `data` statement also names two data sets and the `keep` option specifies the variables they are to contain.

To begin, we shall graph the data by plotting the box plots of each of the five repeated measures separately for each treatment group:

```
proc sgpanel data=btbl;
  panelby treatment/spacing=10 novarname;
  vbox bdi/category=time;
run;
```

The resulting diagram is shown in Figure 13.11.

Figure 13.11 shows that there is decline in BDI values in both groups with perhaps the values in the BtB group lower at each postrandomisation visit. We shall fit both random intercept and random intercept and slope models to the data, including the pre-BDI values, treatment group, drugs, and duration as fixed-effect covariates.

The data contain a number of missing values and, in applying proc mixed to the long form of the data set, these will be dropped from the analysis. But notice that only the missing values are removed, *not* participants that have at least one recorded value. *All* the available data are used in the model fitting process.

We begin by fitting the random intercept and slope model:

```
proc mixed data=btbl covtest noclprint=3;
 class drug duration treatment sub;
 model bdi=drug duration treatment time/s cl ddfm=bw;
 random int time/subject=sub type=un;
run;
```

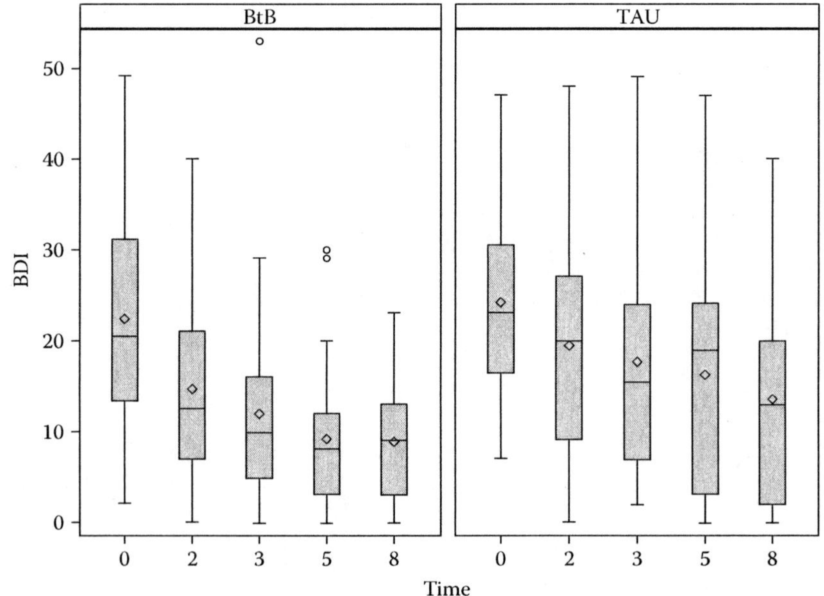

FIGURE 13.11
Box plots for the repeated measures by treatment group for the BtB data.

The random effects (covariance parameters) estimates and associated Wald tests for this model are

Covariance Parameter Estimates					
Cov Parm	Subject	Estimate	Standard Error	Z Value	Pr Z
UN(1,1)	sub	78.8941	15.1932	5.19	<.0001
UN(2,1)	sub	0.08138	1.9103	0.04	0.9660
UN(2,2)	sub	0.2573	0.2823	0.91	0.1811
Residual		38.1343	3.6849	10.35	<.0001

Clearly, a simpler model with only a random intercept is adequate for these data. This model can be fitted by amending the `random` statement to

```
random int /subject=sub;
```

The results from fitting this model are given in Table 13.7. The treatment and time effects are significant but those for drugs and duration are not.

TABLE 13.7

Results from the Random Intercept Model Fitted to the BtB Data

Solution for Fixed Effects								
Effect	drug	Duration	Treatment	Estimate	Standard Error	DF	t Value	Pr > |t|
Intercept				26.4177	2.3184	96	11.39	<.0001
drug	n			−2.0513	2.0474	96	−1.00	0.3189
drug	y			0				
Duration		<6 m		−3.4439	1.9473	96	−1.77	0.0801
Duration		>6 m		0				
Treatment			BtB	−4.2928	2.0172	96	−2.13	0.0359
Treatment			TAU	0				
time				−1.3882	0.1354	279	−10.26	<.0001

Solution for Fixed Effects						
Effect	drug	Duration	Treatment	Alpha	Lower	Upper
Intercept				0.05	21.8157	31.0197
drug	n			0.05	−6.1153	2.0127
drug	y					
Duration		<6 m		0.05	−7.3092	0.4215
Duration		>6 m				
Treatment			BtB	0.05	−8.2969	−0.2888
Treatment			TAU			
time				0.05	−1.6547	−1.1218

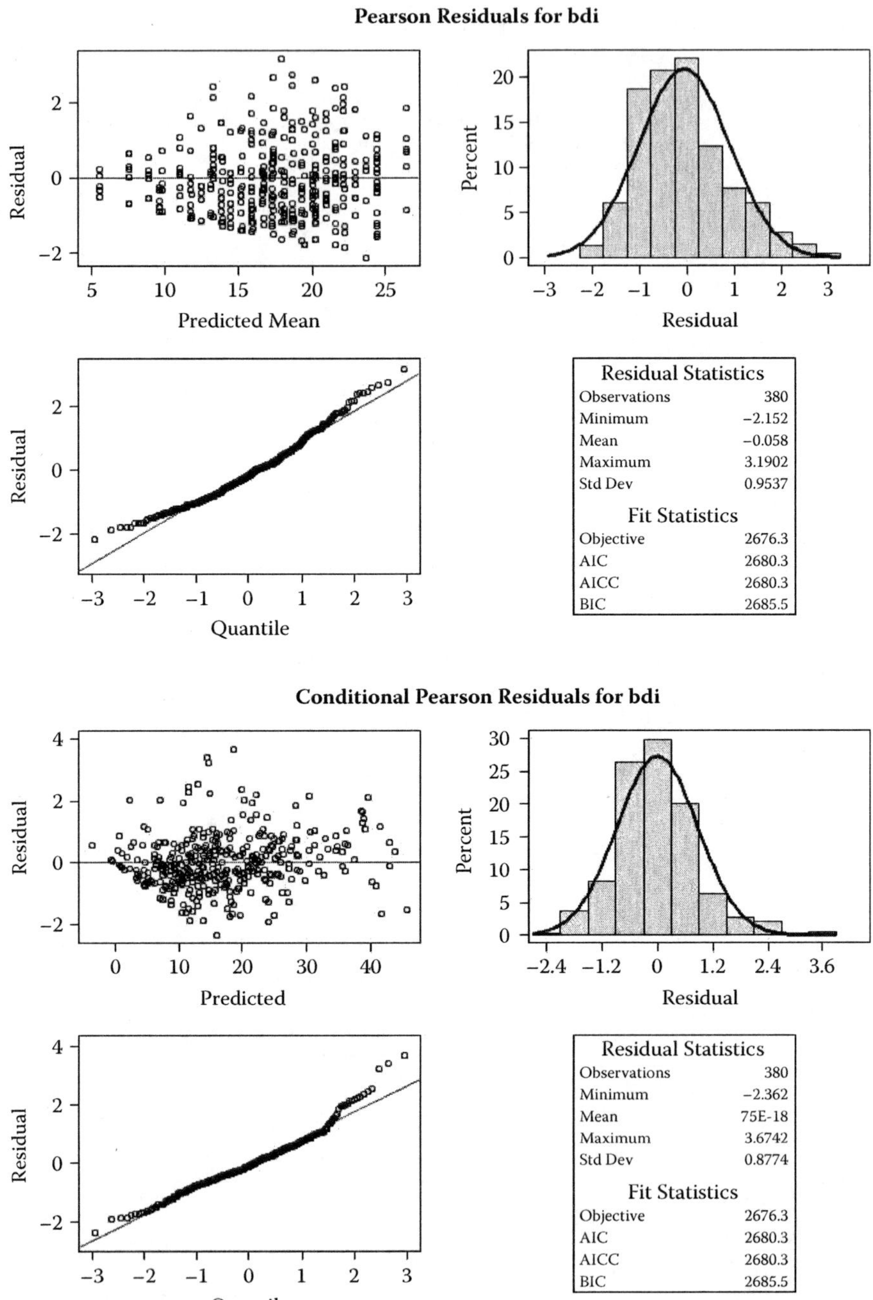

FIGURE 13.12
Conditional residuals from fitting random intercept model to BtB data.

The confidence interval for the treatment effect implies that treatment with BtB reduces the depression score on average by about one fifth of a point to eight points, conditional on the values of the other covariates. Clearly, the lower end of the interval would not represent a decrease that was of any clinical use, but the value at the upper end represents a considerable decrease in a patient's depression.

Various plots of the conditional residuals from fitting the random intercept model are shown in Figure 13.12. Some residuals are a little extreme, but on the whole they are well behaved and no obvious problems with the model are suggested.

How the dropouts may affect the analyses reported previously will be taken up in Chapter 18.

13.4 Summary

Linear mixed-effects models are extremely useful for modelling longitudinal data in particular and repeated measures data more generally. The models allow the correlations between the repeated measurements to be accounted for so that correct inferences can be drawn about the effects of covariates of interest on the repeated response values. In this chapter, we have concentrated on responses that are continuous and conditional on the explanatory variables, and random effects have a normal distribution. Models with random effects can also be applied to non-normal responses, as we shall see in the next chapter.

14

Analysis of Longitudinal Data III: Non-Normal Responses

14.1 Introduction

In many longitudinal studies carried out in medicine, it will be clear that the assumption of normality for the response variable is simply not justified. Two examples are shown in Tables 14.1 and 14.2. The one in Table 14.1 results from a clinical trial comparing two treatments for a respiratory illness (Davis 1991). In each of two centres, eligible patients were randomly assigned to active treatment or placebo. During treatment, the respiratory status (categorised as 0 = poor, 1 = good) was determined at each of four monthly visits. A total of 111 patients were entered into the trial, 54 into the active group and 57 into the placebo group. The sex and age of each participant were also recorded and a baseline respiratory status. Here the response variable is binary, making the models described in the previous chapter inappropriate for these data. (These data were used previously in Chapter 12.) The observations for the first five patients in the data set are shown in Table 14.1.

The data in Table 14.2 also arise from a clinical trial reported in Thall and Vail (1990). Here, 59 patients with epilepsy were randomised to receive either the antiepileptic drug progabide or a placebo in addition to standard chemotherapy. The number of seizures was counted over four 2-week periods. In addition, a baseline seizure rate was recorded for each patient, based on the 8-week prerandomisation seizure count. Finally, the age of each patient was recorded. Data for the first five patients are given in Table 14.2. In this example, the observations are counts which can take only positive values and thus again make the normality assumption needed for the linear mixed-effects models of Chapter 13 difficult to justify.

In the models for Gaussian responses described in Chapter 13, estimation of the regression parameters linking explanatory variables to the response variable and their standard errors needed to take account of the correlational structure of the data, but their interpretation could be undertaken *independently* of this structure. When modelling non-normal responses, this independence of estimation and interpretation no longer holds; different

TABLE 14.1

Respiratory Disorder Data for First Five Patients

Patient	Centre	Treatment	Sex	Age	BL	V1	V2	V3	V4
1	1	1	1	46	0	0	0	0	0
2	1	1	1	28	0	0	0	0	0
3	1	2	1	23	1	1	1	1	1
4	1	1	1	44	1	1	1	1	0
5	1	1	2	13	1	1	1	1	1

Notes: Treatment: 1 = placebo; 2 = active. Sex: 1 = male; 2 = female.

TABLE 14.2

Data for Five Patients from a Clinical Trial of Patients Suffering from Epilepsy

Subject ID	Period 1	Period 2	Period 3	Period 4	Treatment	Baseline	Age
1	5	3	3	3	0	11	31
2	3	5	3	3	0	11	30
3	2	4	0	5	0	6	25
4	4	4	1	4	0	8	36
5	7	18	9	21	0	66	22

Source: Thall, P. F. and Vail, S. C. 1990. *Biometrics*, 46:657–671.

assumptions about the source of the within-subject correlation (the term correlation is not entirely satisfactory here, particularly for a repeated binary response, as we shall see later) can lead to regression coefficients with quite distinct interpretations (for the reasons why, see Fitzmaurice, Laird, and Ware 2004). The essential difference is between *marginal models* (also known as *population-average models*) and *conditional models* (also known as *subject-specific models*). There is no automatic way of choosing between these two types of models for the analysis of non-normal longitudinal data; instead, the choice has to be made on subject-matter considerations, knowing that the different model types have different inferential targets and address often subtly different scientific questions, as we shall attempt to make clear in the following section.

14.2 Marginal Models and Conditional Models

14.2.1 Marginal Models

Marginal models are essentially an extension of generalised linear models (GLMs) to longitudinal data. The 'marginal' term is used in this context to describe that the mean response depends only on the covariates of interest and not on any random effects. This is in contrast to the linear mixed-effects models of the previous chapter, where the mean response depends not only on the covariates but also on a number of random effects. In essence, longitudinal data can be considered as a series of cross sections, and marginal models for such data use the generalised linear model to fit each cross section.

In such models, the relationship of the marginal mean response to the covariates is modelled separately from the within-subject correlation among the repeated responses and the goal when fitting these models is to make inferences about population means; the within-subject correlation is regarded as a 'nuisance' characteristic of the data that nevertheless has to be accounted for properly to make correct inferences about changes in the population mean response. The marginal regression coefficients have the same interpretation as coefficients from a cross-sectional analysis, and marginal models are natural analogues for correlated data of generalised linear models for independent data.

A marginal model for longitudinal data can be specified in terms of the following three components:

- The expectation or mean of each response is conditional on the covariates, which is assumed to depend on these covariates through a known link function.

- As in conventional generalised linear models, the variances of the responses given the covariates are assumed to be of the form $V(y) = \phi V(\mu)$, where the variance function is determined by the choice of distribution family (see Chapter 10). The dispersion or scale parameter ϕ may be known or may have to be estimated. Because overdispersion is common in longitudinal data, estimation of ϕ is often needed even if the distribution requires $\phi = 1$.

- The conditional within-subject correlation among the repeated responses, given the covariates, is assumed to be a function of an additional set of association parameters.

The third component is needed to take care of the characteristic lack of independence of the repeated measurements of the response variable in longitudinal data. It should be noted that, for a binary response, the correlation is not the most useful measure of departure from independence because its values for such responses are restricted to ranges determined by the means of the response (i.e., the probability of a 'success'). The odds ratio (or log odds ratio) is a much more preferable measure of association among pairs of binary responses. (For more details, see Fitzmaurice et al. 2004.)

The problem with applying a direct analogue of the generalised linear model to longitudinal data with non-normal responses is that there is usually no suitable likelihood function with the required combination of the appropriate link function, error distribution, and correlation structure to allow maximum likelihood to be used. To overcome this problem, Liang and Zeger (1986) introduced a general method for incorporating within-subject association in GLMs, which is essentially an extension of the quasi-likelihood approach mentioned briefly in Chapter 10. The feature of this approach that differs from the usual generalised linear model is that, given the covariates, different responses on the same individual are allowed to depart from independence with a relatively small number of parameters defining a relatively simple pairwise correlation structure for the repeated measurements.

The covariance matrix of the repeated measurements implied by the assumed correlation structure is known as a 'working' covariance matrix for the repeated measures, with the implication that it may not accurately represent the variances and within-subject associations of the repeated measures. The estimated regression coefficients; are 'robust' in the sense that any misspecification of the model for the covariance has very little impact on the estimates of the regression coefficients; in particular they remain both unbiased and consistent assuming that the mean structure is correctly specified. However, misspecification of the covariance leads to incorrect values for the estimated standard errors of the estimates of the regression coefficients and can lead to misleading inferences about the regression coefficients with confidence intervals which are too narrow (or in some cases too wide) and p-values that are too small (or sometimes too large).

Where there is some doubt about the model used for the covariance structure of the repeated measurements, valid estimates of the standard errors can be obtained using the so-called *sandwich estimator*; standard error estimates obtained in this way are robust to misspecification of the covariance model. Details of the sandwich estimator are given, for example, in Fitzmaurice et al. (2004). Given that the sandwich estimator of the standard errors is available, an obvious questions arises, 'Why not use the estimator in all cases and thus avoid the effort to model the within-subject association?' For example, why not simply assume that the repeated measurements of the response are independent and then use the sandwich estimators of the standard errors of the estimated regression coefficients? Fitzmaurice et al. give two main reasons for modelling the covariance structure:

- In general, the more closely the 'working' covariance matrix approximates the true underlying covariance matrix, the greater is the efficiency or precision with which the regression coefficients can be estimated.

- The robustness property of the sandwich estimator is a large sample (or asymptotic) property, so the use of the estimator is best suited to balanced longitudinal data where the number of subjects is relatively large and the number of repeated measures relatively small. Reliance on the sandwich estimator is not to be recommended when the number of subjects is modest or the design is unbalanced.

Therefore, in general, modelling the correlation structure of the repeated measurements will be worthwhile and the following four possibilities are commonly used:

- An identity matrix leads to the independence working model in which the generalised estimating equation reduces to the univariate estimating equation given in Chapter 10, obtained by assuming that the repeated measurements are independent

- An *exchangeable* correlation matrix with a single parameter similar to that described in Chapter 13; here, the correlation between each pair of repeated measurements is assumed to be the same—that is, $\text{corr}(Y_{ij}, Y_{ik}) = \alpha$, where Y_{ij} is the jth repeated measurement for the ith individual

- An AR-1 *autoregressive* correlation matrix, also with a single parameter, but in which $\text{corr}(Y_{ij}, Y_{ik}) = \alpha^{|k-j|}$, $j \neq k$; this can allow the correlations of measurements taken further apart to be less than those taken closer to one another

- An unstructured correlation matrix with $T(T-1)/2$ parameters in which $(Y_{ij}, Y_{ik}) = \alpha_{jk}$

For binary responses it is usually preferable to specify the lack of independence part of a marginal model in terms of the log odds ratios, as we shall see in a later example.

For given values of the regression parameters $\beta_1, \ldots, \beta_p$, the α-parameters of the working correlation matrix can be estimated along with the dispersion parameter ϕ (see Zeger and Liang 1986 for details). These estimates can then be used in the so-called *generalised estimating equations* (GEEs) to obtain estimates of the regression parameters. The GEE algorithm proceeds by iterating between estimation of (1) the regression parameters using the correlation and dispersion parameters from the previous iteration and (2) the correlation and dispersion parameters using the regression parameters from the previous iteration. (For more details, see Fitmaurice et al. 2004.)

The regression parameters in a marginal model describe features of the mean response in the population and how these features relate to the covariates. This interpretation is not altered by the assumptions made about the nature or the magnitude of the lack of within-subject independence.

14.2.2 Conditional Models

In Chapter 13 we saw how the incorporation of random effects for individuals introduces correlations among the repeated measurements at the population level. In this section, we describe briefly how a generalised linear modelling approach can be applied to longitudinal data with a non-normal response by allowing some of the regression coefficients in a model to vary randomly from one individual to another. Such *generalised linear mixed-effects models*, however, can be difficult to estimate because the likelihood involves integrals over the random-effects distribution that generally do not have closed forms; the integrals have to be evaluated numerically, which in some cases may involve substantial computational effort. A consequence is that it is often only possible to fit relatively simple models.

As an illustration of a generalised linear mixed-effects model, we will look at a logistic regression model for longitudinal data with a binary response. Therefore, we consider a set of longitudinal data in which Y_{ij} is the value of a binary response for individual i at, say, time t_j. The logistic regression model (see Chapter 9) for the response is now written as

$$\text{logit}\left[\Pr\left(Y_{ij} = 1 \mid u_i\right)\right] = \beta_0 + \beta_1 t_j + u_i \tag{14.1}$$

where u_i is a random effect assumed to be normally distributed with zero mean and variance σ_u^2.

The model is a simple logistic regression model with randomly varying intercepts and can be considered as a discrete data analogue of the random intercept model described in the previous chapter. The model allows for natural heterogeneity in individuals' propensity to respond positively, a propensity that persists in all the repeated binary responses for an individual. In this model, the regression parameter β_1 represents the change in the log odds per unit change in time, as in the usual logistic regression model, but now it is *conditional* on the random effect u_i. In other words, β_1 represents the change in the log odds per unit change in time for any given individual having an unobservable underlying propensity to respond positively, u_i. The regression parameter represents the influence of the covariate on a *specific subject's* mean response. We can illustrate the conditional nature of the model graphically by simulating the model in (14.1); the result is shown in Figure 14.1.

In Figure 14.1, thin curves represent subject-specific relationships between the probability that the response equals one and a covariate x for model (14.1). The horizontal shifts are due to different values of the random intercept. The thick curve represents the population averaged relationship, formed by averaging the thin curves for each value of x. It is, in effect, the thick curve that would be estimated in a marginal model. The population averaged regression parameters tend to be attenuated (closer to zero) relative to the subject-specific regression parameters. A marginal regression model does not address questions concerning heterogeneity between individuals. Estimating the parameters in a generalised linear mixed-effects model is undertaken by some form of maximum likelihood, but for details readers are referred to Fitzmaurice et al. (2004).

The important point to reiterate here is that, in conditional models, estimated regression coefficients have to be interpreted conditional on the random effects. The regression parameters in the model are said to be *subject specific* and such effects will differ from the marginal or population averaged

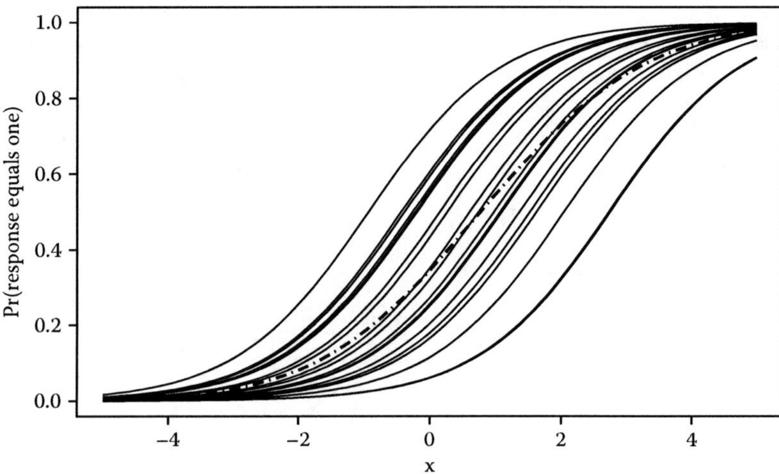

FIGURE 14.1
Simulation of random effects logistic regression model.

effects estimated using GEE, except when using an identity link function and a normal error distribution.

14.3 Analysis of the Respiratory Data

In this section we shall apply both the generalised estimating equations approach and the generalised linear mixed-effects approach to the respiratory data in Table 14.1. This will enable us to compare the population averaged and subject-specific regression estimates. We begin by fitting two marginal models to the data.

14.3.1 Marginal Models

First, we will fit a marginal model that includes only the covariate age. As we are dealing with a binary response, we shall assume that the probability of a good respiratory response is related to age by a logit link function and thus the logistic regression model will be

$$\log\left\{\frac{\Pr(Y_{ij}=1)}{\Pr(Y_{ij}=0)}\right\} = \beta_0 + \beta_1 \text{age}_i \tag{14.2}$$

where $Y_{ij}=1$ if the ith individual has good respiratory status on visit V_j and $Y_{ij}=0$ if respiratory status is poor.

To compare with later results, we will begin by fitting a model that assumes that the pairwise repeated measurements are independent. As explained in the previous chapter, we need to work with the 'long' form of the data and can produce this from their 'wide' form as follows:

```
data respw;
  infile 'c:\amsus\data\resp.dat';
  input id centre treat sex age bl v1-v4;
run;

data respl;
  set respw;
  array vs {4} v1-v4;
  do time=1 to 4;
  status=vs{time};
  output;
  end;
run;
```

We can now apply the required logistic regression model using `proc genmod` as follows:

```
proc sort data=respl;
  by id time;
run;
proc genmod data=respl desc;
  class id;
  model status=age/d=b;
repeated subject=id/type=ind modelse;
run;
```

The use of `proc genmod` to fit generalised linear models was described in Chapter 10. Extending the procedure to cover GEE models is done by including the `repeated` statement and specifying the variable which identifies the subjects, `id` in this case. This variable must be named on a `class` statement. The structure of the working correlation matrix is specified with `type=` option. Other structures commonly used for longitudinal data are autoregressive (`ar`) and unstructured (`un`). The order in which the repeated measurements were made could be specified with the `withinsubject` (`within=`) option and, if so, the variable must also be named on a `class` statement. Even when the data are in the correct order, as they are here, this option might still be important if subjects had measurements missing in the middle of a sequence. For GEE models, `proc genmod` gives the sandwich estimators by default (although it refers to them as 'empirical standard error estimates'). The model-based standard errors can be requested in addition by using the `modelse` option on the `repeated` statement.

The results giving both the sandwich estimators of the standard errors and the model-based standard errors are shown in Table 14.3. For age, the estimated

TABLE 14.3

Results from Fitting a Logistic Regression Model to the Respiratory Data with
Age as the Only Covariate and Assuming Independence between
the Repeated Measurements

GEE Fit Criteria	
QIC	616.7298
QICu	610.0202

Analysis of GEE Parameter Estimates						
Empirical Standard Error Estimates						
Parameter	Estimate	Standard Error	95% Confidence Limits		Z	Pr > |Z|
Intercept	0.6458	0.3957	−0.1297	1.4213	1.63	0.1027
age	−0.0120	0.0117	−0.0350	0.0110	−1.02	0.3059

Analysis of GEE Parameter Estimates						
Model-Based Standard Error Estimates						
Parameter	Estimate	Standard Error	95% Confidence Limits		Z	Pr > |Z|
Intercept	0.6458	0.2553	0.1454	1.1461	2.53	0.0114
age	−0.0120	0.0071	−0.0259	0.0018	−1.70	0.0888
scale	1.0000					

regression coefficient is −0.0120, but of more interest are the two estimates of
the standard error of this parameter estimate; the sandwich estimate is 0.0117
and the model-based estimate is 0.0071. Here, we know the independence
model is unrealistic and the standard error estimate based on the unrealistic
model is too optimistic about the precision of the parameter estimate.

The two fit criteria, QIC and QICu, are described in Pan (2001). The former
is a modification of the Akaike information criterion developed for models
that have been fitted using GEE. The QIC is appropriate for selecting models and working correlations, whereas the QICu is only of use for selecting
regression models (see Pan for more details). Models can be compared using
the QIC; the preferred model is the one with the lower QIC.

The assumption of independence is usually unrealistic for repeated measures data and we need to consider a marginal model that allows for departures from independence. As we are dealing here with a binary response, we
will specify lack of independence amongst the repeated measurements in
terms of pairwise log odds ratios—specifically that

$$\log OR(Y_{ij}, Y_{ik}) = \alpha_{jk} \tag{14.3}$$

where

$$\mathrm{OR}\,(Y_{ij}, Y_{ik}) = \frac{\Pr(Y_{ij} = 1, Y_{ik} = 1)\,\Pr(Y_{ij} = 0, Y_{ik} = 0)}{\Pr(Y_{ij} = 1, Y_{ik} = 0)\,\Pr(Y_{ij} = 0, Y_{ik} = 1)} \qquad (14.4)$$

To begin, we will again fit this new model to the data with the single covariate, age. To fit this model, we use the following SAS code:

```
proc genmod data=respl desc;
 class id;
 model status=age / d=b;
repeated subject=id / logor=fullclust modelse;
run;
```

The results are shown in Table 14.4.

Comparing the values of the empirical and model-based estimates of the standard error of the age regression coefficient in this model, we find that they are very similar (0.0116 and 0.0113) and also very similar to the empirical estimate in the previous 'independence' model (0.0117). The estimates of the parameters defining the covariance structure are of little real interest, although they are all highly significant and indicate the positive relationships between the pairs of repeated measurements.

Now we will fit a marginal model again with the association structure shown in (14.3) but with treatment, time, sex, age, centre, and baseline respiratory status as covariates. Using an obvious nomenclature to label the covariate values for the ith individual and where time$_j$ takes the value j for $j = 1, 2, 3, 4$, the logistic regression model we shall fit is

$$\log\left\{\frac{\Pr(Y_{ij} = 1)}{\Pr(Y_{ij} = 0)}\right\} = \beta_0 + \beta_1 \mathrm{age}_i + \beta_2 \mathrm{time}_j + \beta_3 \mathrm{baseline}_i \qquad (14.5)$$

$$+ \beta_4 \mathrm{center}_i + \beta_5 \mathrm{treatment}_i + \beta_6 \mathrm{sex}_i$$

The SAS code required to fit this model is as follows:

```
proc genmod data=respl desc;
class id;
 model status=centre treat sex age time bl / d=b;
repeated subject=id / logor=fullclust modelse;
run;
```

The results are shown in Table 14.5.

First, we might compare the empirical estimates of the standard errors and those derived from the fitted model. If we do this, we find that the two sets of standard error estimates are very similar, suggesting that the

TABLE 14.4

Results from Fitting a Logistic Regression Model to the Respiratory Data with a Single Covariate, Age, and the Dependence Structure Specified in Equation (14.3)

Log Odds Ratio Parameter Information	
Parameter	**Group**
Alpha1	(1, 2)
Alpha2	(1, 3)
Alpha3	(1, 4)
Alpha4	(2, 3)
Alpha5	(2, 4)
Alpha6	(3, 4)

GEE Fit Criteria	
QIC	616.6598
QICu	610.0499

Analysis of GEE Parameter Estimates						
Empirical Standard Error Estimates						
Parameter	**Estimate**	**Standard Error**	**95% Confidence Limits**		**Z**	**Pr > |Z|**
Intercept	0.6338	0.3948	−0.1400	1.4076	1.61	0.1084
age	−0.0113	0.0116	−0.0341	0.0116	−0.97	0.3334
Alpha1	2.2440	0.4441	1.3737	3.1143	5.05	<.0001
Alpha2	1.9214	0.4294	1.0798	2.7630	4.47	<.0001
Alpha3	2.3449	0.4492	1.4645	3.2252	5.22	<.0001
Alpha4	2.6370	0.4695	1.7169	3.5571	5.62	<.0001
Alpha5	2.4557	0.4554	1.5632	3.3482	5.39	<.0001
Alpha6	2.7506	0.4769	1.8159	3.6852	5.77	<.0001

Analysis of GEE Parameter Estimates						
Model-Based Standard Error Estimates						
Parameter	**Estimate**	**Standard Error**	**95% Confidence Limits**		**Z**	**Pr > |Z|**
Intercept	0.6338	0.4097	−0.1692	1.4368	1.55	0.1219
age	−0.0113	0.0113	−0.0335	0.0110	−0.99	0.3205
Alpha1	2.2440					

(Continued)

TABLE 14.4 (*Continued*)

Results from Fitting a Logistic Regression Model to the Respiratory Data with a Single Covariate, Age, and the Dependence Structure Specified in Equation (14.3)

Analysis of GEE Parameter Estimates					
Model-Based Standard Error Estimates					
Parameter	Estimate	Standard Error	95% Confidence Limits	Z	Pr > |Z|
Alpha2	1.9214				
Alpha3	2.3449				
Alpha4	2.6370				
Alpha5	2.4557				
Alpha6	2.7506				
Scale	1.0000				

chosen nonindependence structure adequately describes the departures from independence in the data. The covariate of most interest in this study is, of course, treatment, and the estimated regression coefficient for this covariate is 1.297 with a 95% confidence interval [0.635, 1.960] (using the model standard errors). Exponentiating the limits of the confidence interval leads to the conclusion that the odds in favour of a good respiratory response in the active treatment group are between about two and seven times the corresponding odds in the placebo group. (It is of some interest to note that this confidence interval is very similar to the confidence interval arrived at from the simpler summary measure overdispersed model fitted to the respiratory data in Chapter 12.)

The values of the fit criteria in Table 14.5 are much lower than the corresponding values in Tables 14.4 and 14.3, demonstrating that the model specified in (14.5) is, not surprisingly, far better than the model defined by (14.2). (Other correlation structures could be considered but this will be left as an exercise for the reader.)

14.3.2 Generalised Linear Mixed-Effects Models

In this section, we will fit the following conditional model to the respiratory data:

$$\log\left\{\frac{\Pr(Y_{ij}=1\,|\,u_i)}{\Pr(Y_{ij}=0\,|\,u_i)}\right\} = \beta_0 + \beta_1 \text{age}_i + \beta_2 \text{time}_j + \beta_3 \text{baseline}_i + \beta_4 \text{center}_i \tag{14.6}$$

$$+\,\beta_5 \text{treatment}_i + \beta_6 \text{sex}_i + u_i$$

where u_i is a random effect assumed to be normally distributed with zero mean and variance σ_u^2.

TABLE 14.5

Results from Fitting Logistic Regression Model Specified in Equation (14.5) to the Respiratory Data Using the Dependence Structure Specified in Equation (14.3)

Log Odds Ratio Parameter Information	
Parameter	Group
Alpha1	(1, 2)
Alpha2	(1, 3)
Alpha3	(1, 4)
Alpha4	(2, 3)
Alpha5	(2, 4)
Alpha6	(3, 4)

GEE Fit Criteria	
QIC	508.6969
QICu	496.9675

Analysis of GEE Parameter Estimates

Empirical Standard Error Estimates

Parameter	Estimate	Standard Error	95% Confidence Limits		Z	Pr > |Z|
Intercept	−2.8383	0.8955	−4.5934	−1.0832	−3.17	0.0015
Centre	0.6472	0.3524	−0.0435	1.3378	1.84	0.0663
Treat	1.2974	0.3446	0.6221	1.9727	3.77	0.0002
Sex	0.0869	0.4396	−0.7746	0.9484	0.20	0.8433
Age	−0.0154	0.0126	−0.0401	0.0093	−1.22	0.2219
Time	−0.0710	0.0801	−0.2279	0.0860	−0.89	0.3755
BI	1.9386	0.3446	1.2631	2.6141	5.63	<.0001
Alpha1	1.6208	0.4930	0.6545	2.5871	3.29	0.0010
Alpha2	1.0557	0.4879	0.0995	2.0119	2.16	0.0305
Alpha3	1.6813	0.4874	0.7260	2.6366	3.45	0.0006
Alpha4	2.0995	0.5038	1.1122	3.0869	4.17	<.0001
Alpha5	1.9482	0.4761	1.0151	2.8812	4.09	<.0001
Alpha6	2.2137	0.5040	1.2258	3.2015	4.39	<.0001

Analysis of GEE Parameter Estimates

Model-Based Standard Error Estimates

Parameter	Estimate	Standard Error	95% Confidence Limits		Z	Pr > |Z|
Intercept	−2.8383	0.9266	−4.6544	−1.0222	−3.06	0.0022
centre	0.6472	0.3458	−0.0306	1.3249	1.87	0.0613

(Continued)

TABLE 14.5 (*Continued*)

Results from Fitting Logistic Regression Model Specified in Equation (14.5) to the Respiratory Data Using the Dependence Structure Specified in Equation (14.3)

Analysis of GEE Parameter Estimates						
Model-Based Standard Error Estimates						
Parameter	**Estimate**	**Standard Error**	**95% Confidence Limits**		**Z**	**Pr > |Z|**
Treat	1.2974	0.3382	0.6345	1.9602	3.84	0.0001
Sex	0.0869	0.4267	−0.7494	0.9232	0.20	0.8386
Age	−0.0154	0.0128	−0.0404	0.0096	−1.21	0.2277
Time	−0.0710	0.0815	−0.2307	0.0887	−0.87	0.3838
BI	1.9386	0.3451	1.2622	2.6150	5.62	<.0001
Alpha1	1.6208					
Alpha2	1.0557					
Alpha3	1.6813					
Alpha4	2.0995					
Alpha5	1.9482					
Alpha6	2.2137					
Scale	1.0000					

To fit this model, we use the following SAS code:

```
proc glimmix data=respl noclprint;
 class id;
 model status(desc)=centre treat sex age time bl/d=binary s
 ddfm=bw;
 random int/subject=id;
run;
```

Proc glimmix has a similar syntax to proc mixed with additional options to cover distributions other than the normal distribution. The distribution is specified with the d= option on the model statement. The solution (s) option gives the parameter estimates for the fixed effects and ddfm=bw specifies the between–within method of calculating the denominator degrees of freedom, which is suitable for longitudinal data. For binary responses, the desc option can be specified in parentheses after the response variable to reverse the default ordering. The noclprint option on the proc statement is used to suppress the listing of the patient ids.

The results are shown in Table 14.6. The estimated regression coefficients and their estimated standard errors are not too different from the corresponding coefficients and standard errors derived from the marginal model fitted to the data and given in Table 14.5. Concentrating on the estimated treatment effect from the random-effects model—namely, 1.535, with estimated

TABLE 14.6

Results from Fitting the Logistic Regression Model Specified
in Equation (14.7) to the Respiratory Data

Fit Statistics	
−2 Res Log Pseudo-Likelihood	2108.37
Generalised Chi-Square	281.75
Generalised Chi-Square/DF	0.64

Covariance Parameter Estimates			
Cov Parm	Subject	Estimate	Standard Error
Intercept	id	2.0433	0.5305

Solutions for Fixed Effects					
Effect	Estimate	Standard Error	DF	t Value	Pr > |t|
Intercept	−3.3772	1.0369	105	−3.26	0.0015
Centre	0.7563	0.4110	105	1.84	0.0686
Treat	1.5350	0.3911	105	3.92	0.0002
Sex	0.1426	0.5127	105	0.28	0.7814
Age	−0.01891	0.01513	105	−1.25	0.2142
Time	−0.08012	0.1018	332	−0.79	0.4317
BI	2.1967	0.4003	105	5.49	<.0001

standard error 0.391—leads to a 95% confidence interval for the odds ratio
of approximately [2, 10]. In this model, the treatment effect describes the
effect of treatment on a specific patient's probability of a positive respiratory
response. The variance of the random effects in the model is estimated to be
2.04 with a standard error of 0.53.

14.4 Analysis of Epilepsy Data

Here we will begin by constructing a useful graphic of the data—namely,
box plots of the number of epileptic seizures before and after treatment separately for the two treatment groups (the before count is the 2-week average).
The necessary code is

```
data epiw;
  infile 'c:\AMSUS\data\epi.dat';
  input id p1-p4 treat bl age;
```

```
run;
data epil;
  set epiw;
  bl=bl/4;
  lbl=log(bl);
  array ps {*} bl p1-p4;
  do time=1 to 5;
  nsz=ps{time};
  output;
  end;
run;

proc format;
  value visits 1='Baseline' 2='Week 2' 3='Week 4' 4='Week 6'
  5='Week 8';
run;
proc sgpanel data=epil;
  panelby treat/columns=2 spacing=10;
  vbox nsz/category=time datalabel=id labelfar;
  format time visits.;
run;
```

The resulting graph is shown in Figure 14.2. There is little evidence for a convincing treatment effect from this graph, but there is evidence that some of the patients have some very large seizure rates, particularly patient 49. This patient, who could have an unreasonably large influence on any analysis of the data, should perhaps be considered for removal prior to any such analysis. Here, however, we shall model *all* the data, *including* the observations with very high seizure rates. Readers are encouraged to repeat the analysis with at least observation number 49 removed and then compare the results with the ones that follow.

It is also useful to look at the means and variances of seizure rates at baseline and at the post-treatment times; these can be found using the following code:

```
proc means data=epil mean var;
  class time;
  var nsz;
run;
```

The results are given in Table 14.7. The variances are far larger than the corresponding means—a point we will return to in the next subsection.

Now we shall move on to fit a number of marginal models to these data.

14.4.1 Marginal Models

Count data are usually modelled as Poisson random variables using a log link function and that is what we shall do here. Using all available covariates, the model for the mean response is therefore

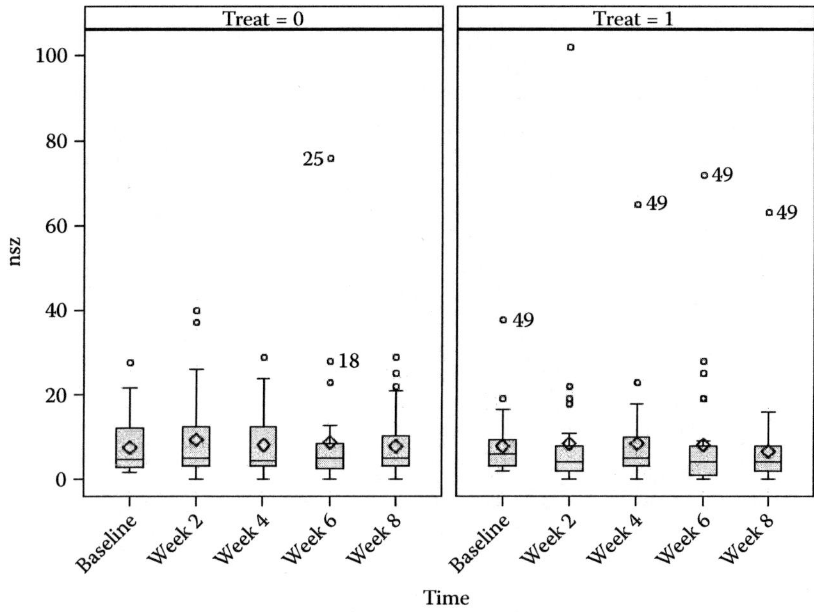

FIGURE 14.2
Box plots of seizure counts at each time point for each treatment group.

TABLE 14.7

Means and Variances of Seizure Rates at
Baseline and for the Post-treatment Times

Analysis Variable: nsz			
Time	*N* obs.	Mean	Variance
1	59	7.8050847	45.1488530
2	59	8.9491525	220.0835769
3	59	8.3559322	103.7849211
4	59	8.4406780	200.1817650
5	59	7.3050847	93.1122151

$$\log\left[E(N_{ij})\right] = \beta_0 + \beta_1 \text{time}_j + \beta_2 \log(\text{baseline}_i) + \beta_3 \text{treatment}_i \qquad (14.7)$$

where N_{ij} is the observed number of seizures for individual i in time period
time_j and $\text{time}_j = j$, $j = 1, 2, 3, 4$.

We use log(baseline) rather than baseline itself so that the exponentiated regression coefficient for the covariate represents the effect of the number of baseline seizures on subsequent seizure rates. We shall assume an exchangeable correlational structure—namely, that

$$\text{Corr}(Y_{ij}, Y_{ik}) = \alpha \qquad\qquad (14.8)$$

The descriptive statistics given in Table 14.7 show that the variances are substantially greater than the corresponding means. As a result, the Poisson assumption that the means and variances are the same is not appropriate for these data; this overdispersion will be accounted for by allowing for the scale parameter to be estimated and not fixed at one. The model is fitted using the following code:

```
data epil;
  set epil;
  if time>1;
run;

proc genmod data=epil;
class id;
 model nsz= treat age time lbl/d=p;
 repeated subject=id/type=exch modelse;
run;
```

The results are shown in Table 14.8.

The model-based standard errors and the corresponding empirical values are very similar. There is no evidence of a treatment effect. Clearly, the baseline seizure rate influences the subsequent seizure rates and age also has an effect just significant at the 5% level. The exponentiated confidence interval limits for the age effect given in Table 14.8 indicate that the seizure rate for an increase in age of 1 year is about 1.008 to 1.04 times that of the younger age. Here, it might be more useful to give the corresponding confidence interval for a 10-year age difference; this can be calculated simply as $[\exp(10 \times 0.02 - 1.96 \times 0.008), \exp(10 \times 0.02 + 1.96 \times 0.008)]$—that is, $[1.04, 1.43]$.

The scale parameter is estimated to be 2.2, indicating the overdispersion, relative to that predicted by Poisson variability, in these data.

14.4.2 Generalised Linear Mixed-Effects Models

We begin by fitting a random intercept model, namely,

$$\log\left[E(N_{ij} \mid u_i)\right] = \beta_0 + \beta_1 \text{time}_j + \beta_2 \log(\text{baseline}_i) + \beta_3 \text{treatment}_i + u_i \qquad (14.9)$$

where u_i is a random effect assumed to be normally distributed with zero mean and variance σ_u^2. To fit the model, we use the following code:

```
proc glimmix data=epil noclprint method=mspl;
  class id;
  model nsz= treat age time lbl/s ddfm=bw d=p;
  random int/subject=id;
run;
```

TABLE 14.8

Results from Fitting the Model Specified by Equation (14.8) to the Epilepsy
Data Using the Dependence Structure in Equation (14.9)

GEE Fit Criteria	
QIC	−1195.7698
QICu	−1214.9370

Analysis of GEE Parameter Estimates						
Empirical Standard Error Estimates						
Parameter	Estimate	Standard Error	95% Confidence Limits		Z	Pr > |Z|
Intercept	−0.8166	0.4722	−1.7420	0.1089	−1.73	0.0837
Treat	−0.0242	0.1911	−0.3987	0.3503	−0.13	0.8992
Age	0.0200	0.0098	0.0008	0.0392	2.04	0.0412
Time	−0.0587	0.0350	−0.1273	0.0099	−1.68	0.0934
Lbl	1.2247	0.1557	0.9196	1.5298	7.87	<.0001

Analysis of GEE Parameter Estimates						
Model-Based Standard Error Estimates						
Parameter	Estimate	Standard Error	95% Confidence Limits		Z	Pr > |Z|
Intercept	−0.8166	0.5358	−1.8668	0.2336	−1.52	0.1275
Treat	−0.0242	0.1553	−0.3286	0.2802	−0.16	0.8761
Age	0.0200	0.0125	−0.0045	0.0445	1.60	0.1098
Time	−0.0587	0.0346	−0.1265	0.0091	−1.70	0.0896
Lbl	1.2247	0.1055	1.0178	1.4316	11.60	<.0001
Scale	2.1959					

The results are shown in Table 14.9.

Of most interest here is that the treatment effect is marginally significant at the 5% level. An approximate 95% confidence interval for the effect of treatment on seizure count is given by [exp(−0.3172 − 2*0.1542), exp(−0.3172 + 2*0.1542)—that is, [0.53,0.99]. The seizure count with progabide is estimated to be between just over 50% and 99% of the seizure rate on the placebo; this describes the effect of treatment on a specific patient's seizure count. The treatment effect in the marginal model fitted to these data in the previous section describes the effect of treatment in the population of patients assigned to placebo versus progabide. The random effects in the model are estimated to have variance 0.285.

TABLE 14.9

Results from Fitting Model in Equation (14.8) to Epilepsy Data

Fit Statistics	
–2 Log Pseudo-Likelihood	568.24
Generalised Chi-Square	411.39
Generalised Chi-Square/DF	1.74

Covariance Parameter Estimates			
Cov Parm	Subject	Estimate	Standard Error
Intercept	id	0.2606	0.05921

Solutions for Fixed Effects					
Effect	Estimate	Standard Error	DF	t Value	Pr > |t|
Intercept	–0.06650	0.4365	55	–0.15	0.8795
treat	–0.3135	0.1485	55	–2.11	0.0393
age	0.01063	0.01202	55	0.88	0.3804
time	–0.05872	0.02028	176	–2.90	0.0043
lbl	1.0104	0.09998	55	10.11	<.0001

Now we will fit a model that includes random effects for intercept and slope:

$$\log\left[E(N_{ij}\,|\,\mathbf{u})\right] = \beta_0 + (\beta_1 + u_{i2})\text{time}_j + \beta_2\log(\text{baseline}_i)$$
$$+ \beta_3\text{treatment}_i + u_{i1} \tag{14.10}$$

where $\mathbf{u}' = [u_{i1}, u_{i2}]$ and the random effects are assumed to have a bivariate normal distribution with zero mean and a covariance matrix $\Sigma_\mathbf{u}$ given by

$$\Sigma_\mathbf{u} = \begin{pmatrix} \sigma_{u_1} & \sigma_{u_1 u_2} \\ \sigma_{u_1 u_2} & \sigma_{u_2} \end{pmatrix} \tag{14.11}$$

Here, the model is a log-linear regression model with randomly varying intercept and slopes used to describe the heterogeneity among individuals in both their baseline seizure level and in the expected number of seizures over time.

When initially fitting the previous random intercept model, a procedure called *residual pseudolikelihood* was used; this is the default estimation procedure in SAS. But using this method to fit the more complex model with random intercepts and slopes resulted in problems of convergence, so an alternative estimation procedure, *maximum pseudolikelihood,* was used. The required SAS code to fit the new model becomes

```
proc glimmix data=epil noclprint method=mspl;
 class id;
 model nsz= treat age time lbl/s ddfm=bw d=p;
 random int time/subject=id type=un;
run;
```

The results are shown in Table 14.10. The parameter estimates in this table are very similar to those in Table 14.9. If we compare the log likelihood values for the two models, we see that the decrease when fitting the random intercept and random slope effects is 20.38 for the addition of two parameters: the variance of the slope random effect and the covariance of the two random effects. Testing the decrease as a chi-squared variable with two degrees of freedom suggests that the more complicated model gives a far better fit here.

TABLE 14.10

Results from Fitting Model Specified in Equations (14.10) and (14.11) to Epilepsy Data

Fit Statistics	
−2 Log Pseudo-Likelihood	547.86
Generalised Chi-Square	360.04
Generalised Chi-Square/DF	1.53

Covariance Parameter Estimates			
Cov Parm	Subject	Estimate	Standard Error
UN(1,1)	Id	0.5322	0.1755
UN(2,1)	Id	−0.07580	0.03635
UN(2,2)	Id	0.02088	0.008960

Solutions for Fixed Effects					
Effect	Estimate	Standard Error	DF	t Value	Pr > |t|
Intercept	−0.07339	0.4425	55	−0.17	0.8689
treat	−0.3095	0.1478	55	−2.09	0.0409
age	0.009909	0.01197	55	0.83	0.4113
time	−0.05130	0.03106	176	−1.65	0.1004
lbl	1.0077	0.09952	55	10.13	<.0001

The random effects for the intercept have estimated variance of 0.53 and, for the slope random effects, the corresponding value is 0.021; the covariance of the two types of random effects is −0.076.

14.5 Summary

In this chapter, the generalised linear model has been extended to deal with longitudinal data in two different ways: marginal models and conditional or generalised linear mixed-effects models. Marginal models are used to make inferences about population means on some transformed scale—for example, the logit or log scale—by modelling the mean conditional on the covariates but not on unobserved random effects. The model for the mean and the model to account for lack of pairwise independence in the repeated measurements are specified separately.

In generalised linear mixed-effects models, by contrast, random effects are used to model heterogeneity in some of the regression coefficients (e.g., slopes and intercepts); however, conditional on these random effects, the repeated measurements for an individual are independent. The regression coefficients in these models have subject-specific effects that describe changes in an individual's mean response and how these changes are related to covariates. Conditional models are of most use when the aim of the investigator is to make inferences about individuals rather than the study population.

It should perhaps be said that fitting generalised linear mixed-effects models in SAS requires some care as convergence and other problems can occur. More details are given in Fitzmaurice et al. (2004), who also give an excellent and more detailed account of marginal and conditional models for longitudinal data than that given in this chapter, which is of necessity relatively brief.

15

Survival Analysis

15.1 Introduction

In many medical studies, the main outcome variable is the time to the occurrence of a particular event. In a randomised controlled trial of treatment for cancer, for example, surgery, radiation, and chemotherapy might be compared with respect to time from randomisation and the start of therapy until death. In this case, the event of interest is the death of a patient, but in other situations, it might be remission from a disease, relief from symptoms, or the recurrence of a particular condition. Such observations are generally referred to by the generic term *survival data*, even when the endpoint or event being considered is not death but something else. Such data generally require special techniques for their analysis for two main reasons:

- Survival data are generally not symmetrically distributed; such data are often positively skewed, with a few individuals surviving a very long time compared to the majority. Consequently, basing the analysis of survival data on, say, the assumption that they have a normal distribution would not be sensible.

- At the completion of the study, some individuals may not have reached the endpoint of interest (death, relapse, etc.) so, for these individuals, their exact survival times will not be known, although they will be greater than the times the individuals have been in the study. The survival times of these individuals are said to be *censored*. More precisely, the survival times are *right censored:* The right-censored survival time is less than the actual, but unknown, survival time. (Other forms of censoring are possible—for example, *left censoring* and *interval censoring;* see Collett 2003b. However, we shall not be concerned with either of these in this chapter.)

An important assumption made by the methods for the analysis of survival times to be described later in this chapter is that the actual survival time of an individual, t, is independent of any mechanism that causes that individual's survival time to be censored at time c, where $c < t$. For example, in a treatment trial, where the survival time of an individual may be censored because treatment is withdrawn as a result of deterioration in the individual's health, actual survival time is not independent of the mechanism that has caused the censoring; here we have what is known as *informative censoring*. This type of censoring makes the survival analysis methods described later largely invalid.

15.2 Survivor Function and the Hazard Function

The first step in the analysis of a set of survival times is the calculation of numerical summaries and the construction of hopefully informative graphics. Central to this first step are two functions used to describe the distribution of survival times—namely, the *survivor* (or *survival*) function and the *hazard* function.

15.2.1 Survivor Function

The survivor function, $S(t)$, is defined as the probability that the survival time, T, is greater than or equal to t—that is,

$$S(t) = \Pr(T > t) \tag{15.1}$$

We will first examine what the survivor function looks like for two distributions often used to model survival time data: the *exponential distribution* and the *Weibull distribution*. First, the exponential with probability density function is

$$f(t) = \lambda e^{-\lambda t}, \ 0 \le t < \infty \tag{15.2}$$

for which the survivor function is given by

$$S(t) = \int_t^\infty \lambda e^{-\lambda u} du = e^{-\lambda t} \tag{15.3}$$

Plots of the survivor functions of the exponential distribution for different values of λ are shown in Figure 15.1.

The Weibull probability density function is given by

$$f(t) = \lambda \gamma t^{\gamma-1} \exp(-\lambda t^\gamma), 0 \le t < \infty \tag{15.4}$$

The survivor function of the Weibull is given by

$$S(t) = \int_t^\infty \lambda \gamma u^{\gamma-1} \exp(-\lambda u^\gamma) du = \exp(-\lambda t^\gamma) \tag{15.5}$$

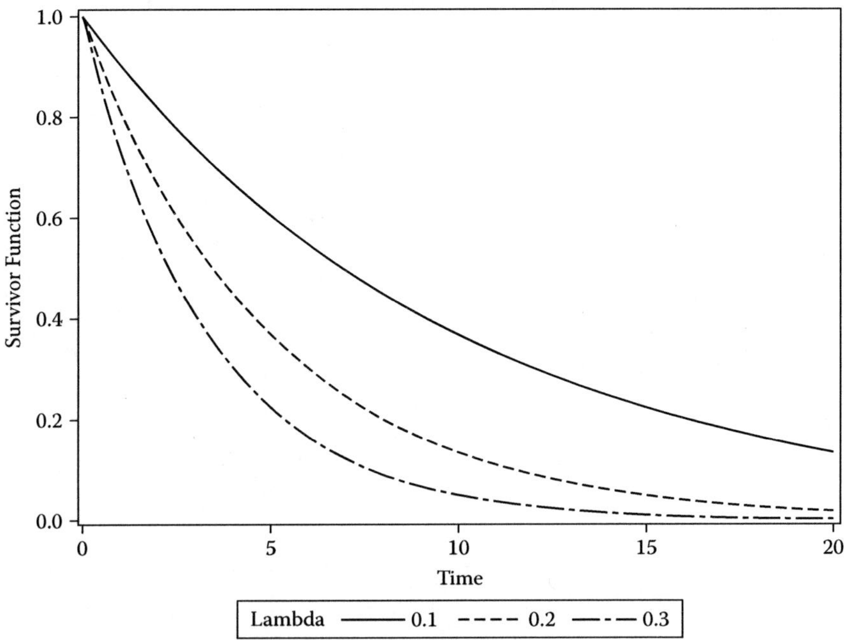

FIGURE 15.1
Survival functions for a number of exponential distributions.

Plots of the survivor function of the Weibull distribution for different values of the scale parameter, λ, and the shape parameter, γ, are shown in Figure 15.2.

When we have a sample of survival times, a plot of an estimate of $S(t)$ against t is often a useful way of describing the survival experience of the individuals in the sample. When there are no censored observations in a sample of n survival times, a *nonparametric estimate* (i.e., does not require specific assumptions about the distribution of the survival times) of the survivor function is given by

$$\hat{S}(t) = \frac{\text{number of individuals with survival times} \geq t}{\text{number of individuals in the data set}} \qquad (15.6)$$

with the convention that $\hat{S}(t) = 1$ for t less than the smallest observed survival time. Because this is simply a proportion, confidence intervals can be obtained for each time t by using the variance estimate

$$\hat{S}(t)\left(1 - \hat{S}(t)\right) / n \qquad (15.7)$$

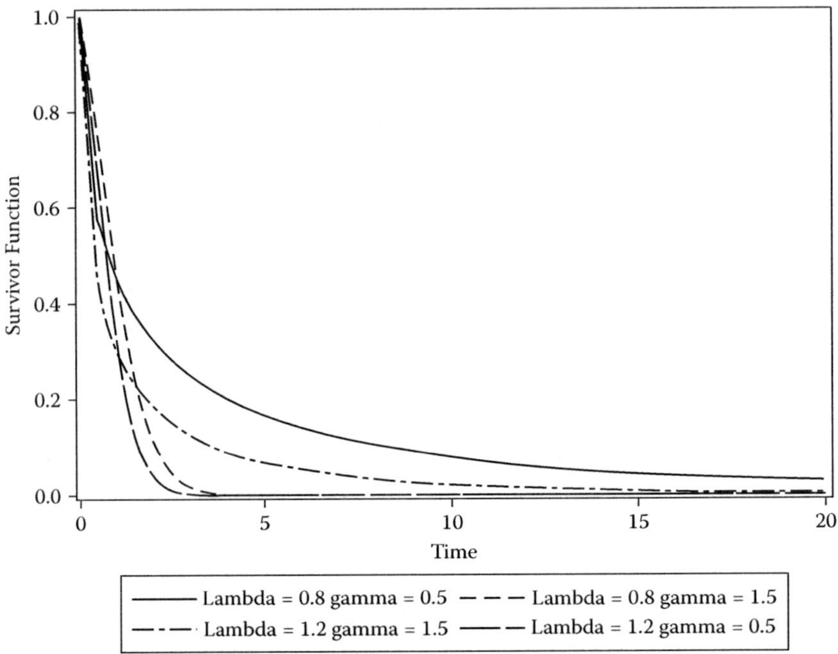

FIGURE 15.2
Survival functions for a number of Weibull distributions.

The estimated survivor function, $\hat{S}(t)$, is assumed to be constant between two adjacent death times, with the consequence that a plot of t against $\hat{S}(t)$ is a *step function* which decreases immediately after each observed survival time.

This simple method cannot be used to estimate the survivor function when the data contain censored observations, and such observations are the quintessential feature of survival data. In the presence of censoring, the survivor function is generally estimated using the *Kaplan–Meier estimator* (also known as the *product-limit estimator*), which again is nonparametric. This estimator is based on the calculation and use of conditional probabilities and incorporates information from all the observations available, both censored and uncensored, by considering survival to any point in time as a series of 'steps', which are intervals defined by a rank ordering of the survival times. Therefore, we denote by $t_1 < t_2...$ the times when 'deaths' occurred and by d_j the number of individuals who die at time t_j. Then, the Kaplan–Meier estimator for the survivor function is given by

$$\hat{S}(t) = \prod_{t_j \leq t}\left(1 - \frac{d_j}{r_j}\right) \tag{15.8}$$

where r_j is the number of individuals at risk (i.e., alive and not censored) just prior to time t_j. If there are no censored observations, the estimator in (15.8) reduces to that in (15.6). The estimated variance of the Kaplan–Meier estimator is given by

$$V\left[\hat{S}(t)\right] = [\hat{S}(t)]^2 \sum_{t_j \le t} \frac{d_j}{r_j(r_j - d_j)} \tag{15.9}$$

When there is no censoring, this reduces to the variance estimator given in (15.7). A $100(1 - \alpha)\%$ confidence interval for $S(t)$ for a given value of t is given by the interval $\hat{S}(t) \pm z_{\alpha/2}\sqrt{V\left[\hat{S}(t)\right]}$ where $z_{\alpha/2}$ is the upper $\alpha/2$ value of the standard normal distribution. These intervals can be superimposed on a graph of the estimated survivor function, as we shall see later.

Collett (2003b) points out a potential problem with this procedure that arises from the fact that the confidence intervals are symmetric and, when the survivor function is close to zero or unity, symmetric intervals are inappropriate because they can lead to confidence intervals for the survivor function that lie outside the interval (0,1). Collett offers as a pragmatic solution replacing any limit that is greater than unity by 1.0 and any limit that is less than zero by 0.0. He also describes some alternative approaches to constructing confidence intervals for the survivor function.

To illustrate the use of the Kaplan–Meier estimator, we shall use the small data set shown in Table 15.1, which gives survival times in weeks for 20 patients with stage 3 and 4 melanoma. We can find and plot the estimated survivor function and its 95% confidence interval for these data using the following SAS code:

```
data melanoma34;
   infile 'c:\AMSUS\data\melanoma34.dat';
   input weeks status$;
   if status='alive' then censor=1;
      else censor=0;
run;

ods graphics on;
proc lifetest data=melanoma34 plots=(survival(cl));
   time weeks*censor(1);
run;
```

`Proc lifetest` is used to estimate and plot the survivor function as well as to test differences in survival between groups. A range of plots are available with the `plots=` option; here, we request the survivor function plot with confidence limits. The `time` statement is used to specify survival time and censoring. The variable containing the survival times comes first and then an asterisk and the censoring variable with a value, or list of values,

TABLE 15.1

Survival Times for Patients with Stage 3
and Stage 4 Melanoma and Status of the
Patient at the End of the Study

Survival Time (weeks)	Status
12.8	Dead
15.6	Dead
24.0	Alive
26.4	Dead
29.2	Dead
30.8	Alive
39.2	Dead
42.0	Dead
58.4	Alive
72.0	Alive
77.2	Dead
82.4	Dead
87.2	Alive
94.4	Alive
97.2	Alive
106.0	Alive
114.8	Alive
117.2	Alive
140.0	Alive
168.0	Alive

indicating censored observations in parentheses. The censoring variable
needs to be numeric, so a new variable is computed for the purpose in the
preceding data step. The resulting plot is shown in Figure 15.3.

As the distribution of survival times tends to be skewed positively, the
median is the preferred summary measure of the location of the distribution. Once the survivor function has been estimated, it is simple to find the
required estimate of the *median survival time*. The median survival time is
the time beyond which 50% of the individuals in the population of interest
are expected to survive and is given by the value $t_{50\%}$ for which $S(t_{50\%}) = 0.5$.
As the estimated survivor function is a step function, it will generally not
be possible to find an estimated survival time that makes the estimated survivor function exactly equal to 0.5. Instead, the estimated median survival
time, $\hat{t}_{50\%}$, is defined to be the smallest observed survival time for which
the estimated survivor function is less than 0.5. Confidence intervals for
the median survival time can be found using the variance estimator given
in (15.5).

On occasion, the estimated survivor function is greater than 0.5 for all values of t; in these cases, the data can be summarised by estimated survival

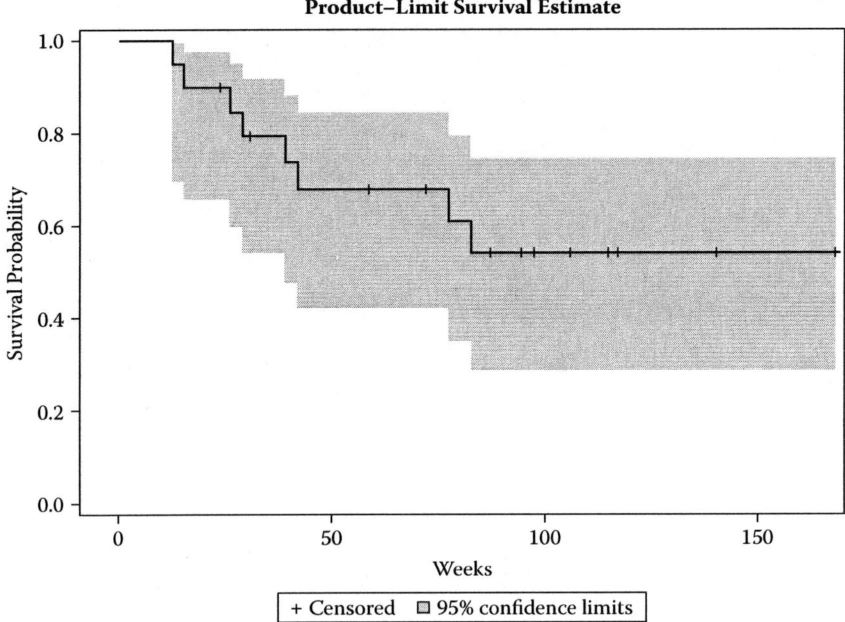

FIGURE 15.3
Estimated survivor function and 95% confidence limits for the melanoma survival times in Table 15.1.

probabilities at particular time points. For the data in Table 15.1, we cannot estimate the median survival time because more than half the observations are censored.

15.2.2 Hazard Function

In the analysis of survival data, it is often of interest to assess which periods have high or low chances of death (or whatever the event of interest may be) among those still active at the time. A suitable approach to characterise such risks is the hazard function, $h(t)$. This is defined as the probability that an individual experiences the event in a small time interval s, given that the individual has survived up to the beginning of the interval, when the size of the time interval approaches zero; mathematically this is written as

$$h(t) = \lim_{s \to 0} \frac{\Pr(t \leq T \leq t+s \,|\, T \geq t)}{s} \tag{15.10}$$

where T is the individual's survival time. The conditioning feature of this definition is very important. For example, the probability of dying at age 100 is very small because most people die before that age; in contrast, the probability of a person who has reached age 100 dying at that age is much greater.

The hazard function is a measure of how likely an individual is to experience an event as a function of the age of the individual; it is often known as the *instantaneous death rate*. Collett (2004) shows that the hazard function can be given in terms of a probability density function and the corresponding survivor function as

$$h(t) = \frac{f(t)}{S(t)} \tag{15.11}$$

It follows from (15.11) that

$$h(t) = -\frac{d}{dt}\left\{\log S(t)\right\} \tag{15.12}$$

so

$$S(t) = \exp\{-H(t)\} \tag{15.13}$$

where

$$H(t) = \int_0^t h(u)\,du \tag{15.14}$$

The function $H(t)$ is called the *integrated* or *cumulative hazard*.

Applying (15.11) first to the exponential distribution, we obtain its hazard function:

$$h(t) = \frac{\lambda e^{-\lambda t}}{e^{-\lambda t}} = \lambda \tag{15.15}$$

Here, the hazard function is a constant; the hazard of death at any time after the time origin of the study remains the same no matter how much time has elapsed.

Next, we can apply (15.11) to the Weibull distribution to obtain its hazard function:

$$h(t) = \frac{\lambda \gamma t^{\gamma-1} \exp(-\lambda t^{\gamma})}{\exp(-\lambda t^{\gamma})} = \lambda \gamma t^{\gamma-1} \tag{15.16}$$

By plotting this hazard function for different values of λ and γ (see Figure 15.4), we see that the Weibull distribution can accommodate

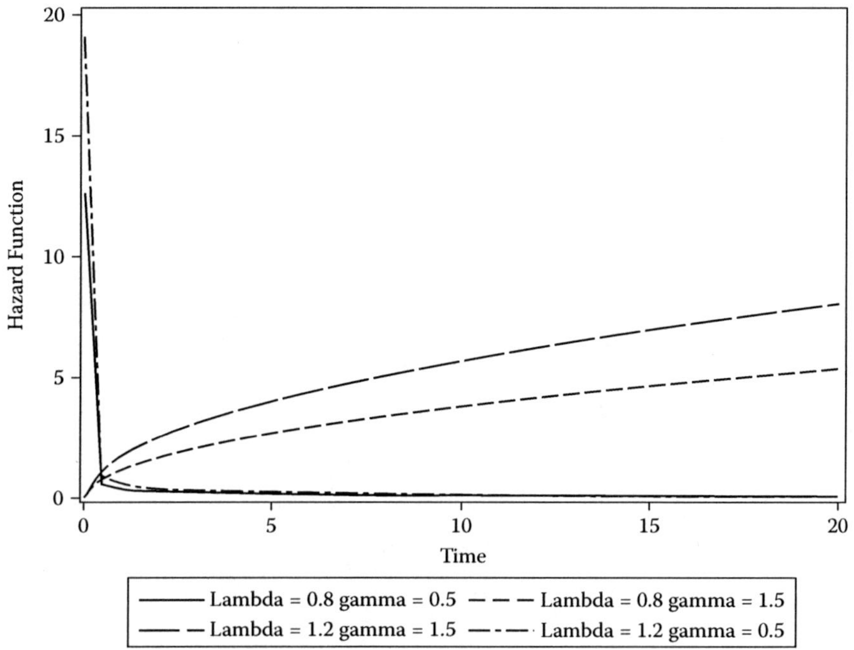

FIGURE 15.4
Weibull hazard functions.

increasing, decreasing, and constant hazard functions. In practice, constant hazard functions are uncommon, making the exponential distribution less useful than the Weibull distribution for modelling survival times. However, even the Weibull distribution may not be flexible enough for many examples of survival data, as we can see from the hazard function for death in human beings given in Figure 15.5, which has a 'bathtub' shape: It is relatively high immediately after birth, declines rapidly in the early years, and then remains relatively constant before beginning its inexorable rise in the later years. Why we should be concerned about the shape of hazard functions when dealing with survival data will become clear in the next chapter.

The hazard function can be estimated from sample data as the proportion of individuals experiencing the event of interest in an interval per unit time, given that they have survived to the beginning of the interval—that is,

$$\hat{h}(t) = \frac{\text{number of individuals 'dying' in the interval beginning at time } t}{(\text{number of individuals alive at time } t)(\text{interval width})} \quad (15.17)$$

The sampling variation in the estimate of the hazard function within each interval is usually considerable and a 'smoothed' version is produced by

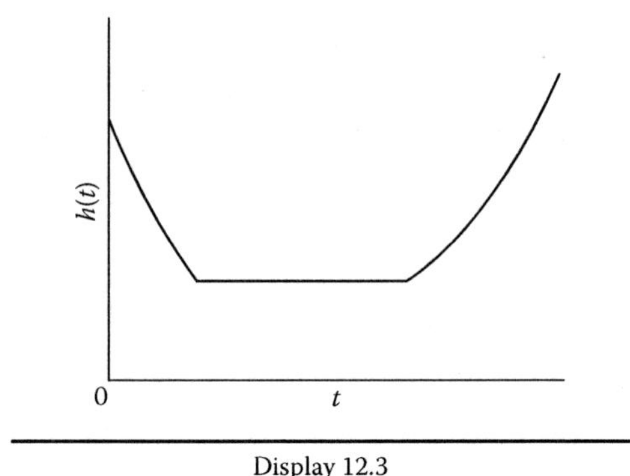

Display 12.3

FIGURE 15.5
Bathtub hazard.

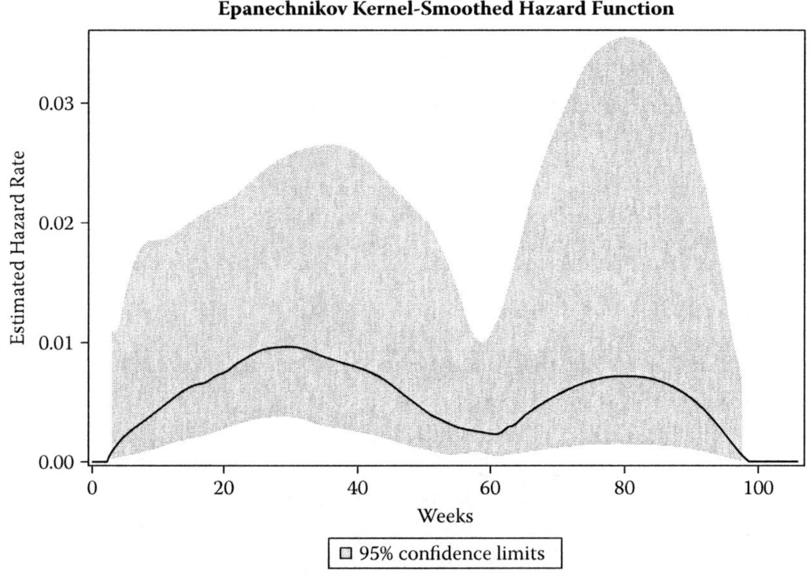

Bandwidth = 21.80363

FIGURE 15.6
Estimated hazard function for data in Table 15.1.

default when ODS graphics are on so that the following code produces the result shown in Figure 15.6:

```
ods graphics on;
proc lifetest data=melanoma34 plots=(h(cl));
  time weeks*censor(1);
run;
```

Plots of the cumulative hazard function, obtained by summing the interval estimates over time, are often easier to interpret. The result is shown in Figure 15.7. For the data in Table 15.1, the cumulative hazard function can be plotted as follows:

```
proc lifetest data=melanoma34 outsurv=ltout method=lt
intervals=1 to 170 noprint;
   time weeks*censor(1);
run;
data ltout;
   set ltout;
   cumhaz+hazard;
run;
proc sgplot data=ltout;
   series y=cumhaz x=weeks;
run;
```

Hazard functions become of more importance when we come to discuss regression models for survival data in the next chapter.

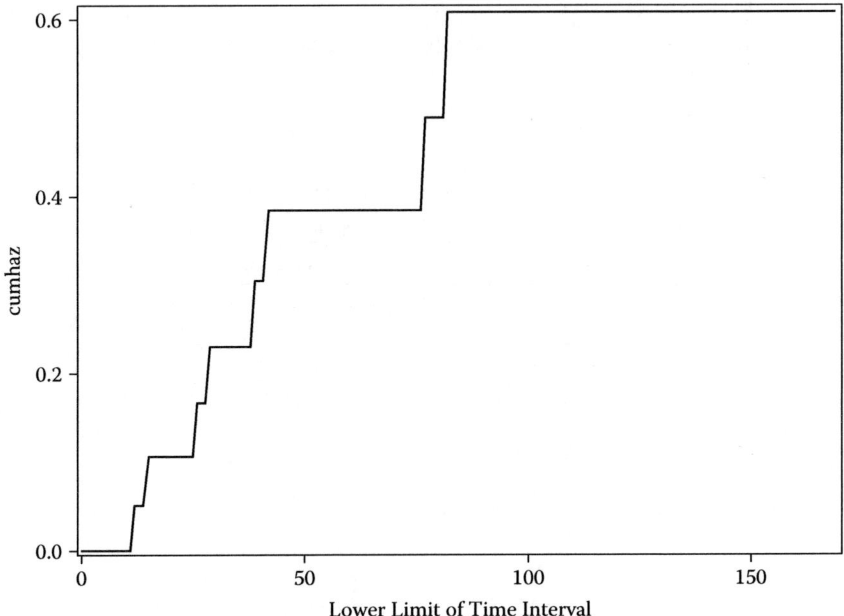

FIGURE 15.7
Estimated cumulative hazard function for data in Table 15.1.

15.3 Comparing Groups of Survival Times

Although the survivor function of a single group of patients is a useful description of their survival times, it is often the comparison of the survivor functions of different groups of patients that is of greater interest. For example, a clinician may wish to compare the survival times of males and females suffering from some particular condition. Again, a researcher may need to compare the retinopathy-free time of two groups of diabetic patients, and, in a clinical trial, the survival times of patients given an active treatment may need to be compared with those of patients receiving a placebo.

A very useful initial step in comparing the survival times of two groups of individuals is to plot the two estimated survivor functions on the same axes—perhaps along with their respective confidence intervals, although this sometimes makes the plot less rather than more useful. We will use the data in Table 15.2 to illustrate this type of plot. These data are the results of an investigation reported in Leathem and Brooks (1987) designed to evaluate a histochemical marker which discriminates between primary breast cancer that has metastasized and that which has not. The marker was a lectin from the albumin gland of the Roman snail, *Helix pomatia*, known as *Helix pomatia* agglutinin, or HPA. The marker binds to those breast cancer cells associated with metastasis to local lymph nodes and the HPA stained cells can be identified by microscopic examination. What the investigator wants to know from the data in Table 15.2 is whether or not there is any compelling evidence

TABLE 15.2

Survival Times (Weeks) of Women Who Received Surgical Treatment for Breast Cancer Grouped by the Result of HPA Staining of Their Tumours

Negative Staining		Positive Staining	
23	5	48	143
47	8	50	154[a]
69	10	59	162[a]
70[a]	13	68	188[a]
100[a]	18	71	212[a]
101[a]	24	76[a]	
148	26	105[a]	
181	26	107[a]	
198[a]	31	109[a]	
208[a]	35	113	
212[a]	40	116[a]	
224[a]	41	118	

[a] Observations are censored.

that women with negative HPA staining tend to live longer after surgery than those with positive staining.

We can construct and plot the survivor functions of the women with negative HPA staining and those with positive HPA staining and the appropriate confidence intervals using the following SAS code:

```
data HPA;
  infile 'c:\AMSUS\data\hpa.dat';
  input staining weeks censor;
run;

ods graphics on;
proc lifetest data=HPA plots=(s(cl));
  time weeks*censor(1);
  strata staining;
run;
```

The resulting plot is shown in Figure 15.8.

Plotting the survivor functions of the two groups of women gives an informal (but useful) comparison of the survival experiences of the two groups, and the two survivor functions plotted in Figure 15.8 give a strong indication that women with negative staining survive longer than those with positive staining. But in most cases, this informal appraisal of the survivor functions

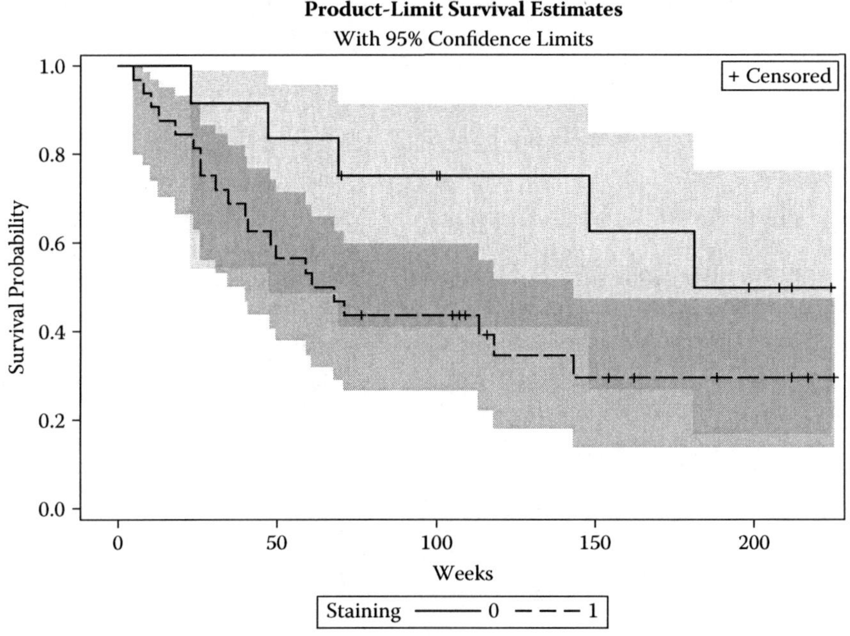

FIGURE 15.8
Plots of survivor functions and the respective confidence intervals for the data in Table 15.2.

would need to be followed up by a more formal test of the null hypothesis that the two population survivor functions are the same—that is, a test of

$$H_0: S_1 = S_2$$

A variety of tests have been suggested to assess this hypothesis, but here we shall describe only one: the *log-rank test*.

15.3.1 Log-Rank Test

We begin by supposing that there are r distinct death times in the two groups and the ordered death times are represented as $t_{(1)} < t_{(2)} < \cdots < t_{(r)}$. A 2×2 table is constructed for each of these r death times giving the number of individuals dying and the number remaining alive *and* at risk. The resulting table for the jth death time is shown in Table 15.3.

Unless two or more individuals have the same recorded death time, the values of d_{1j} and d_{2j} will be either zero or unity. Assuming that there is no difference in the survival experience of the two groups or, in other words, that the probability of death at time $t_{(j)}$ is the same in the two groups, the expected number of individuals who die at time $t_{(j)}$ can be calculated from the appropriate row and column marginal totals as when testing for independence in a 2×2 table. That is, the expected number of deaths in group 1 is $e_{2j} = n_{2j}d_j/n_j$ and, in group 2, is $e_{1j} = n_{1j}d_j/n_j$. The observed and expected number of deaths for each group, at each time point, are then summed to give values O_1, O_2, E_1, and E_2, which form the basis of the test for assessing the null hypothesis that the survivor functions of the two groups are the same; the test statistic is

$$X^2 = \frac{(O_1 - E_1)^2}{E_1} + \frac{(O_2 - E_2)^2}{E_2} \tag{15.18}$$

If the null hypothesis is true, this has a chi-squared distribution with a single degree of freedom.

Alternatives to the log-rank test include the Wilcoxon test and the likelihood ratio test (described in Collett 2003b). All three are produced by default when the strata statement is used and thus result from the preceding code used to generate the survival plot. The various test statistics and their p-values are shown in Table 15.4.

TABLE 15.3

Number of Deaths and Number Surviving at the jth Death Time

Group	Number of Deaths at $t_{(j)}$	Number Surviving Beyond $t_{(j)}$	Number at Risk Just Before $t_{(j)}$
1	d_{1j}	$n_{1j} - d_{1j}$	n_{i1}
2	d_{2j}	$n_{2j} - d_{2j}$	n_{i2}
Total	d_j	$n_j - d_j$	n_j

TABLE 15.4

Tests for the Equality of the Survival
Function of the Two Groups in Table 15.2

Test of Equality over Strata			
Test	Chi-Square	DF	Pr > Chi-Square
Log-Rank	2.9722	1	0.0847
Wilcoxon	3.5737	1	0.0587
−2Log(LR)	3.9361	1	0.0473

In any statistical analysis in which more than one significance test is available, we need to make a decision about which test to use and to report. In the analysis of the HPA breast cancer data, there is not really a great problem because all the tests give rather similar results, although the likelihood ratio test is just significant at the 5% level whereas the other two tests are not. A reasonable conclusion here is that there is no convincing evidence of a difference in the survival experience of the two groups.

But for other data sets, the tests might give more conflicting results and we then have to decide between the tests in some way. It is known that the log-rank test is the most suitable test when the alternative to the equality of survivor functions null hypothesis is that the hazard of death at any given time for an individual in one group is proportional to the hazard at that time for a similar individual in the other group. This is the assumption of *proportional hazards,* which is the basis of a number of methods of analysing survival data and about which we will have much more to say in the next chapter. If the hazard functions *are* proportional, it implies that the survivor functions of the two groups do not cross one another (see Collett 2003b for details).

Consequently, an informal assessment of whether or not the data satisfy the proportional hazards assumption can be made from a plot of the two estimated survivor functions; if these do not cross, then the assumption is likely to be reasonable, making the log-rank test the test of choice. In the case of the breast cancer survivor function in Figure 15.8, we see that the one for the negatively stained women always lies above the one for the positively stained women. This suggests that proportional hazards hold and that we should therefore use the results from the log-rank test when assessing the null hypothesis that the survivor functions of the two groups are the same.

It should be noted that when the survivor functions of two groups cross (e.g., when they have the same median and cross each other at that value), but one group has more favourable survival experience at early times and the other group at later times, then none of the tests are of much use because they are unable to detect this type of difference.

The log-rank tests (and the other tests mentioned before) can be extended to deal with testing the equality of the survivor functions of more than two groups. Details are given in Collett (2003b). Here, we will simply give

                                    Applied Medical Statistics Using SAS

TABLE 15.5

Initial Remission Times (Days) for Leukaemia Patients

Treatment 1:
4, 5, 9, 10, 11, 12, 13, 23, 28, 28, 28, 29, 31, 32, 37, 41, 41, 57, 62, 74, 100, 139, 200+, 258+, 269+
Treatment 2:
8, 10, 10, 12, 14, 20, 48, 70, 75, 99, 103, 162, 169, 195, 220, 161+, 199+, 217+, 245
Treatment 3:
8, 10, 11, 23, 25, 25, 28, 28, 31, 31, 40, 48, 89, 124, 143, 12+, 159+, 190+, 196+, 197+, 205+, 219+

Note: + indicates right censoring.

an example using the data shown in Table 15.5; these data are initial remission times in days for individuals suffering from leukaemia who had been randomly allocated to three different treatments. We wish to test the hypothesis that the survivor functions of the three treatments are the same.

With a small data set like that in Table 15.5, it would be easy to reformat with a text editor (e.g., the SAS editor) so that it can be read relatively simply. Here, however, we read the data directly as it appears in Table 15.5 for illustrative purposes:

```
data leukemia;
  infile cards dsd missover;
    treatment=_n_;
    do until(days=.);
      input number$ @;
      censor=0;
      if indexc(number,'+') then censor=1;
      number=compress(number,'+');
      days=input(number,3.);
      if days~=. then output;
    end;
cards;
4, 5, 9, 10, ... 74, 100, 139, 200+, 258+, 269+
8, 10, 10, ... 195, 220, 161+, 199+, 217+, 245
8, 10, 11, ... 12+, 159+, 190+, 196+, 197+, 205+, 219+
;

proc lifetest data=leukemia plots=(s);
  time days*censor(1);
  strata treatment / test=(all);
run;
```

Using proc lifetest to compare the survival functions of different groups is achieved by including the strata statement and specifying the variable(s) that define the subgroups on it. The test=(all) option gives all the available nonparametric tests. The results are shown in Table 15.6.

The conclusions from all the tests are the same; there is no evidence of a difference in the survivor functions of the three treatments. With such small sample sizes, the power of all the tests will, of course, be rather low.

TABLE 15.6

Tests of the Equality of the Survival Functions
of the Three Groups in Table 15.5

Test of Equality over Strata			
Test	**Chi-Square**	**DF**	**Pr > Chi-Square**
Log-Rank	2.2797	2	0.3199
Wilcoxon	3.0028	2	0.2228
Tarone	3.1466	2	0.2074
Peto	2.8168	2	0.2445
Modified Peto	2.8666	2	0.2385
Fleming(1)	2.7208	2	0.2566

15.3.2 Stratified Tests

In a multicentre clinical trial comparing survival times for two treatments for
cancer, individual log-rank tests can be calculated for the data from each centre. However, a more sensitive test for a treatment difference might be possible
if the information from each centre could be combined in some way. Such data
are said to be *stratified* by clinic. Other examples of stratification might involve
age group, sex, etc.; an example in a different context is given in Chapter 4.

A stratified version of the log-rank test can be applied to such data; the
relevant test statistic is

$$X^2 = \sum_{k=1}^{r} \frac{\left[\sum_{l=1}^{k} (O_{kl} - E_{kl}) \right]^2}{\sum_{l=1}^{k} E_{kl}} \tag{15.19}$$

where r is the number of groups that are being compared and l is the number of strata. Under the null hypothesis that the survival experience of the r
groups is the same, the test statistic has a chi-squared distribution with $r - 1$
degrees of freedom.

An example of a stratified set of survival data is shown in Table 15.7 (the
data are given in Lee, 1992, and Collett 2003b). The data arise from a study
in which two immunotherapy treatments were compared for their ability
to prolong the life of patients suffering from melanoma. For each patient,
the tumour was surgically removed before allocation to *Bacillus* Calmette–
Guerin (BCG) vaccine or to a vaccine based on the bacterium *Corynebacterium
parvum* (*C. parvum*). The survival times of the patients (in months) in each
treatment group were also classified according to the age of the patient
(grouped into 21–40, 41–60, and 61–).

TABLE 15.7

Survival Times of Melanoma Patients in Two Treatment
Groups Stratified by Age Group

21–40		41–60		61–	
BCG	*C. parvum*	BCG	*C. parvum*	BCG	*C. parvum*
19	27[a]	34[a]	8	10	25[a]
24[a]	21[a]	4	11[a]	5	8
8	18[a]	17[a]	23[a]		11[a]
17[a]	16[a]		12[a]		
17[a]	7[a]		15[a]		
34[a]	12[a]		8[a]		
	24		8[a]		
	8				
	8[a]				

Source: Lee, E. T. 1992. *Statistical Methods for Survival Data
Analysis.* New York: Wiley.

[a] Observations are censored.

To apply the relevant test, we can use the following SAS code:

```
data melanoma;
 infile 'c:\AMSUS\data\melanoma.dat';
 input agegrp treatment censor survtime;
run;

proc lifetest data=melanoma plots=(s);
  time survtime*censor(1);
  strata treatment agegrp;
run;
```

The result is shown in Table 15.8. The three tests give quite different *p*-values
in this case, but all tests indicate that there is no difference in the survival
experience of the two treatment groups.

TABLE 15.8

Tests of the Equality of the Survival Experience
of the Two Treatment Groups in Table 15.7

Test of Equality over Strata			
Test	Chi-Square	DF	Pr > Chi-Square
Log-Rank	9.5298	5	0.0897
Wilcoxon	8.3444	5	0.1383
−2Log(LR)	4.8785	5	0.4309

15.4 Sample Size Estimation

As with the other types of studies described in earlier chapters, an important part of a study involving survival data is the determination of the sample size needed to achieve a particular power. Sample sizes in survival analysis can be calculated in a variety of ways (see, for example, Collett 2003b). Here, we shall illustrate a method due to Lakatos (1988), which can be applied to find the required sample sizes for a given power when applying the log-rank test; survival curves that would be expected under very general conditions are modelled by using a stochastic process. The asymptotic expectation and variance of the log-rank statistic applied to these curves are then used to calculate sample size (for full technical details, see Lakatos's original paper).

We can assume that the study of interest is a comparison of two treatments: one the standard and the other one new. (Schoenfeld 1983 shows that the expression for calculating the required number of deaths is the same whether or not account is taken of covariates other than treatment group.)

To calculate the actual number of individuals needed in the study, we first need to specify the length of the accrual period during which individuals are recruited into the study and the length of the follow-up period after recruitment is complete. Thereafter, we can specify the expected survival of the two groups in a number of ways. Perhaps the simplest of these is to give the median survival times, as follows:

```
proc power;
   twosamplesurvival
       power=.8
       accrualtime = 12
       followuptime = 24
       groupmedsurvtimes=15 | 20 22 24
       npergroup = .;
run;
```

The default test for `twosamplesurvival` is the log-rank test. The median survival times for the two groups are separated by a bar (|). In this example, we expect that the median survival for the control group would be 15 months and wish to calculate sample sizes needed if the treatment group median survival time is 20, 22, or 24 months. The results are shown in Table 15.9. The example demonstrates that relatively large sample sizes are needed to detect even quite substantial differences in median survival times.

TABLE 15.9

An Example of Sample Size Estimation in Survival Analysis

Log-Rank Test for Two Survival Curves	
Fixed Scenario Elements	
Method	Lakatos normal approximation
Form of Survival Curve 1	Exponential
Form of Survival Curve 2	Exponential
Accrual Time	12
Follow-up Time	24
Group 1 Median Survival Time	15
Nominal Power	0.8
Number of Sides	2
Number of Time Sub-intervals	12
Group 1 Loss Exponential Hazard	0
Group 2 Loss Exponential Hazard	0
Alpha	0.05

Computed N per group			
Index	Med Surv Time 2	Actual Power	N Per Group
1	20	0.801	273
2	22	0.800	158
3	24	0.802	108

It can be informative to display the relationship between an effect size and sample size in the form of a plot. The following example shows the sample sizes corresponding to a range of hazard ratios:

```
proc power plotonly;
  twosamplesurvival
      power=.8
      accrualtime = 12
      followuptime = 24
      curve('md12')=12:.5
      curve('md15')=15:.5
      curve('md18')=18:.5
      refsurv='md12' 'md15' 'md18'
      hazardratio=.4 to .8 by .1
      npergroup = .;
  plot x=effect;
run;
```

The `groupmedsurvtimes` option cannot be used to specify the median survival time of just one of the two groups. Instead, this is done with one

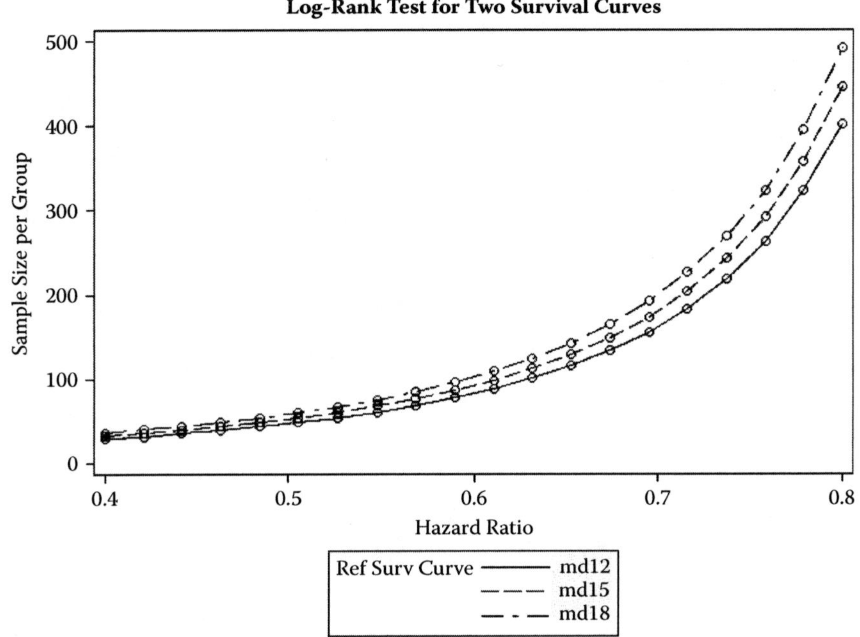

FIGURE 15.9
Sample sizes needed to achieve a power of 0.8 for varying hazard ratios.

or more `curve` options and a `refsurv` option. The `curve` option defines a curve in terms of pairs of points separated by a colon. The first value is the survival time and the second the proportion surviving to that point. For an exponential survival curve, only one point is required. Thus, the three curves defined above correspond to median survival times of 12, 15, and 18 months. A range of hazard ratios is specified and a plot statement is included. The resulting plot is shown in Figure 15.9.

15.5 Summary

Survival analysis is the study of times to some terminating event, death, relapse, etc. A distinguishing feature of survival data is the presence of censored observations for which the only information on the time to the event of interest is that it is greater than some value. In this chapter, methods for describing a sample of survival times have been described along with methods of comparing survival times of a number of distinct groups—for example, males and females. In the next chapter, we shall consider models that allow the dependence of survival times on a number of explanatory variables (covariates) to be investigated.

16

Cox's Proportional Hazards Models for Survival Data

16.1 Introduction

The methods described in the previous chapter are useful in the analysis of a single sample of survival times or when there are survival times for the categories of a categorical variable that the investigator wishes to compare. But in most survival investigations in medicine, there will be many other explanatory variables (covariates) that have been recorded and whose effects on survival time will be of interest. We need a suitable model that links the survival times to the covariates, but because of the special features of such data, something different from the multiple regression model described in Chapter 8 is necessary. In this chapter, we describe the most widely used approach to modelling survival data: Cox's proportional hazards models.

16.2 Modelling the Hazard Function: Cox's Regression

In considering models for survival data, the first question that needs to be addressed and satisfactorily answered is 'What are we going to model?' More specifically, what is going to play the role of the systematic component in a regression model? According to Hosmer and Lemeshow (2000), it is the inherent aging process that is present when individuals are followed over time that distinguishes survival times from other response (dependent) variables, and it is the hazard function that most directly captures the essence of this aging process. Consequently, it is natural to consider regression models for the hazard function in the analysis of survival time data. And the most common of these models are proportional hazards models, a term encountered briefly in the previous chapter but one which we shall now consider in more detail.

To begin, we will suppose that survival data have been collected on n individuals in the context of a clinical trial and that there is only a single covariate of interest and that is treatment group coded 0 for the standard treatment group and 1 for the new treatment group. Suppose that $h_0(t)$ and $h_1(t)$ are the corresponding hazard functions for the two groups; then, the proportional hazards assumption implies that

$$h_1(t) = \psi h_0(t) \tag{16.1}$$

where ψ is a constant giving the ratio of the hazards of death at any time for an individual on the new treatment relative to one on the standard treatment; ψ is known as the relative hazard or the hazard ratio. If $\psi < 1$, the hazard of death at t is smaller for an individual on the new treatment, relative to an individual on the standard treatment; if $\psi > 1$, the reverse is the case. Taking logarithms of both sides of (16.1) produces the following equation:

$$\log[h_1(t)] = \log(\psi) + \log[h_0(t)] \tag{16.2}$$

The proportional hazards function means that if graphs were drawn of $\log[h_1(t)]$ and $\log[h_0(t)]$, then regardless of how complex (or, indeed, how simple) the baseline hazard function was, the vertical distance between the two curves at any point in time will be $\log(\psi)$. An implication of the proportional hazards assumption is that the population survivor functions for the two groups do not cross as mentioned in the previous chapter. (Proportionality of hazards is an assumption that needs to be checked; suitable methods will be described later.)

As ψ cannot be negative, we can write it as $\exp(\beta)$, where the parameter β is the log of the hazard ratio. Note that with the coding used for treatment group, positive values of β are obtained when ψ is greater than one—that is, when the new treatment is inferior to the standard. By introducing an explanatory variable, x_i, for treatment group for the ith individual and with values one and zero for new and standard treatment, respectively, the hazard function for this individual, $h_i(t)$, can be written as

$$h_i(t) = e^{\beta x_i} h_0(t) \tag{16.3}$$

This model can be extended to the situation where there are p covariates measured at the start of the study (we shall deal with so-called time-varying covariates later), which for the ith individual take the values $x_i' = [x_{i1}, x_{i2}, \ldots, x_{ip}]$; these covariates are allowed to be a mixture of continuous and binary variables (and also categorical variables with more than two categories if suitably coded as a series of dummy variables). The model is now

$$h_i(t) = e^{[\beta_1 x_{i1} + \beta_2 x_{i2} + \ldots + \beta_p x_{ip}]} h_0(t) \tag{16.4}$$

In this model, the regression coefficient, $\exp(\beta_j)$, gives the relative hazard for two individuals differing by one unit on the jth covariate, with all other covariates being the same for the two individuals. Now, $h_0(t)$ is known as the baseline hazard function and is the hazard function for an individual with zero values for all covariates or, if the covariates are reexpressed as differences from their mean values, the hazard function of an individual with the mean value of each covariate. The model in (16.4) can be written in the form of

$$\log\left[\frac{h_i(t)}{h_0(t)}\right] = \beta_1 x_{i1} + \beta_2 x_{i2} + \ldots + \beta_p x_{ip} \tag{16.5}$$

Thus, the proportional hazards function may be regarded as a linear model for the logarithm of the hazard ratio.

Before the model can be of any use in the analysis of survival data, we will, of course, need to estimate its parameters, $\boldsymbol{\beta}' = [\beta_1, \beta_2, \ldots, \beta_p]$. If we are willing to assume that the observed survival times are taken from a population with a particular distribution, then we can use maximum likelihood estimation. For example, if we assume that the survival times arise from a Weibull distribution for which the hazard function is $\lambda \gamma t^{\gamma-1}$ (see previous chapter), then the hazard function for the ith individual will be

$$h_i(t) = e^{\left[\beta_1 x_{i1} + \beta_2 x_{i2} + \ldots + \beta_p x_{ip}\right]} \lambda \gamma t^{\gamma-1} \tag{16.6}$$

Maximum likelihood estimation can now be applied to find estimates of the regression coefficients, $\boldsymbol{\beta}$, and the parameters, λ and γ; see, for example, Collett (2003b). But there are two problems with this approach:

- Small or even moderate-sized samples of survival times often give little evidence about the form that it is reasonable to assume for their distribution.
- Hazard functions met in practice are unlikely always to be of the simple increasing or decreasing types implied by the Weibull assumption. They may often be more complex (see, for example, the 'bathtub' hazard function in the previous chapter).

For these reasons, Sir David Cox in his classic 1972 paper developed an approach, now generally called simply Cox's regression, in which the regression coefficients in (16.6) can be estimated without making any assumptions about the form of the baseline hazard. Therefore, inferences about the effects of the covariates on the relative hazard can be made without the need for an estimate of $h_0(t)$. (If required, an estimate of $h_0(t)$ can be constructed using the estimated regression coefficients, as we shall see later.)

Cox's regression is a semiparametric model: It makes a parametric assumption concerning the effect of the predictors on the hazard function, but makes no assumption regarding the nature of the hazard function itself. In many situations, the form of the true hazard function is unknown or it is complex and most interest centres on the effects of the covariates rather than the exact nature of the hazard function. Cox's regression allows the shape of the hazard function to be ignored when making inferences about the regression coefficients in the model.

Estimation for Cox's regression involves a procedure known as partial likelihood; the essence of this approach is that the partial likelihood function depends only on the vector of regression coefficients, β—not on the baseline hazard. Details are given in Kalbfeisch and Prentice (1980) and Collett (2003b). Here, we shall content ourselves with describing some examples of the application of Cox's regression.

16.2.1 Examples of Cox's Regression

We begin by returning to the data on HPA staining and breast cancer described in Chapter 15. We can use proc phreg to apply Cox's regression to these data with the single covariate, staining or no staining, as follows:

```
proc phreg data=HPA;
  model weeks*censor(1)=staining/rl;
run;
```

As with proc lifetest in the previous chapter, the model statement has the survival time variable followed by an asterisk and then the censoring variable with the value, or values, indicating censored observations in parentheses. The rl (risklimits) option requests confidence limits for the hazard ratios. The results are shown in Table 16.1. There is no evidence for a difference in the survival experiences of members of the two groups. The confidence interval for the hazard ratio contains the value one.

Our second example of Cox's regression will use data that arise from a randomised clinical trial investigating the effects of hormonal treatment

TABLE 16.1

Results from Applying Cox's Regression to the HPA Staining Data

Analysis of Maximum Likelihood Estimates					
Parameter	DF	Parameter Estimate	Standard Error	Chi-Square	Pr > ChiSq
staining	1	0.84032	0.50167	2.8058	0.0939

Analysis of Maximum Likelihood Estimates			
Parameter	Hazard Ratio	95% Hazard Ratio Confidence Limits	
staining	2.317	0.867	6.194

TABLE 16.2

Subset of the German Breast Cancer Data

Id	Horm	Age	Menstat	Tsize	Tgrade	Pnodes	Progrec	Estrec	Time	Cens
1	No	70	Post	21	II	3	48	66	1814	1
2	Yes	56	Post	12	II	7	61	77	2018	1
3	Yes	58	Post	35	II	9	52	271	712	1
4	Yes	59	Post	17	II	4	60	29	1807	1
5	No	73	Post	35	II	1	26	65	772	1
6	No	32	Pre	57	III	24	0	13	448	1
7	Yes	59	Post	8	II	2	181	0	2172	0
8	No	65	Post	16	II	1	192	25	2161	0
9	No	80	Post	39	II	30	0	59	471	1
10	No	66	Post	18	II	7	0	3	2014	0
11	Yes	68	Post	40	II	9	16	20	577	1
12	Yes	71	Post	21	II	9	0	0	184	1
13	Yes	59	Post	58	II	1	154	101	1840	0
14	No	50	Post	27	III	1	16	12	1842	0
15	Yes	70	Post	22	II	3	113	139	1821	0
16	No	54	Post	30	II	1	135	6	1371	1
17	No	39	Pre	35	I	4	79	28	707	1
18	Yes	66	Post	23	II	1	112	225	1743	0
19	Yes	69	Post	25	I	1	131	196	1781	0
20	No	55	Post	65	I	4	312	76	865	1

Notes: The variables are horm: dichotomous variable indicating whether hormonal therapy was applied, 0 = no, 1 = yes; age: age in years; menstat: menopausal status, post or pre; tsize: tumour size; tgrade: tumour grade; pnodes: number of positive lymph nodes; progrec: progesterone receptor; estrec: estrogen receptor; time: survival time in days; status: whether alive (0) or dead (1) at end of study.

with Tamoxifen in women suffering from node-positive breast cancer (Schumacher et al. 1994). Data from randomised patients from this trial and additional nonrandomised patients from the German Breast Cancer Study group 2 (GBSG2) make up the 686 women in the data set. Seven covariates are available for each of the women in the study (Sauerbrei and Royston 1999): age at the start of the study, menopausal status, tumour size, tumour grade, number of positive lymph nodes, progesterone receptor, and estrogen receptor and whether or not the patient received hormonal therapy. A small subset of the data is given in Table 16.2.

To fit a Cox's regression model to the data, we use the following SAS code:

```
data GBSG2;
 infile 'c:\amsus\data\GBSG2.dat' expandtabs;
 input id onhorm $ age menstat $ tsize tgrade $ pnodes progrec
 estrec time status;
```

```
 horm=onhorm='yes';
 mnths=time/30.5;
run;

proc phreg data=GBSG2;
  class menstat tgrade;
  model mnths*status(0)=horm age menstat tsize tgrade pnodes
  estrec/rl;
run;
```

The default coding for categorical variables listed on the `class` statement is reference (dummy variable) coding with the last value as the reference category, so the three categories of tumour grade are coded by two dummy variables with tumour grade III being the reference category (see later for more details). The results are shown in Table 16.3.

The results show that the hazard of death for patients having the hormonal therapy is estimated to be 0.705 times the hazard of death for patients not having the treatment with a 95% confidence interval of [0.55,0.91]. And having a tumour of grade I implies a hazard of death of between 0.22 and 0.63 of the hazard for a patient with a tumour of grade III. But, as in multiple regression, interpreting coefficients in this way in the search for explanatory variables that we can remove from the model is problematic because of the probable lack of independence of the explanatory variables; dropping one particular explanatory variable, for example, and then reestimating the model will likely lead to different coefficient estimates and different standard errors. Instead, we should try to find a parsimonious model for the data by comparing models including different subsets of the explanatory variables. Again, as in multiple regression, there are automatic procedures for doing this. Here we look at a backward elimination process (see Chapter 8) using the results from Wald's test to decide which variables to eliminate. Wald's test is essentially equivalent to using the ratio of the estimated regression parameter to its estimated standard error.

To apply the backward elimination procedure, we can use the following SAS code:

```
proc phreg data=GBSG2;
  class menstat tgrade;
  model mnths*status(0)=horm age menstat tsize tgrade pnodes
  estrec/rl selection=b;
run;
```

The results are shown in Table 16.4.

The variables `estrec`, `age`, `menstat`, and `tsize` are found not to contribute to predicting the hazard of death. The interpretation of the hormone therapy variable and tumour grade variables is much the same as that given for the full model. The other variable included in the reduced model is number of

TABLE 16.3

Results from Fitting Cox's Regression Model to the German Breast Cancer Data

Type 3 Tests			
Effect	**DF**	**Wald Chi-Square**	**Pr > ChiSq**
horm	1	7.3140	0.0068
age	1	1.2468	0.2642
menstat	1	3.3569	0.0669
tsize	1	3.2901	0.0697
tgrade	2	14.0360	0.0009
pnodes	1	45.2587	<.0001
estrec	1	1.2200	0.2694

Analysis of Maximum Likelihood Estimates						
Parameter		**DF**	**Parameter Estimate**	**Standard Error**	**Chi-Square**	**Pr > ChiSq**
horm		1	−0.34886	0.12900	7.3140	0.0068
age		1	−0.01031	0.00923	1.2468	0.2642
menstat	Post	1	0.33176	0.18107	3.3569	0.0669
tsize		1	0.00706	0.00389	3.2901	0.0697
tgrade	I	1	−0.98144	0.26325	13.8987	0.0002
tgrade	II	1	−0.23162	0.13432	2.9734	0.0846
pnodes		1	0.04999	0.00743	45.2587	<.0001
estrec		1	−0.0005088	0.0004607	1.2200	0.2694

Analysis of Maximum Likelihood Estimates					
Parameter		**Hazard Ratio**	**95% Hazard Ratio Confidence Limits**		**Label**
horm		0.705	0.548	0.908	
age		0.990	0.972	1.008	
menstat	Post	1.393	0.977	1.987	menstat Post
tsize		1.007	0.999	1.015	
tgrade	I	0.375	0.224	0.628	tgrade I
tgrade	II	0.793	0.610	1.032	tgrade II
pnodes		1.051	1.036	1.067	
estrec		0.999	0.999	1.000	

TABLE 16.4

Results of Backwards Elimination Applied to the Cox's Model Fitted to the German Breast Cancer Data

		Type 3 Tests	
Effect	DF	Wald Chi-Square	Pr > ChiSq
horm	1	7.2227	0.0072
tgrade	2	15.5575	0.0004
pnodes	1	66.4346	<.0001

Analysis of Maximum Likelihood Estimates					
Parameter		DF	Parameter Estimate	Standard Error	Chi-Square	Pr > ChiSq
horm		1	−0.33739	0.12554	7.2227	0.0072
tgrade	I	1	−1.02709	0.26243	15.3180	<.0001
tgrade	II	1	−0.25250	0.13348	3.5786	0.0585
pnodes		1	0.05531	0.00679	66.4346	<.0001

Analysis of Maximum Likelihood Estimates					
Parameter		Hazard Ratio	95% Hazard Ratio Confidence Limits		Label
horm		0.714	0.558	0.913	
tgrade	I	0.358	0.214	0.599	tgrade I
tgrade	II	0.777	0.598	1.009	tgrade II
pnodes		1.057	1.043	1.071	

positive lymph nodes; an increase of one in this variable produces an increase in the hazard of death of between 4% and 7%.

16.2.2 Estimating the Baseline Hazard Function

The estimated hazard function for the ith individual with vector of covariates $\mathbf{x}_i$ is given by

$$\hat{h}_i(t) = e^{\hat{\beta}'\mathbf{x}_i}\hat{h}_0(t) \tag{16.7}$$

where $\hat{\beta}$ is the vector of estimated regression coefficients from fitting a Cox's regression model and $\hat{h}_0(t)$ is the estimated baseline function.

But how do we find an estimate of the baseline hazard function? Kalbfleisch and Prentice (1973) show that the baseline hazard function can be estimated using a maximum likelihood approach. In the particular case when there are no tied survival times, the baseline hazard function at ordered survival time $t_{(i)}$ is estimated as

$$\hat{h}_0(t_{(i)}) = 1 - \hat{\xi}_i \tag{16.8}$$

where

$$\hat{\xi}_j = \left[1 - \frac{\exp(\hat{\beta}'\mathbf{x}_{(i)})}{\sum_{l \in R(t_{(i)})} \exp(\hat{\beta}'\mathbf{x}_{(i)})} \right]^{\exp(-\hat{\beta}'\mathbf{x}_{(i)})} \tag{16.9}$$

where $\mathbf{x}_{(i)}$ is the vector of explanatory variables for the individual who dies at time $t_{(i)}$ and $R(t_{(i)})$ is the set of individuals at risk at time $t_{(i)}$. Collett (2003b) shows that if we assume that the hazard of death of death is constant between adjacent death times, then can be regarded as an estimate of the probability that an individual survives through the interval from $t_{(i)}$ to $t_{(i+1)}$. The baseline survivor function can then be estimated by

$$\hat{S}_0(t) = \prod_{i=1}^{k} \hat{\xi}_i \tag{16.10}$$

for $t_{(k)} \leq t < t_{(k+1)}$, $k = 1, 2 \dots r - 1$. Note that the estimate is a step function.

The relationships between the hazard, cumulative hazard, and the survivor function demonstrated in Chapter 15 can now be used to give estimates of, in particular, the survivor functions for the individuals in the sample. For example, the estimated survivor function for the ith individual is

$$\hat{s}(t) = \left[\hat{s}_0(t) \right]^{\exp(\hat{\beta}'x_i)} \tag{16.11}$$

for $t_{(k)} \leq t < t_{(k+1)}$, $k = 1, 2 \dots r - 1$. (See Collett 2003b for full details.)

For the German breast cancer data, the selected Cox model contained the explanatory variables hormonal therapy, tumour grade, and number of positive lymph nodes. Tumour grade was coded in the form of two dummy variables (D1 and D2) as follows:

	Tumour Grade		
	I	II	III
D1	1	0	0
D2	0	1	0

The model for the hazard function was found to be

$$\hat{h}_i(t) = \exp\left(-0.34\text{horm} - 1.03\text{D1} - 0.25\text{D2} + 0.06\text{pnodes}\right)\hat{h}_0(t) \quad (16.12)$$

Consequently, the estimated baseline function is the estimated hazard of death at time t for an individual who is not on hormonal therapy, has a grade III tumour, and has no positive lymph nodes. We can find the baseline hazard, the baseline survivor function, and the cumulative hazard using the following SAS code:

```
data covs;
  retain horm 0 tgrade 'III' pnodes 0;
run;
proc phreg data=GBSG2;
  class tgrade;
  model mnths*status(0)=horm tgrade pnodes/rl;
  baseline covariates=covs out=phout survival=surv
  cumhaz=cumhaz;
run;
data phout;
 set phout;
 lch=lag(cumhaz);
 hazd=cumhaz-lch;
run;
proc print noobs;
 var mnths hazd surv cumhaz;
 format mnths 4.1 hazd surv cumhaz 4.3;
run;
```

The `baseline` statement creates a data set with baseline function estimates. By default, these are calculated at the mean values of continuous covariates and reference categories of categorical predictors. To have the calculations made for other values of the predictors, a data set needs to be created with the required values and then referenced with the `covariates=` option on the `baseline` statement. A short data step calculates the hazard from the cumulative hazard.

The results are shown in Table 16.5. We see that the estimated baseline hazard stays relatively constant for a long period and then gradually increases. The estimates only apply at the death times of the patients in the study. From Table 16.5, we can estimate the median survival time, which is the smallest observed survival time for which the estimated survivor function is less than or equal to 0.5. From Table 16.5, we find that the estimated median survival time for patients who are not on hormonal therapy, have a grade III tumour, and have no positive lymph nodes is 66.7 months.

By raising the estimate of the baseline survivor function to a suitable power, we can find the estimated survivor function for patients with other

TABLE 16.5

Estimates of the Baseline Hazard, the Baseline Survivor Function, and the Cumulative Hazard for the Breast Cancer Data

Mnths	Hazd	Surv	Cumhaz
0.0	.	1.00	.000
2.4	.001	.999	.001
3.2	.001	.998	.002
3.7	.001	.997	.003
3.9	.001	.996	.004
5.2	.001	.995	.005
5.5	.001	.994	.006
5.6	.001	.993	.007
5.7	.001	.991	.009
5.7	.001	.990	.010
5.8	.002	.988	.012
5.9	.001	.987	.013
5.9	.001	.986	.014
6.0	.001	.985	.015
6.3	.001	.984	.016
6.4	.001	.983	.017
6.7	.001	.982	.018
7.3	.001	.981	.020
7.4	.001	.980	.021
7.6	.001	.978	.022
7.8	.001	.977	.023
7.9	.001	.976	.024
7.9	.001	.975	.025
8.1	.001	.974	.026
8.2	.001	.973	.027
8.2	.001	.972	.029
8.9	.002	.970	.031
9.0	.001	.969	.032
9.2	.002	.966	.034
9.3	.002	.964	.037
9.4	.001	.963	.038
9.4	.001	.962	.039
9.6	.001	.961	.040
10.0	.001	.960	.041
10.1	.001	.959	.042
10.1	.002	.956	.045
10.4	.001	.955	.046
10.8	.001	.954	.047

(Continued)

TABLE 16.5 (*Continued*)

Estimates of the Baseline Hazard, the Baseline Survivor Function, and the Cumulative Hazard for the Breast Cancer Data

Mnths	Hazd	Surv	Cumhaz
11.0	.001	.953	.048
11.1	.004	.950	.052
11.2	.001	.948	.053
11.3	.001	.947	.054
11.4	.001	.946	.055
11.5	.001	.945	.057
11.6	.001	.944	.058
11.7	.001	.943	.059
11.7	.001	.942	.060
11.8	.002	.939	.063
11.8	.001	.938	.064
12.1	.001	.937	.065
12.1	.002	.935	.067
12.2	.001	.934	.069
12.2	.001	.933	.070
12.3	.001	.931	.071
12.3	.001	.930	.072
12.4	.001	.929	.074
12.4	.001	.928	.075
12.6	.001	.927	.076
12.9	.001	.926	.077
12.9	.001	.924	.079
13.2	.001	.923	.080
13.4	.001	.922	.081
13.6	.001	.921	.082
13.7	.001	.920	.084
13.8	.003	.918	.086
14.0	.003	.915	.089
14.3	.001	.914	.090
14.4	.001	.913	.091
14.6	.001	.912	.092
14.7	.001	.911	.094
14.7	.001	.909	.095
14.9	.001	.908	.096
15.0	.001	.907	.098
15.1	.001	.906	.099
15.2	.001	.905	.100
15.4	.001	.903	.102
15.5	.001	.902	.103

TABLE 16.5 (*Continued*)

Estimates of the Baseline Hazard, the Baseline Survivor Function, and the Cumulative Hazard for the Breast Cancer Data

Mnths	Hazd	Surv	Cumhaz
15.6	.001	.901	.104
15.6	.003	.899	.107
15.8	.001	.897	.108
15.9	.001	.896	.110
16.1	.001	.895	.111
16.1	.004	.891	.115
16.2	.001	.890	.116
16.3	.001	.889	.118
16.4	.001	.888	.119
16.5	.001	.887	.120
16.5	.001	.885	.122
16.5	.001	.884	.123
16.9	.001	.883	.124
17.0	.001	.882	.126
17.2	.001	.881	.127
17.3	.001	.879	.129
17.4	.001	.878	.130
17.5	.001	.877	.131
17.5	.001	.876	.133
17.6	.001	.874	.134
17.6	.001	.873	.136
17.7	.001	.872	.137
17.8	.001	.871	.138
17.8	.003	.868	.141
17.9	.001	.867	.143
17.9	.001	.866	.144
18.0	.004	.862	.148
18.0	.003	.860	.151
18.1	.003	.857	.154
18.2	.003	.855	.157
18.3	.001	.853	.159
18.3	.001	.852	.160
18.5	.001	.851	.162
18.5	.001	.850	.163
18.7	.001	.848	.164
18.8	.001	.847	.166
18.9	.001	.846	.167
18.9	.001	.845	.169
19.0	.001	.843	.170

(Continued)

TABLE 16.5 (*Continued*)

Estimates of the Baseline Hazard, the Baseline Survivor Function, and the Cumulative Hazard for the Breast Cancer Data

Mnths	Hazd	Surv	Cumhaz
19.0	.001	.842	.172
19.2	.002	.841	.173
19.5	.003	.838	.176
19.5	.002	.837	.178
19.6	.002	.836	.180
19.7	.002	.834	.181
20.1	.002	.833	.183
20.4	.002	.832	.184
20.5	.003	.829	.187
20.6	.002	.828	.189
20.7	.002	.827	.190
20.9	.002	.825	.192
21.2	.002	.824	.194
21.2	.002	.823	.195
21.3	.002	.821	.197
21.7	.002	.820	.198
22.0	.002	.819	.200
22.1	.002	.817	.202
22.3	.002	.816	.203
22.5	.002	.815	.205
22.9	.002	.813	.207
23.2	.002	.812	.208
23.3	.002	.811	.210
23.4	.002	.809	.212
23.7	.002	.808	.213
23.8	.002	.806	.215
23.9	.002	.805	.217
23.9	.002	.804	.219
24.0	.002	.802	.220
24.0	.002	.801	.222
24.3	.002	.800	.224
24.4	.002	.798	.225
24.5	.002	.797	.227
24.5	.002	.795	.229
24.7	.002	.794	.231
24.8	.002	.793	.232
25.0	.002	.791	.234
25.2	.002	.790	.236
25.3	.002	.788	.238

TABLE 16.5 (*Continued*)

Estimates of the Baseline Hazard, the Baseline
Survivor Function, and the Cumulative Hazard for
the Breast Cancer Data

Mnths	Hazd	Surv	Cumhaz
25.4	.002	.787	.240
25.7	.002	.785	.242
25.9	.002	.784	.244
26.1	.002	.782	.246
26.1	.004	.779	.249
26.2	.002	.778	.251
26.3	.002	.776	.253
26.4	.002	.775	.255
26.9	.002	.773	.257
27.1	.002	.772	.259
27.4	.002	.770	.261
27.5	.002	.769	.263
27.6	.002	.767	.265
28.0	.004	.764	.269
28.1	.002	.763	.271
28.2	.004	.759	.275
28.2	.002	.758	.277
28.4	.002	.756	.279
28.4	.002	.755	.281
28.4	.002	.753	.283
28.7	.002	.752	.286
29.0	.002	.750	.288
29.1	.002	.748	.290
29.2	.002	.747	.292
29.2	.002	.745	.294
29.3	.002	.744	.296
30.1	.002	.742	.298
31.0	.002	.740	.300
31.3	.004	.737	.305
31.4	.002	.736	.307
31.5	.002	.734	.309
31.6	.002	.732	.312
32.2	.002	.730	.314
32.2	.002	.729	.316
32.2	.002	.727	.319
32.5	.002	.725	.321
32.9	.002	.724	.324
34.0	.002	.722	.326
34.2	.002	.720	.328

(*Continued*)

TABLE 16.5 (*Continued*)

Estimates of the Baseline Hazard, the Baseline
Survivor Function, and the Cumulative Hazard for
the Breast Cancer Data

Mnths	Hazd	Surv	Cumhaz
34.7	.002	.718	.331
35.4	.002	.717	.333
35.7	.002	.715	.336
35.8	.003	.713	.338
35.9	.003	.711	.341
36.2	.005	.708	.346
36.3	.003	.706	.349
36.7	.003	.704	.351
37.4	.003	.702	.354
37.6	.003	.700	.357
37.7	.003	.698	.359
37.9	.003	.696	.362
38.1	.003	.694	.365
38.2	.003	.692	.368
38.4	.003	.691	.370
38.5	.003	.689	.373
38.8	.003	.687	.376
39.1	.003	.685	.379
39.1	.003	.683	.382
39.6	.003	.681	.385
39.9	.003	.679	.388
40.0	.003	.677	.391
40.2	.003	.675	.394
40.9	.003	.673	.397
41.1	.003	.670	.400
41.9	.003	.668	.403
42.0	.006	.664	.409
42.5	.003	.662	.413
42.8	.003	.660	.416
43.6	.003	.658	.419
43.8	.003	.656	.422
44.0	.003	.653	.426
44.3	.003	.651	.429
44.7	.004	.649	.433
44.8	.004	.646	.436
45.0	.004	.644	.440
45.5	.004	.642	.443
45.5	.004	.639	.447
46.6	.004	.637	.451

TABLE 16.5 (*Continued*)

Estimates of the Baseline Hazard, the Baseline
Survivor Function, and the Cumulative Hazard for
the Breast Cancer Data

Mnths	Hazd	Surv	Cumhaz
47.5	.004	.635	.455
47.8	.004	.632	.458
47.9	.004	.630	.462
48.0	.004	.627	.466
48.6	.004	.625	.470
49.0	.004	.622	.474
49.2	.004	.620	.478
49.9	.004	.617	.483
50.0	.004	.614	.487
50.1	.004	.612	.491
52.0	.004	.609	.496
52.1	.005	.606	.500
52.5	.005	.604	.505
53.8	.005	.601	.510
54.9	.005	.598	.515
55.0	.005	.595	.520
55.2	.005	.592	.525
55.8	.005	.588	.530
56.7	.006	.585	.536
57.5	.006	.581	.543
57.8	.006	.577	.549
59.2	.007	.574	.556
59.2	.007	.570	.563
59.5	.014	.562	.577
62.9	.010	.556	.587
64.8	.011	.550	.598
64.8	.011	.544	.609
65.2	.012	.537	.621
65.2	.012	.531	.633
66.1	.014	.524	.647
66.2	.014	.516	.661
66.6	.015	.509	.675
66.7	.015	.501	.690
66.9	.015	.494	.706
68.6	.019	.485	.725
75.0	.042	.465	.767
77.8	.056	.439	.823
80.5	.106	.395	.929

values of the covariates using (16.11). The estimated survivor function for individual i is

$$\hat{S}_i(t) = \left[\hat{S}_0(t)\right]^{\exp\left(-0.34\,\mathrm{horm}_i - 1.03\mathrm{D1}_i - 0.25\mathrm{D2}_i + 0.06\,\mathrm{pnodes}_i\right)} \tag{16.13}$$

Thus, for an individual with a grade III tumour and no positive lymph nodes and on hormonal therapy, the estimated survivor function for the individual is $\left[\hat{S}_0(t)\right]^{\exp(-0.34)}$; for example, the estimated survivor function for such an individual at the median survival for a baseline individual is $(0.5)^{\exp(-0.34)}$, giving the value 0.61. Therefore, it is estimated that 61% of individuals with grade III tumour and no positive lymph nodes but having the hormonal treatment will survive nearly 67 months as opposed to the 50% estimated to survive amongst those individuals with the same tumour grade and number of positive lymph nodes but not having hormonal therapy. (Note that, as the value of the baseline survivor function is always between zero and one, it follows that if $\exp(\boldsymbol{\beta}'\mathbf{x}_i) > 1$, then $\hat{S}_i(t) < \hat{S}_0(t)$ and, conversely, $\exp(\boldsymbol{\beta}'\mathbf{x}_i) < 1$ if, then $\hat{S}_i(t) > \hat{S}_0(t)$.)

We can plot the estimated baseline survivor function and the survivor function for individuals with grade III tumour and no positive lymph nodes but on hormonal therapy by adding a second observation to the covs data set for those on hormone therapy and repeating the proc step with ODS graphics on and plots(overlay)=s on the proc statement:

```
data covs;
   retain tgrade 'III' pnodes 0;
   horm=1; output;
   horm=0; output;
run;

ods graphics on;
proc phreg data=GBSG2 plots(overlay)=s;
   class tgrade;
   model mnths*status(0)=horm tgrade pnodes /rl;
   baseline covariates=covs;
run;
```

The result graph is shown in Figure 16.1. The survivor function for the individuals on hormonal therapy is always greater than for the corresponding function of those not on hormonal therapy.

16.2.3 Checking Assumptions in Cox's Regression

After any statistical model has been fitted to a data set and the parameters of the model estimated, the adequacy of the model needs to be assessed to

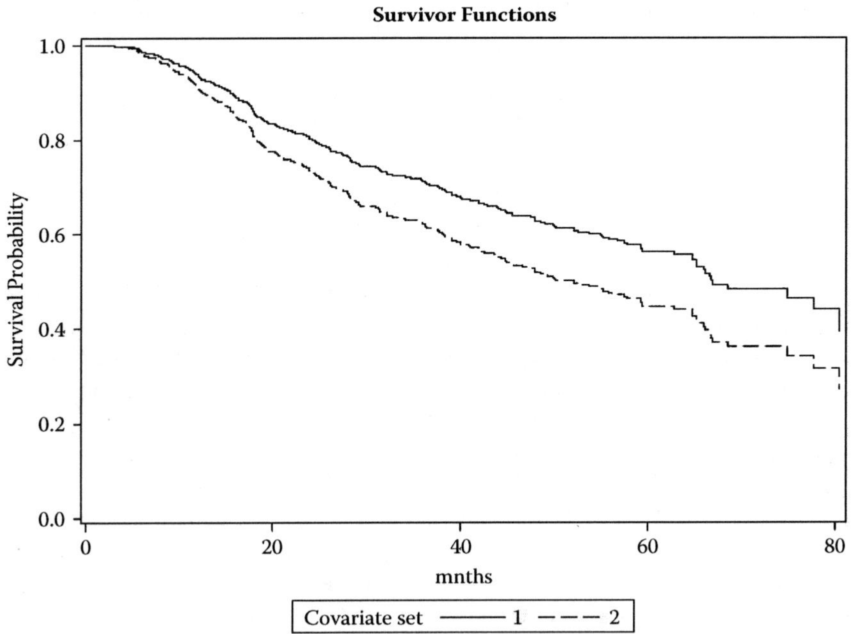

FIGURE 16.1
Estimated survivor functions for the breast cancer data; the continuous line is for grade III tumour, no positive lymph nodes, and receiving hormonal therapy; the dashed line is for grade III tumour, no positive lymph nodes, and not receiving hormonal therapy.

ensure that inferences drawn are defendable and valid. A thorough examination of how well the assumptions made by a model are met is just as important as systematic development of a model. When modelling survival data, similarly to dealing with the multiple linear regression model (see Chapter 8), assessment of model adequacy is based on the use of residuals. But the residuals for survival data are not nearly as obvious as those used in multiple regression, and the absence of an obvious residual has led to several having been proposed; we shall look at three of these.

Cox–Snell residual (Cox and Snell 1968):

$$r_i^{(CS)} = \exp\left(\beta' x_i\right) \hat{H}_0(t_i) \tag{16.14}$$

where $\hat{H}_0(t_i)$ is the integrated hazard function at time t_i, the observed survival time of the ith subject. If the correct model has been fitted, the Cox–Snell residuals for the n individuals will be n observations from a unit exponential distribution. (In fact, if an observed survival time is right censored, then the corresponding residual is also right censored and the residuals will be a censored sample from the exponential distribution.)

Deviance residual (Therneau, Grambsch, and Fleming 1990):
This type of residual is defined as follows:

$$r_i^{(D)} = \text{sign}\left(r_i^{(M)}\right)\left(\sqrt{-2\left\{r_i^{(M)} + \delta_i \log\left(\delta_i - r_i^{(M)}\right)\right\}}\right) \qquad (16.15)$$

where
sign is the sign function taking the value +1 if its argument is positive and
−1 if it is negative

$r_i^{(M)} = \delta_i - r_i^{(CS)}$ is known as a Martingale residual (see Fleming and
Harrington 1991)

δ_i is a censoring indicator that takes the value 0 if the observed survival
time of the ith individual is censored and 1 if it is uncensored

Such residuals are used to assess whether any particular individuals are poorly fitted by the model where a large negative or positive value of the residual indicates a lack of fit. Deviance residuals can also be plotted against the corresponding values of a continuous covariate to investigate the appropriate functional form of the variable in the model.

Score residual (Schoenfeld residual) (Schoenfeld 1982):

$$r_{ij}^{(S)} = \delta_i \left\{ x_{ij} - \frac{\sum_{k \in R(t_i)} x_{kj} \exp\left(\beta' x_k\right)}{\sum_{k \in R(t_i)} \exp(\beta' x_k)} \right\} \qquad (16.16)$$

where $R(t_i)$ is the set of all individuals at risk at time t_i.

These residuals are based on the individual contributions to the derivative of the logarithm of the partial likelihood function; see Hosmer and Lemeshow (1999) for details. In essence, the residuals compare the vector of covariate values for the ith subject with its estimated expected value among all those subjects at risk. The score residual is the covariate value for the person who actually died at time t_i minus the estimated expected value of the covariate for the risk set at t_i, so there are separate residuals for each individual for each covariate; these residuals are not defined for censored individuals. Plots of these residuals against survival time, or a rank order of the survival times, for each covariate should show a random scatter of points, centred on zero, if the fitted model is adequate. Substantial trends in such data indicate that the proportional hazards assumption is suspect.

We will now demonstrate briefly how these various residuals can be used by finding their values and constructing a number of plots for the model selected by backward elimination for the German breast cancer data (see Equation 16.12).

First, we will consider the Cox–Snell residuals and assess whether or not they have a unit exponential distribution. Collett (2004) shows that if the

Kaplan–Meier estimate of the survivor function of the residuals is computed (denoted by $\hat{S}(r_i^{(CS)})$; residuals from censored observations are themselves regarded as censored) and the values of $\log\{-\log\hat{S}(r_i^{(CS)})\}$ are plotted against the values of $\log r_i^{(CS)}$, then a straight line plot with unit slope and zero intercept will indicate that the fitted model is correct. Systematic departures from this straight line or a straight line that does not have unit slope or zero intercept suggests that the model needs to be modified in some way. The required plot can be constructed from the following SAS code:

```
proc phreg data=GBSG2;
   class tgrade;
   model mnths*status(0)=horm tgrade pnodes;
   output out=phout logsurv=ls;
run;
data phout;
   set phout;
   rcs=ls*-1;
run;
proc phreg data=phout noprint;
   class tgrade;
   model rcs*status(0)=horm tgrade pnodes;
   output out=phout2 survival=srcs/method=pl;
run;
data phout2;
   set phout2;
   llsrcs=log(-1*log(srcs));
   lrcs=log(rcs);
run;
proc sgplot data=phout2;
  reg y=llsrcs x=lrcs;
  refline 0 ;
  refline 0/axis=x;
run;
```

The resulting plot is shown in Figure 16.2. The plot gives no concerns about the fitted model.

Next, we will use the output statement to calculate the deviance and Schoenfeld residuals. We begin by plotting the deviance residuals against the values of each of the covariates in the model:

```
proc phreg data=GBSG2;
   class tgrade;
   model mnths*status(0)=horm tgrade pnodes/rl;
   output out=phout logsurv=ls resdev=dres resch=sres;
run;

proc sgscatter data=phout;
  plot dres*(pnodes horm tgrade)/columns=2;
run;
```

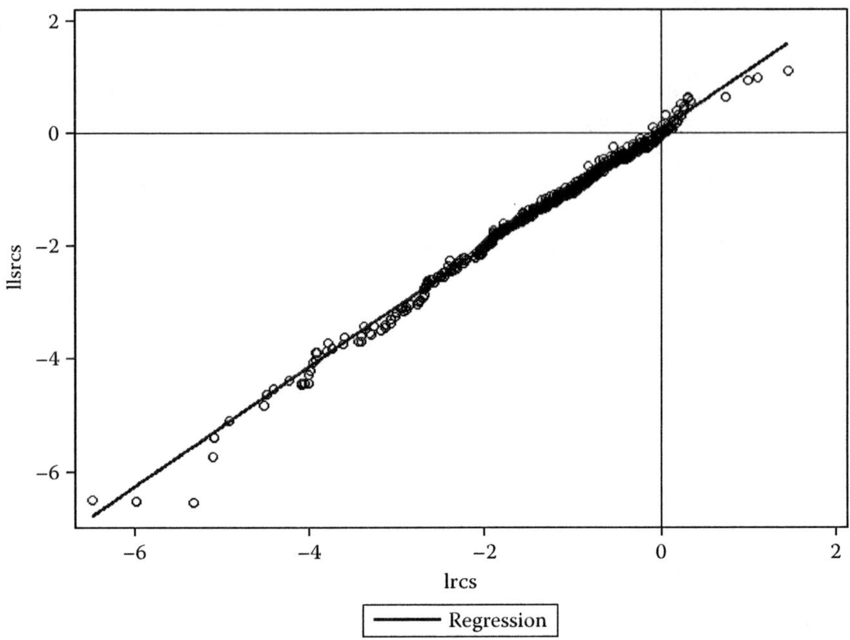

FIGURE 16.2
Plot of Cox–Snell residuals for the breast cancer data.

The plot is shown in Figure 16.3. The plot for the number of positive lymph nodes shows no discernible pattern and there are no residuals that stand out from the rest. The residuals for the two treatment groups appear to have very similar distributions, as do those for the three tumour grades. Overall, the deviance residual plots suggest that the fitted model is satisfactory.

The Schoenfeld residuals can be plotted in the same way and are shown in Figure 16.4. The plots for treatment and tumour grade show the type of pattern that is typical in plots of this type of residual for categorical variables (see Collett 2003b). The plot for the number of positive lymph nodes shows no pattern that would give cause for concern for the fitted model.

16.2.4 Stratified Cox's Regression

For some sets of survival data, a suspected lack of proportionality among hazard functions may be the result of the baseline hazard function differing among the levels of some categorical variable. In such a case, a simple approach to the analysis of the data is to apply Cox's regression within each category or strata of this variable. A more efficient procedure is to fit a model in which each stratum has a different baseline hazard function, but all the other covariates satisfy the proportional hazards function within each

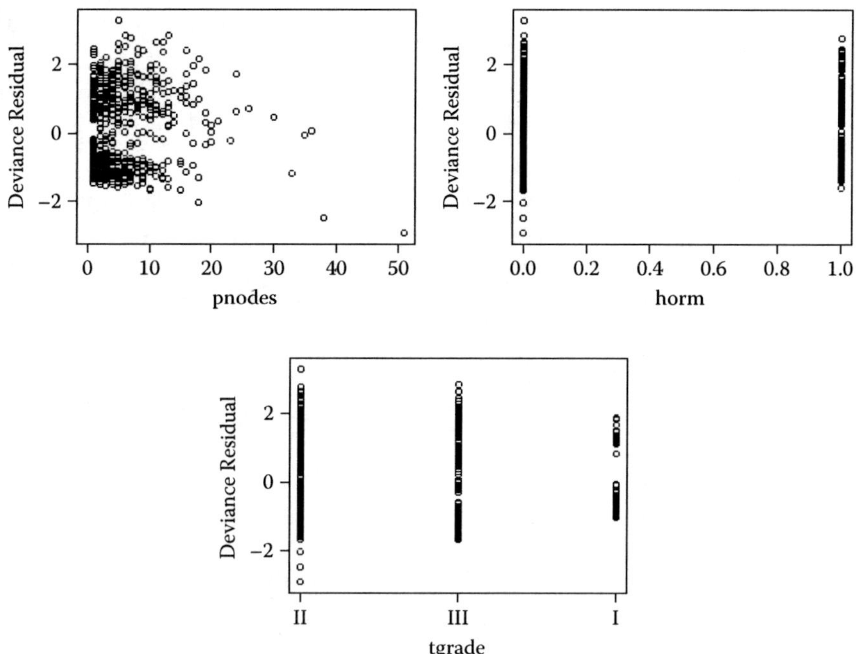

FIGURE 16.3
Plots of deviance residuals for the breast cancer data.

stratum. This leads to the following stratified proportional hazards model (stratified Cox's regression):

$$h_{ij}(t) = h_{0j}(t)\exp(\boldsymbol{\beta}'\mathbf{x}_{ij}) \tag{16.17}$$

where
  $h_{ij}(t)$ is the hazard function of the ith individual in the jth stratum where
      $i = 1,2\ldots,n_j$ and $j = 1,2\ldots,s$
  $h_{0j}(t)$ is the baseline hazards function in the jth stratum
  $\mathbf{x}_{ij}$ is the vector of covariate values for the ith individual in the jth stratum
  $\boldsymbol{\beta}$ is the vector of regression coefficients assumed to be the same in each
      stratum

To begin, we need to check the validity of the proportional hazards model. For this, we can use a method suggested in Lin, Wei, and Ying (1993). This involves the use of the Martingale residuals and is invoked via the assess statement, which can also be used to check the appropriate functional form of covariates. In this case, we reran the previous proc phreg step, adding

```
assess ph/resample;
```

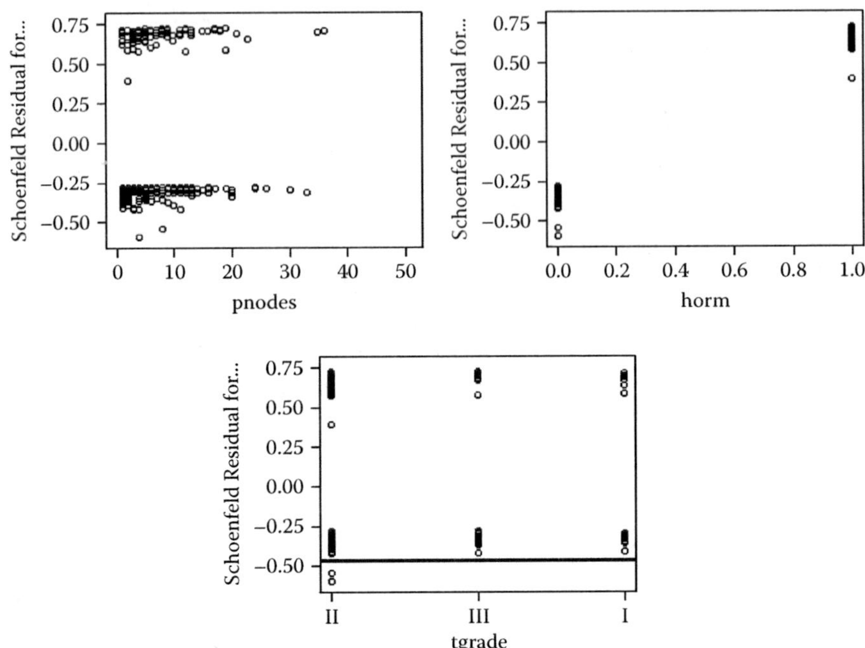

FIGURE 16.4
Schoenfeld (score) residuals for the breast cancer data.

in place of the output statement. The `resample` option requests Kolmogorov supremum tests based by default on 1000 simulations but which can be controlled with `resample =n`. Using `ph` on the `assess` statement tests the proportional hazards assumption for all variables in the model. With ODS graphics on, plots are produced for each of the tests. The plot for tgrade I is shown in Figure 16.5 and the table of test results in Table 16.6. To test the linearity of one or more variables `var=(<variable list>)` could be used—for example,

```
assess ph var=(pnodes) / resample;
```

Now we will apply the stratified Cox's regression model stratifying on `tgrade`:

```
proc phreg data=GBSG2;
  class tgrade;
  model mnths*status(0)=horm pnodes/rl;
  strata tgrade;
run;
```

The results are shown in Table 16.7 and are very similar to those for the non-stratified analysis described earlier in this chapter.

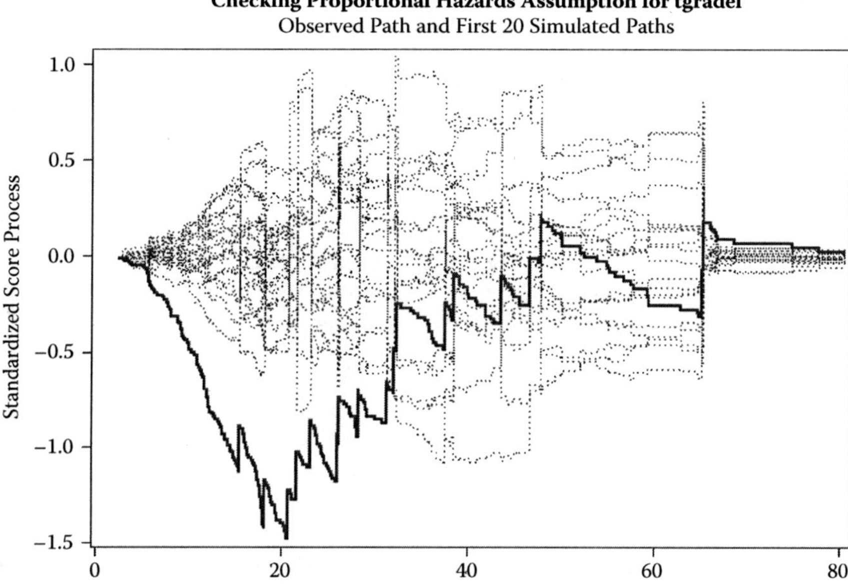

FIGURE 16.5

Testing the assumption of proportional hazards for tgrade in the breast cancer data.

TABLE 16.6

Results of Testing the Proportional Hazards Assumption in the Breast Cancer Data

Supremum Test for Proportionals Hazards Assumption				
Variable	Maximum Absolute Value	Replications	Seed	Pr > MaxAbsVal
Horm	0.7028	1000	899906001	0.6350
tgradei	1.4745	1000	899906001	0.0360
tgradeii	1.2835	1000	899906001	0.0790
Pnodes	0.6263	1000	899906001	0.3560

16.3 Time-Varying Covariates

In previous sections, we have implicitly assumed that the values of all covariates were determined at the time at which follow-up began on each subject and that these values remain constant over the period that the study takes place. But in many survival studies, individuals are monitored over the course of the study and the values of some potentially prognostic

TABLE 16.7

Results from Stratified Cox Regression on Breast Cancer Data

Analysis of Maximum Likelihood Estimates					
Parameter	DF	Parameter Estimate	Standard Error	Chi-Square	Pr > ChiSq
Horm	1	−0.33922	0.12558	7.2970	0.0069
Pnodes	1	0.05439	0.00686	62.8613	<.0001

Analysis of Maximum Likelihood Estimates			
Parameter	Hazard Ratio	95% Hazard Ratio Confidence Limits	
horm	0.712	0.557	0.911
pnodes	1.056	1.042	1.070

variables will change with time—for example, laboratory measurements made repeatedly on the individual. If there are time-varying covariates, then the observations for the ith individual at time t_j can be represented as the vector $\mathbf{x}_i(t_j) = [x_{i1}(t_j), x_{i2}(t_j), \dots, x_{ip}(t_j)]$. This notation can accommodate non-time-varying covariates if, for such covariates, we set $x_{ik}(t_j) = x_{ik}(t = 0) = x_{ik}$. The generalisation of Cox's regression to include both time-varying and non-time-varying covariates is now

$$h_i(t) = h_0(t)\exp\left[\boldsymbol{\beta}'\mathbf{x}_i(t)\right] \tag{16.18}$$

An important assumption in this model is that the effect of any time-varying coefficient given by the appropriate regression coefficients does not depend on time; models with time-varying coefficients are more complex and readers are referred to Hosmer and Lemeshow (1999) for details. It is also important to note that, in the model given in (16.18), the values of at least some of the covariates depend on time, so the relative hazard is also time dependent. Consequently, the hazard of death at time t is now not proportional to the baseline hazard and the model is now not a proportional hazards model.

The parameters in (16.18) are again estimated using the partial likelihood approach; details are given in Collett (2003b). But for the time-varying covariates, the survival period of each patient has to be divided up into a sequence of shorter survival spells, each characterised by an entry time and an exit time and within which the covariate value remains fixed. Thus, the data for each patient on a time-varying covariate are represented by a number of shorter censored spells and possibly one spell ending in the event of interest (for example, death). To illustrate the necessary arrangement, we can use the small data set shown in Table 16.8. In Table 16.9, the data in Table 16.8 are

TABLE 16.8

Hypothetical Survival Data with a Time-Varying Covariate

| Individual | Laboratory Measurement (day) | | | Survival Time | Status |
	0	60	120		
1	0.5	0.7	0.8	130	1
2	0.2	0.6	0.3	190	1
3	0.2	0.4	—	70	0

Notes: Status: 1 = dead; 2 = censored.

TABLE 16.9

Rearranged Data from Table 16.8

Individual	Interval (T_1, T_2)	Lab Measurement	Status
1	0, 60	0.5	0
1	61, 120	0.7	0
1	121, 130	0.8	1
2	0, 60	0.2	0
2	61, 120	0.6	0
2	121, 130	0.3	1
3	0, 60	0.2	0
3	61, 170	0.4	1

rearranged in the manner described earlier in this paragraph. The survival time for each interval is calculated as $t_2 - t_1$.

It may be thought that the observations in Table 16.9 that arise from the same individual are 'correlated' and thus not suitable for Cox's regression as described in the previous chapter. Fortunately, this is not an issue, since the partial likelihood on which estimation is based has a term for each unique death or event time and involves sums over those observations that are available or at risk at the actual event date. Since the intervals for a particular individual do not overlap, the likelihood will involve, at most, only one of the observations for the individual, and thus will still be based on independent observations. The values of the covariates between event times do not enter the partial likelihood. Thus, applying Cox's model to survival data with time-varying covariates is little more complex than for time-fixed covariates.

One circumstance where the use of time-varying covariates may be helpful is where the timing of the delivery of one or both treatments is not under complete experimental control. Such circumstances frequently arise in organ and tissue transplantation, where, at the time of randomisation, no suitably well-matched donors may be available for all patients. Two comparisons then become of interest. The first essentially defines the treatment as that given (i.e., a waiting time of unknown duration followed by transplantation) and compares survival over both waiting and post-transplant survival periods combined. The second defines the treatment as transplantation, for which only the post-transplant survival is relevant. These correspond to the two rather different clinical circumstances of considering the treatment alternatives of a patient for whom a well-matched donor is already available (the second case) and a patient for whom one is yet to be found (the first case).

Without a very rigorous protocol, it is often unreasonable to assume that the waiting time to find a well-matched donor is independent of transplant survival, since matching criteria are likely to be relaxed as the waiting time increases and transplantation may only be possible if the patient is fit enough to survive surgery. Despite this potential difficulty, we shall now illustrate the use of Cox's regression with time-varying covariates with an example of this type, using the well-known set of survival times of potential heart transplant recipients from their date of acceptance into the Stanford heart transplant program.

Part of the data is shown in Table 16.10 in the form described previously. For example, patient 3 waited a single day for a transplant and then died after 15 days. In these data, patients change treatment status during the course of the study. Specifically, a patient is part of the control group until a suitable donor is located and transplantation takes place, at which time he joins the treatment group. Thus, treatment is a time-dependent covariate. The other covariates to be considered are age (in years minus 48), whether the patient had had previous heart surgery, and waiting time for acceptance into the program (years since October 1, 1967).

The necessary SAS code to read in the data and apply a series of Cox's regression model—the first with a single covariate, transplant, the second

TABLE 16.10

A Subset of the Heart Transplant Data

ID	Start	Stop	Event	Age	Year	Surgery	Transplant
1	0.0	50.0	1	−17.155	0.123	0	0
2	0.0	6.0	1	3.836	0.255	0	0
3	0.0	1.0	0	6.297	0.266	0	0
3	1.0	16.0	1	6.297	0.266	0	1
4	0.0	36.0	0	−7.737	0.490	0	0
4	36.0	39.0	1	−7.737	0.490	0	1
5	0.0	18.0	1	−27.214	0.608	0	0
6	0.0	3.0	1	6.5955	0.701	0	0
7	0.0	51.0	0	2.8693	0.780	0	0
7	51.0	675.0	1	2.8693	0.780	0	1
8	0.0	40.0	1	−2.650	0.835	0	0
9	0.0	85.0	1	−0.838	0.857	0	0
10	0.0	12.0	0	−5.498	0.862	0	0
10	12.0	58.0	1	−5.498	0.862	0	1

Notes: Surgery: 0 = no previous surgery, 1 = previous surgery; transplant: 0 = no transplant, 1 = transplant; event: 0 = censored, 1 = died.

with all four covariates, and the third with an interaction between year and transplant—is as follows:

```
data SHTD;
infile 'c:\AMSUS\data\shtd.dat';
input ID Start Stop Event Age Year Surgery Transplant;
duration=stop-start;
run;

proc phreg data=SHTD;
  model (start,stop)*event(0)=Transplant/rl;
run;

proc phreg data=SHTD;
  model (start,stop)*event(0)=Age Year Surgery Transplant/rl;
run;

proc phreg data=SHTD;
  model (start,stop)*event(0)=Age Year Surgery Transplant
  year*transplant/rl;
run;
```

Proc phreg has an alternative version of the model statement designed for data in this format, which SAS refers to as the 'counting process style of input'. Instead of a single variable for the survival time, two variables are named (in parentheses) which define the beginning and end of a period during which the subject is at risk.

Selected output from these three models is shown in Table 16.11. In the first model, there is no evidence that transplantation affects the hazard function. In the second model, the regression coefficients for both age and year are significant, implying that each is associated with survival. The results from the last

TABLE 16.11

Results from Fitting Three Cox Regression Models to the Heart Transplant Data

Analysis of Maximum Likelihood Estimates					
Parameter	DF	Parameter Estimate	Standard Error	Chi-Square	Pr > ChiSq
Transplant	1	0.12567	0.30108	0.1742	0.6764
Age	1	0.02715	0.01372	3.9158	0.0478
Year	1	−0.14611	0.07047	4.2994	0.0381
Surgery	1	−0.63582	0.36721	2.9980	0.0834
Transplant	1	−0.01189	0.31364	0.0014	0.9698
Age	1	0.02988	0.01374	4.7307	0.0296
Year	1	−0.25211	0.10482	5.7848	0.0162
Surgery	1	−0.66270	0.36811	3.2410	0.0718
Transplant	1	−0.62153	0.53092	1.3704	0.2417
Year*transplant	1	0.19697	0.13944	1.9953	0.1578

model appear to imply that survival time depends on the time of acceptance into the study; as this increases, the hazard function for the death of a patient decreases. But this claim become less clear-cut if we examine the transplant × time of acceptance interaction, which approaches significance, with an effect that is in the opposite direction. According to Kalbfleisch and Prentice (1980), taken together these results imply that the overall quality of patients being admitted to the study may be improving with time (possibly due to the relaxation of admission requirements or to improving patient management); however, the survival time of the transplanted patients is not improving at the same rate.

A further model which might be considered is one that allows separate baseline hazards for the after-transplanted and before- or not transplanted patients but common coefficients in each group. To fit this model, we can use the following code:

```
proc phreg data=SHTD plots(cl)=s;
   model (start,stop)*event(0)=Age Year Surgery/rl;
   strata transplant;
run;
```

The results are shown in Table 16.12.

We can plot the graph of the predicted survival curves in each stratum, with all covariates equal to their mean values, using the following code:

```
ods graphics on;
proc phreg data=SHTD plots(cl overlay=row)=s;
```

The resulting plot appears in Figure 16.6 and demonstrates the longer survival experience of patients who have a transplant.

As this example illustrates, time-varying covariates can be introduced into a Cox model for survival data very simply. But this apparent simplicity should not disguise the potential problems. The main one is that the inclusion of such covariates runs the risk of biasing the estimated treatment effect if they themselves reflect the development of the disease process and thus may be partly influenced by treatment. Biochemical or physical measures of disease are obvious examples.

This is well illustrated in an example given by Altman and DeStavola (1994). High levels of bilirubin and low levels of albumin reflect advanced biliary cirrhosis and are highly prognostic. A treatment that leads to an improvement in the cirrhosis will tend to reduce bilirubin levels and increase those of albumin. Altman and DeStavola showed how much of the significant and substantial estimate of treatment effect could be removed by the inclusion into the model of updated values of either of these variables. From the point of view of treatment effect estimation, updating these variables is most unwise, casting unnecessary doubt on treatment differences. From the point of view of a scientific investigation of the development of the process and for constructing prognostic indices, their inclusion will be of more interest.

TABLE 16.12

Results from Stratified Cox Regression for the Heart Transplant Data

Summary of the Number of Event and Censored Values					
Stratum	**Transplant**	**Total**	**Event**	**Censored**	**Percent Censored**
1	0	103	30	73	70.87
2	1	69	45	24	34.78
Total		172	75	97	56.40

Analysis of Maximum Likelihood Estimates					
Parameter	**DF**	**Parameter Estimate**	**Standard Error**	**Chi-Square**	**Pr > ChiSq**
Age	1	0.02931	0.01391	4.4370	0.0352
Year	1	−0.15201	0.07099	4.5849	0.0323
Surgery	1	−0.61681	0.37067	2.7690	0.0961

Analysis of Maximum Likelihood Estimates		
Parameter	**Hazard Ratio**	**95% Hazard Ratio Confidence Limits**
Age	1.030	1.002 1.058
Year	0.859	0.747 0.987
Surgery	0.540	0.261 1.116

Reference Set of Covariates for Plotting		
Age	**Year**	**Surgery**
−2.484017	3.453285	0.168605

Thus, it is important that internal or endogenous variables should be distinguished from external or exogenous variables. External variables are either predetermined (e.g., a patient's age) or vary independently of survival (e.g., the weather). However, for many time-varying variables, their status as internal or external is uncertain, which explains our caution. It is perhaps most helpful to think of internal variables as being those that are 'causally downstream' of treatment, but the link between treatment and the internal variable does not have to be a direct one. Thus, if the poor health of those on the worse or placebo treatment results in their choosing to move to a more pleasant and health-promoting climate, then not even the weather is external!

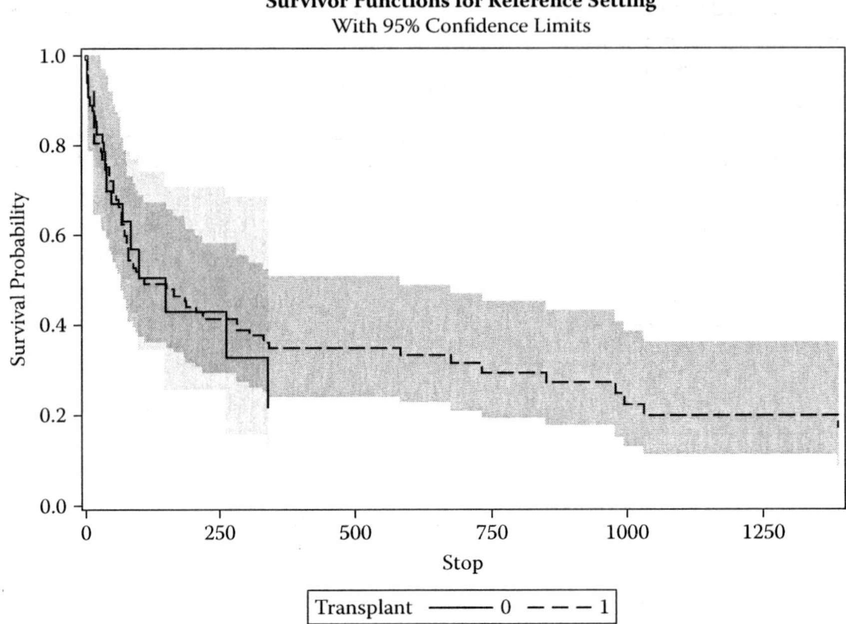

FIGURE 16.6
Predicted survival curves for heart transplant data.

16.4 Random-Effects Models for Survival Data

Cox's proportional hazards model, as described in the previous chapter, has become the workhorse of regression analysis for censored time-to-event data. But one of the implicit assumptions of the method—namely, that the survival times observed are independent of one another—is not necessarily valid in all situations in which survival times are collected. Some types of studies generate correlated survival times, and a suitable model must account for the correlations; some examples of such studies are

- Survival times of individuals that have been formed into matched groups similar on a set of prognostically relevant variables
- Survival times of individuals related, for example, by family membership, marriage, exposure to some agent, etc.
- Recurrent or repeated events, where the same event, for example, myocardial infarction, can happen several times for an individual

The most common way of dealing with correlated survival time data is to use the counterpart of the random-effects models described in Chapter 11. The random effects are again used to generate the dependence between the observations and, conditional on the random effects, the observations are assumed independent. But correlated survival times can also be dealt with by using sandwich estimators of the standard errors of the estimated regression coefficients in a fitted Cox's model to the data, ignoring the lack of dependence of the survival times; both approaches will be used in the example that follows.

As an example of dealing with correlated time-to-event data, we shall use the data consisting of recurrence times to infection at point of insertion of the catheter for kidney patients using portable dialysis equipment; part of the data is shown in Table 16.13. For each patient, two such recurrence times are given. The covariates of interest are age, gender, and the presence/absence of disease types GN, ANN, and PKD. We first fit a Cox regression model to the data, ignoring the possible correlation between the recurrence times of an individual and using the sandwich estimators of the standard errors of the estimated regression coefficients.

The code for fitting the Cox regression to the data and requesting the sandwich estimators of the standard errors is as follows:

```
data catheters;
   infile 'c:\amsus\data\CatheterInfection.dat';
   input Subject Time Status Age Sex Disease;
run;

proc phreg data=catheters covs(aggregate);
 class disease sex /ref=first;
 model time*status(0)=age sex disease/rl;
 id subject;
run;
```

TABLE 16.13

Recurrence Times for Catheter Infection in Five
Kidney Patients

Subject	Time	Status	Age	Sex	Disease
1	8	1	28	1	3
1	16	1	28	1	3
2	23	1	48	2	0
2	13	0	48	2	0
3	22	1	32	1	3
3	28	1	32	1	3
4	447	1	31	2	3
4	318	1	32	2	3
5	30	1	10	1	3
5	12	1	10	1	3

Notes: Time: recurrence time in days; status: 1 = infection
occurs, 0 = censored; disease: 0 = GN, 1 = AN, 2 = PKD,
3 = other; sex: 1 = male, 2 = female; age: age in years.

The `covs` (or `covsandwich`) option on the `proc` statement invokes sandwich estimators and (`aggregate`) specifies that these are for the clusters defined by the variable on the `id` statement. The results are shown in Table 16.14. The standard errors in the table are the sandwich estimates and the column headed 'Std error ratio' is the ratio of the sandwich estimator of an estimated regression coefficient to the corresponding model-based estimate. For some covariates, the sandwich estimators are smaller than the model-based estimates; for others, the reverse is the case. The only significant regression coefficient is that for sex. The hazard for women is between 10% and about 50% of that for males.

Analogous to the random-effects models for longitudinal data described in Chapter 13, random effects can be introduced into the Cox model to account for the likely dependence between time-to-event measures made on the same patient; again, conditional on the random effects, the observations are considered independent. For survival data, the random effects are usually known as frailties—a term first introduced by Vaupel, Manton, and Stallard (1993). Frailty models can be fitted to survival or other time-to-event data by what is known as a penalized partial likelihood approach, details of which are given in Therneau and Grambsch (2000) and Wienke (2010). Here, we content ourselves with an example of such models using the kidney patient data in Table 16.13.

The model that we shall fit to these data is as follows:

$$\log[h_{ij}(t)] = \log[h_0(t)] + \beta_1\text{Age} + \beta_2\text{Sex} + \beta_3\text{D}_1 + \beta_4\text{D}_2 + \beta_5\text{D}_3 + u_i \quad (16.19)$$

where
    $h_{ij}(t)$ is the hazard function of the jth recurrence time for the ith individual
    D_1, D_2, and D_3 are the three dummy variables used to code the four categories of disease
    u_i is the random effect or frailty associated with the ith individual

The random effects are assumed to have a normal distribution with zero mean and a variance that has to be estimated.

The random-effects model specified in (16.19) is applied using the following SAS code:

```
proc phreg data=catheters;
 class subject disease sex /ref=first;
 model time*status(0)=age sex disease/rl;
 random subject;
run;
```

The results are shown in Table 16.15. Some of the estimated standard errors of the estimated regression coefficients differ considerably from the sandwich estimates in Table 16.14, but the conclusion from the random-effects model is much the same—namely, that the hazard for women is between about 7% and 43% of that for men.

TABLE 16.14

Results from a Cox's Regression Fitted to Kidney Patient Data in Table 16.13, Ignoring the Repeated Measures Aspect of the Data

Testing Global Null Hypothesis: BETA = 0			
Test	Chi-Square	DF	Pr > ChiSq
Likelihood Ratio	18.6342	5	0.0022
Score (Model Based)	21.2696	5	0.0007
Score (Sandwich)	10.9436	5	0.0525
Wald (Model Based)	20.9917	5	0.0008
Wald (Sandwich)	17.3897	5	0.0038

Type 3 Tests			
Effect	DF	Wald Chi-Square	Pr > ChiSq
Age	1	0.0787	0.7791
Sex	1	13.6093	0.0002
Disease	3	5.4722	0.1403

Analysis of Maximum Likelihood Estimates							
Parameter		DF	Parameter Estimate	Standard Error	Std Error Ratio	Chi-Square	Pr > ChiSq
Age		1	0.00199	0.00710	0.632	0.0787	0.7791
Sex	2	1	−1.51940	0.41186	1.142	13.6093	0.0002
Disease	1	1	0.28361	0.34419	0.909	0.6790	0.4099
Disease	2	1	−1.55571	0.90654	1.553	2.9450	0.0861
Disease	3	1	−0.15666	0.29053	0.705	0.2908	0.5897

Analysis of Maximum Likelihood Estimates					
Parameter		Hazard Ratio	95% Hazard Ratio Confidence Limits		Label
Age		1.002	0.988	1.016	
Sex	2	0.219	0.098	0.491	Sex 2
Disease	1	1.328	0.676	2.607	Disease 1
Disease	2	0.211	0.036	1.247	Disease 2
Disease	3	0.855	0.484	1.511	Disease 3

TABLE 16.15

Results from Fitting Random-Effects Model to the Kidney Patient Data in Table 16.13

Covariance Parameter Estimates		
Cov Parm	REML Estimate	Standard Error
Subject	0.5923	0.3441

Type 3 Tests					
Effect	Wald Chi-Square	DF	Pr > ChiSq	Adjusted DF	Adjusted Pr > ChiSq
Age	0.0446	1	0.8328	0.4939	0.5710
Sex	13.8088	1	0.0002	0.5804	<.0001
Disease	4.3461	3	0.2264	1.6465	0.0821
Subject	20.2901			13.1557	0.0929

Analysis of Maximum Likelihood Estimates						
Parameter		DF	Parameter Estimate	Standard Error	Chi-Square	Pr > ChiSq
Age		1	0.00328	0.01554	0.0446	0.8328
Sex	2	1	−1.78528	0.48043	13.8088	0.0002
Disease	1	1	0.24241	0.53347	0.2065	0.6495
Disease	2	1	−1.32714	0.79317	2.7996	0.0943
Disease	3	1	−0.29545	0.56628	0.2722	0.6019

Analysis of Maximum Likelihood Estimates					
Parameter		Hazard Ratio	95% Hazard Ratio Confidence Limits		Label
Age		1.003	0.973	1.034	
Sex	2	0.168	0.065	0.430	Sex 2
Disease	1	1.274	0.448	3.625	Disease 1
Disease	2	0.265	0.056	1.255	Disease 2
Disease	3	0.744	0.245	2.258	Disease 3

16.5 Summary

Survival analysis is the study of the distribution of times to some terminating event (death, relapse, etc.). A distinguishing feature of survival data is the presence of censored observations, and this has led to the development of a wide range of methodologies for analysing survival times. Of the available methods, Cox's regression, which allows the investigation of the effects of multiple covariates on the hazard function, is the most commonly applied. The model has been almost universally adopted by statisticians and applied researchers, primarily because it allows inferences about the regression coefficients without making any assumptions about the baseline hazard. Departures from the proportional hazards assumption that is central to the model can often be accommodated by careful use of strata and by the inclusion of suitable time-varying covariates. Repeated measurement time-to-event data can be dealt with by including random effects (frailties) in the Cox model.

17

Bayesian Methods

17.1 Introduction

According to Everitt and Pickles (2004), Bayesian statistics were, until relatively recently, little more than an intellectual curiosity, rich in conceptual insight but of little practical value when it came to actual data analysis. But in the first decade of the twenty-first century, Bayesian methods and applications have become an area of intense activity. The obvious question that arises is 'why?' But before we try to answer this, we need to get clear just what Bayesian methods are. In short, a Bayesian approach has been described in Spiegelhalter, Abrams, and Myles (2004) as 'the explicit quantitative use of external evidence in the design, monitoring, analysis, interpretation and reporting of a health-care evaluation'.

To delve a little deeper into what this means, we must first return to consider the traditional frequentist analysis, which essentially treats each study (a clinical trial, say) as if it were entirely novel; the trial usually is considered as being individually potentially decisive. Scientific progress may occur outside the narrow focus of this particular trial, but the numerical procedures themselves are not formulated to reflect the process of progressive learning or one in which the process itself involves costs and potential beliefs. By contrast, the focus of the Bayesian approach is one of progressive refinement of opinion as data from trials and other sources accumulate. This approach is illustrated in Figure 17.1.

Knowledge prior to a trial is synthesised and formally represented as a distribution over the parameter space of the problem (the *prior distribution*). The trial is undertaken. The data from the trial are then combined with the prior distribution to form a *posterior distribution* over the same parameter space, one that is hopefully more concentrated than the prior. The data collected in the trial are used to update prior beliefs, as defined by parameter or effect distributions. If the prior distribution is diffuse and relatively uninformative, then it is likely that the Bayesian approach will lead to conclusions that are the same as or very similar to those given by the use of the routine procedures of the frequentist statistician.

But differences do occur and the advocates of Bayesian methods claim, with some justification, that their approach is often more flexible than

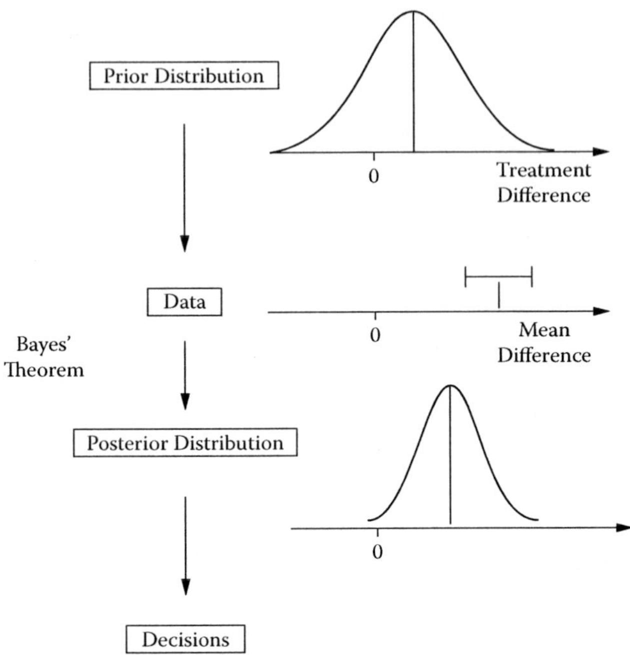

FIGURE 17.1
Conceptual framework for Bayesian analysis.

traditional methods as it can adapt to each unique situation. They may further claim that the Bayesian process is more efficient in that it uses all the available evidence thought to be relevant. Finally, the Bayesian will say that his or her methodology is more useful in providing predictions and inputs for making decisions about individual patients and summarising evidence as direct probability statements that are clinically relevant.

17.2 Bayesian Estimation

Fundamental in both frequentist and Bayesian approaches to statistical inference and estimation is the likelihood function. For the frequentist, the likelihood summarises, for a given value of the unknown parameter(s), how plausible the observed data are. The Bayesian uses the likelihood function to obtain the probability distribution for the unknown parameter(s) conditional on both the data and any background information summarised in the prior distribution. From a Bayesian perspective, both the observed data and the parameters of the model of interest are considered as random quantities. Letting D denote the observed data and Θ the model parameters, a joint probability distribution or *full probability model* $P(D,\Theta)$ is considered. This is decomposed into a prior distribution, $P(\Theta)$, for the parameters and a likelihood, $P(D|\Theta)$, for which

$$P(D,\Theta) = P(D|\Theta)\, P(\Theta) \tag{17.1}$$

Given data from a study (for example, a trial), the posterior distribution of the parameters, given the data $P(D|\Theta)$, is obtained by applying Bayes's theorem as follows:

$$P(\Theta|D) = \frac{P(\Theta)P(D|\Theta)}{\displaystyle\int P(\Theta)P(D|\Theta)} \tag{17.2}$$

Quantities calculated from this posterior distribution of the parameters form the basis of inference. Point estimates of parameters might be found by calculating the mean, median, or mode of a parameter posterior distribution, with parameter precision being estimated by the standard deviation or some suitable interquantile range, for example, from quantiles at p and $1-p$ for a $100(1-2p)\%$ *credible interval* for a parameter. In general, such quantities, $f(\Theta)$, will be estimated by their posterior expectation, given by

$$E[f(\Theta)|D] = \frac{\displaystyle\int f(\Theta)P(\Theta)P(D|\Theta)d\Theta}{\displaystyle\int P(\Theta)P(D|\Theta)d\Theta} \tag{17.3}$$

(When there is more than a single parameter, the integration in this equation will be, of course, a multiple integration.)

As a simple illustration of how Bayesian inference works, we will consider a sequence of Bernoulli trials where the single parameter, θ, is the probability of a 'success'. We will assume that we can characterise any prior knowledge we have as to the likely value of θ in a particular type of prior distribution—namely, a beta distribution with density function

$$P(\theta) = \frac{\Gamma(\alpha+\beta)\theta^{\alpha-1}(1-\theta)^{\beta-1}}{\Gamma(\alpha)\Gamma(\beta)}, \quad 0 \le \theta \le 1 \tag{17.4}$$

This density function has mean $\alpha/(\alpha+\beta)$ and variance $\alpha\beta/[(\alpha+\beta)^2(\alpha+\beta+1)]$. Figure 17.2 shows four beta distributions. Symmetrical unimodal distributions are obtained for $\alpha = \beta > 1$, narrowing as their value increases and becoming asymmetrical when α does not equal β. The beta distribution is what is known as the *conjugate prior* for the Bernoulli parameter, which simply means that the posterior distribution is also a beta distribution, as we shall now demonstrate.

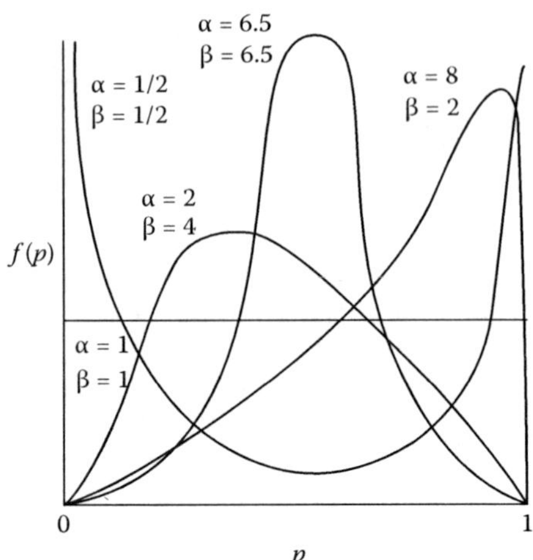

FIGURE 17.2
Four beta distributions.

In a sequence of n Bernoulli trials in which we observe r successes, the likelihood is proportional to $\theta^r(1-\theta)^{n-r}$. The posterior distribution is obtained by multiplying the prior distribution by the likelihood and standardising so that the result is an acceptable density function that integrates to one. The selection of a conjugate prior makes this straightforward and we obtain

$$P(\theta|r,n) \propto \theta^{\alpha+r+1}(1-\theta)^{\beta+n-r-1} \tag{17.5}$$

This is another beta distribution with parameters $\alpha^* = \alpha + r$ and $\beta^* = \beta + n - r$.

The mean of the posterior distribution is $(\alpha+r)/(\alpha+\beta+n)$; as α and β approach zero, corresponding to a prior distribution with the greatest possible variance, so too does the posterior mean approach r/n, the value that would be expected under maximum likelihood. As r and n increase relative to α and β, so too does the variance of the distribution approach the familiar $(r/n)(1-r/n)/n$. Figure 17.2 shows a beta distribution with $\alpha=\beta=6.5$, the posterior distribution that would occur following the observation of six successes in 12 trials with the use of the reasonably uninformative prior in which $\alpha = \beta = 0.5$ (which is also shown in Figure 17.2).

In this hypothetical example, the particular choice of likelihood and prior distribution allowed the required posterior mean to be calculated very simply. With examples encountered in practice, however, this is rarely possible and some other way is needed to tackle the numerical problems posed by the evaluation of the often high-dimensional integrals in (17.3). Much of Bayesian statistics over the last three decades has been concerned with either parameterising models such that the integrals simplify or with the use of approximate methods (Bernado and Smith 1994). Nowadays, the numerical problems have largely been overcome by the use of *Markov chain Monte Carlo* (MCMC) methods.

17.3 Markov Chain Monte Carlo

The most direct way of using (17.3) to evaluate the posterior mean would be to carry out the necessary integrations. But this is usually very difficult to do either analytically or numerically. MCMC methods effectively allow generation of samples from the posterior distribution without requiring the distribution explicitly. By simulating a large enough sample, the mean, variance of any other characteristic of the posterior distribution can be calculated to any degree of accuracy. For example, for a sample of m values of Θ from the posterior distribution, we would estimate the expected value in (17.3) by simply taking the average—that is,

$$\hat{E}[f(\Theta)\,|\,D] = \frac{1}{m}\sum_{i=1}^{m} f(\Theta_i\,|\,D) \tag{17.6}$$

By simply increasing m, the precision of the estimation can be made accurate as required. All that remains is to consider how the required samples are generated and the MCMC approach involves a cleverly constructed *Markov chain* (a sequence of random variables $\{\theta^{(1)},\theta^{(2)},\ldots\}$ such that $\theta^{(i)}$ only depends on $\theta^{(i-1)}$ and not on the rest of the random variables), the stationary distribution of which is precisely the required posterior distribution. The construction of a Markov chain with a stationary distribution that is the posterior distribution of interest is relatively straightforward and was initially proposed by Metropolis et al. (1953) and generalised by Hastings (1970) and is now referred to as the *Metropolis–Hastings algorithm*.

One of the features of the MCMC method is that (in theory at least), regardless of where it is started, in the long run it tends to converge to the required stationary distribution. Application of the method involves what is known as a 'burn-in' period during which it is hoped that the stationary distribution is reached, followed by a period of monitoring during which sample values of the quantities of interest are recorded and tests of convergence are undertaken. Testing for convergence is no formality when using MCMC methods, as some of the material in Gilks, Richardson, and Spiegelhalter (1996) demonstrates. Questions that need to be addressed include

- How long do we need to run the MCMC process to reach the posterior distribution adequately?

- How can we tell if the MCMC process is 'mixing' well where a good chain will have rapid mixing if the stationary distribution is reached quickly from an arbitrary starting point?

An advantage of MCMC estimation is that the parameterisation Θ over which the Markov chain is defined does not constrain the list of quantities, $f(\Theta)$, for which posterior distributions are monitored. Thus, Θ can be chosen for its statistical and estimation properties, while the $f(\Theta)$ can be chosen for their scientific and clinical interest. The additional burden of adding a variety of functions of the parameters into the MCMC sampling cycle is rarely great. As an example, consider a study involving three drug treatments—A, B, and C—and a control treatment; a standard parameterisation would be a mean contrast for the effects of each drug relative to the control group.

We might, however, be more interested in the probability that the pair of drugs that perform best in some small trial actually contains the 'best' drug. This kind of information is extremely valuable in drug development but is not readily calculated from knowledge of the point estimates and covariance matrix of the standard parameters. It is, however, an extremely simple task to monitor the ranks of the effects of each treatment from each MCMC sample and then to obtain and estimate of their distribution, confidence intervals, etc.

We shall not give any of the technical details of MCMC here; for these, readers are referred to Gelman (1996), Roberts (1996), and Gilks et al. (1996).

17.4 Prior Distributions

The Bayesian approach just outlined gives a framework for updating beliefs or evidence. There are several possible types of prior distributions. The *reference prior*, for example, represents minimal prior information and is the least subjective; analyses based on this type of prior act as a useful baseline against which to compare analyses using other priors. An example would be the use of a uniform prior on the interval (0,1) for a binomial proportion. (Such priors are also termed *uninformative*: They have minimal impact on the posterior distribution.)

The *clinical prior* is intended to represent the current state of knowledge. Where possible, it should be based on good evidence, such as a meta-analysis of relevant randomised controlled trials. Where this is not possible, evidence from nonrandomised studies may be needed. Alternatively, subjective clinical opinion may form the basis of a prior distribution. Elicitation of opinion can be carried out using techniques such as interviews or questionnaires (see, for example, Chaloner and Verdinelli 1995 and Chaloner 1996). Such a prior is often referred to as *informative*; an informative prior dominates the likelihood.

Next, the *skeptical prior* formalises the belief that large treatment differences are unlikely. This can be set up, for example, as having a mean of no treatment effect and only a small probability of the effect achieving a clinically relevant value. By contrast, the *enthusiastic prior* can be specified, for example, with a mean equivalent to a clinically relevant effect and only a small probability of no effect, or worse.

17.5 Model Selection When Using a Bayesian Approach

In applying Bayesian statistics to data, so-called *Bayes factors* are often used to choose between competing models. These factors provide a summary of the evidence given by the data D in favour of a model, M_1, relative to another model, M_0. Bayes factors are the ratio of the posterior to prior odds—that is,

$$B_{10} = \frac{P(D \mid M_1)}{P(D \mid M_0)} \tag{17.7}$$

Twice the logarithm of B_{10} is on the same scale as the deviance and the likelihood ratio test statistic. The following is often helpful for interpreting values of Bayes factors:

2lnB10	Evidence for M1
<0	Negative (supports M_0)
0–2.2	Not worth more than a bare mention
2.2–6	Positive
6–10	Strong
>10	Very strong

A further measure of fit when using a Bayesian approach to fit models is the deviance information criterion (DIC) suggested in Spiegelhalter et al. (2002). Lower values of the DIC indicate models that provide a better fit for the data.

In the next section, we will give some examples of the use of MCMC sampling in applying the Bayesian approach.

17.6 Some Examples of the Application of Bayesian Statistics

17.6.1 Psychiatric 'Caseness'

As our first example of the application of Bayesian statistics, we shall return to the example involving psychiatric caseness considered in Chapter 9. The logistic model we will consider is the following:

Logit(Pr (being a case)|gender and GHQ score) = $\beta_0 + \beta_1 \text{Sex} + \beta_2 \text{GHQ}$

where the dummy variable, sex, takes the value one for men and zero for women.

In this model, β_0 represents the logit of the probability of being a case for a woman with GHQ score of zero; if we assume an $N(0,1)$ prior for β_0, it implies that we expect about 95% of its values to lie approximately between $\exp(0-2\times1)/[1 + \exp(0-2\times1)] = 0.12$ and $\exp(0+2\times1)/[1+\exp(0+2\times1)] = 0.88$, which seems reasonable. For β_1 and β_2, we will assume $N(0,0.25)$ priors. This implies that in both cases we expect most of the odd ratio values to be approximately between $\exp(0 - 2 \times \sqrt{0.25}) = 0.37$ and $\exp(0+2\times \sqrt{0.25}) = 2.72$.

Having decided on the priors, we can use proc genmod to apply a Bayesian analysis using MCMC for estimation. We begin by creating a small data set containing the information on the priors to be used. The data set has a variable for each regression coefficient plus a variable, _type_ , to identify the type of prior being specified whose values can be 'mean', 'var' (variance), 'precision' (inverse of the variance), and 'cov' (covariance):

```
data priors;
  input _type_ $ intercept female ghq;
datalines;
Mean 0 0 0
Var 1 .25 .25
;
ods graphics on;
proc genmod data=ghq;
   model cases/total=female ghq /dist=b link=logit;
   bayes seed=12345 cprior=normal(input=priors);
run;
ods graphics off;
```

The use of proc genmod for fitting generalised linear models was introduced in Chapter 10. A Bayesian analysis is invoked with the bayes statement and controlled with its options. Here we specify a seed for the random number generator used in the simulation and normal priors for the regression coefficients with values input from the data set just created. Enabling ODS graphics produces diagnostic plots for the MCMC sampling process.

The output is shown in Table 17.1. The default 'burn-in' of 2000 iterations followed by 10,000 MCMC iterations has been used. The results from using maximum likelihood to estimate the parameters are shown first; this duplicates the results given in Chapter 9. The output provides the mean, standard deviation, and quartiles of the sampled values for each parameter in the model. In addition, the output gives the *highest posterior density* (HPD) interval for each parameter (in this example, we have selected the 95% interval). This interval is such that 95% of the highest area of the posterior density is contained in the interval; in essence, the HPD is the Bayesian equivalent of the frequentist's confidence interval.

TABLE 17.1

Results from Bayesian Analysis of Data on Psychiatric Caseness

Bayesian Analysis	
Model Information	
Data Set	WORK.GHQ
Burn-in Size	2000
MC Sample Size	10,000
Thinning	1
Sampling Algorithm	ARMS
Distribution	Binomial
Link Function	Logit
Response Variable (Events)	cases
Response Variable (Trials)	total

Number of Observations Read	22
Number of Observations Used	22
Number of Events	68
Number of Trials	278

Response Profile		
Ordered Value	**Binary Outcome**	**Total Frequency**
1	Event	68
2	Nonevent	210

Algorithm converged.

Analysis of Maximum Likelihood Parameter Estimates					
Parameter	**DF**	**Estimate**	**Standard Error**	**Wald 95% Confidence Limits**	
Intercept	1	−3.4296	0.4627	−4.3365	−2.5227
female	1	0.9361	0.4343	0.0848	1.7874
ghq	1	0.7791	0.0990	0.5850	0.9732
Scale	0	1.0000	0.0000	1.0000	1.0000
Note: The scale parameter was held fixed.					

(Continued)

TABLE 17.1 (*Continued*)

Results from Bayesian Analysis of Data on Psychiatric Caseness

Bayesian Analysis		
Independent Normal Prior for Regression Coefficients		
Parameter	**Mean**	**Precision**
Intercept	0	1
female	0	4
Ghq	0	4

Algorithm converged.

Initial Values of the Chain				
Chain	**Seed**	**Intercept**	**female**	**ghq**
1	12345	−2.71835	0.339082	0.677575

Fit Statistics	
DIC (smaller is better)	54.648
pD (effective number of parameters)	2.502

Bayesian Analysis						
Posterior Summaries						
			Standard	**Percentiles**		
Parameter	**N**	**Mean**	**Deviation**	**25%**	**50%**	**75%**
Intercept	10,000	−2.7568	0.3213	−2.9677	−2.7550	−2.5353
female	10,000	0.3380	0.2963	0.1380	0.3344	0.5367
ghq	10,000	0.6926	0.0857	0.6336	0.6909	0.7496

Posterior Intervals					
Parameter	**Alpha**	**Equal-Tail Interval**		**HPD Interval**	
Intercept	0.050	−3.3993	−2.1461	−3.3749	−2.1262
female	0.050	−0.2472	0.9134	−0.2272	0.9252
ghq	0.050	0.5323	0.8654	0.5247	0.8567

Posterior Correlation Matrix			
Parameter	**Intercept**	**female**	**ghq**
Intercept	1.000	−0.647	−0.597
Female	−0.647	1.000	0.101
Ghq	−0.597	0.101	1.000

TABLE 17.1 (*Continued*)

Results from Bayesian Analysis of Data on Psychiatric Caseness

Bayesian Analysis			
Posterior Autocorrelations			
Parameter	**Lag 1**	**Lag 5**	**Lag 10**	**Lag 50**
---	---	---	---	---
Intercept	0.1116	0.0082	−0.0019	−0.0002
Female	0.0584	−0.0143	−0.0022	0.0089
Ghq	0.6859	0.1679	0.0526	−0.0268

Geweke Diagnostics		
Parameter	**z**	**Pr > |z|**
Intercept	0.2823	0.7777
female	−0.6851	0.4933
ghq	−0.3550	0.7226

Effective Sample Sizes			
		Autocorrelation	
Parameter	**ESS**	**Time**	**Efficiency**
Intercept	6464.8	1.5468	0.6465
female	9277.2	1.0779	0.9277
ghq	1671.1	5.9842	0.1671

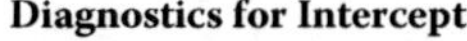

Diagnostics for Intercept

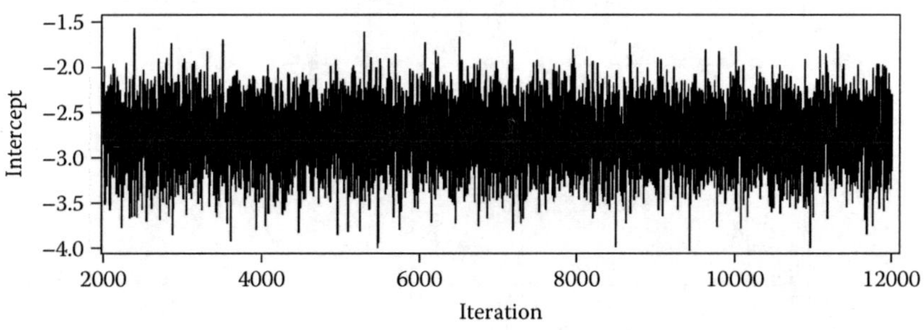

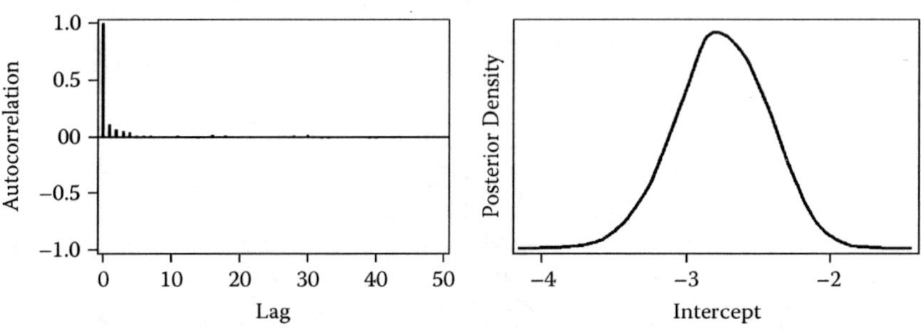

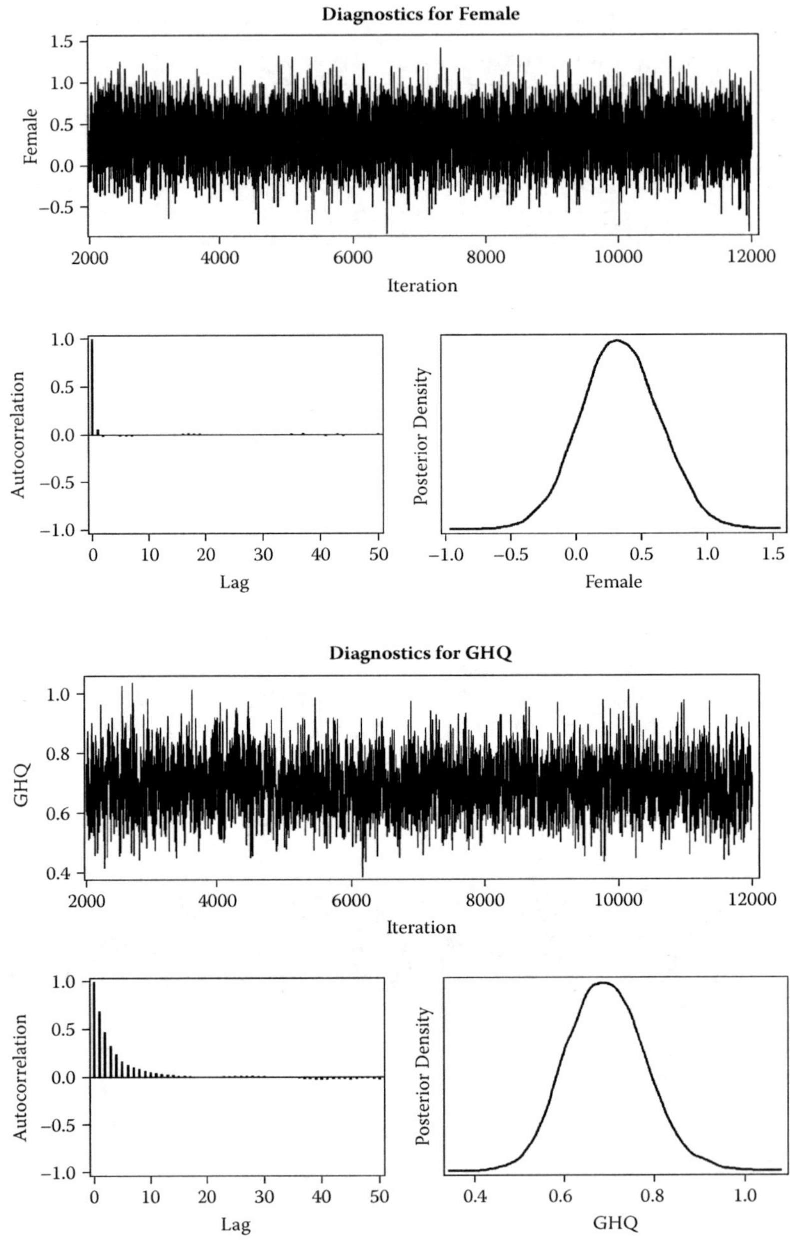

For the regression coefficient of GHQ, the 95% confidence interval from maximum likelihood estimation, (0.58,0.97), is very similar to the HPD from the Bayesian analysis, (0.52,0.86), but the corresponding intervals for the regression coefficient for sex, (0.08,1.79) and (−0.227,0.93), are quite different. In particular, the first suggests a significant effect for sex, with women having an increased risk of being a case, as explained in Chapter 9. However, the HPD interval indicates that there is no evidence of a sex effect. For GHQ, the likelihood is 'stronger' than the prior, but for sex it is not.

Much of the remaining output in Table 17.1 provides diagnostics relating to the MCMC sampling process. For example, the autocorrelations and the effective sample size tell us something about the dependence structure of the sampling; if this is too strong, the effective sample size will be far lower than the nominal sample size set by the investigator. In this example, the latter is 10,000 and the effective sample sizes for the parameters in the model range from 1,671 for GHQ to 9,277 for sex. The former gives perhaps some cause for concern and suggests that a larger sample size might be needed for satisfactory sampling for the corresponding parameter (we leave this to the reader as an exercise). The effective sample sizes reflect the posterior autocorrelations, which are larger for GHQ. The cause of autocorrelation is that the parameters in the model may be highly correlated, so the MCMC process will be slow to explore the entire posterior distribution.

The plots of iterations against sampled value of each variable are generally known as *trace plots*. Any apparent trends in these plots are a clear sign of nonconvergence and suggest that the MCMC process is not working as it should. In Table 17.1, the three trace plots give no cause for concern.

Geweke (1992) proposed a convergence diagnostic for MCMC sampling based on a test of the equality of the means of the first and last part of the Markov chain (by default, the first 10% and the last 50% are used). The Geweke diagnostics in Table 17.1 all have associated p-values much greater than 0.05 and again provide evidence that the MCMC procedure has converged satisfactorily in this example.

To investigate how changing the prior distributions in the caseness example alters the parameter estimates, we will now rerun the Bayesian analysis, in this case using $N(0,0.50)$ priors β_1 and β_2. This now implies that in both cases we expect most of the odd ratio values to be approximately between $\exp(0 - 2 \times \sqrt{0.50}) = 0.24$ and $\exp(0 + 2 \times \sqrt{0.50}) = 4.11$. (We will again assume an $N(0,1)$ prior for β_0.) The required SAS code is

```
data priors;
 input_type_$ intercept female ghq;
datalines;
Mean 0 0 0
Var 1 .5 .5
;
ods graphics on;
proc genmod data=ghq;
  model cases/total=female ghq /dist=b link=logit;
  bayes seed=12345 cprior=normal(input=priors);
run;
ods graphics off;
```

The edited output is shown in Table 17.2. We see that the HPD intervals in this table are similar to those in Table 17.1. Amongst the diagnostics, the Geweke statistic for GHQ is now significant and perhaps underlines the need to investigate the convergence of the MCMC process for this parameter in a little more detail (again, we leave this as an exercise for the reader).

TABLE 17.2

Edited Results from Second Bayesian Analysis of Caseness Data

Bayesian Analysis						
Posterior Summaries						
				Percentiles		
Parameter	N	Mean	Standard Deviation	25%	50%	75%
Intercept	10,000	−2.8303	0.3395	−3.0528	−2.8235	−2.5975
female	10,000	0.4199	0.3275	0.1946	0.4183	0.6483
ghq	10,000	0.7027	0.0867	0.6427	0.7010	0.7593

Posterior Intervals					
		Equal-Tail			
Parameter	Alpha	Interval		HPD Interval	
Intercept	0.050	−3.5076	−2.1820	−3.5078	−2.1830
female	0.050	−0.2167	1.0602	−0.2395	1.0336
ghq	0.050	0.5403	0.8809	0.5263	0.8626

Bayesian Analysis				
Posterior Autocorrelations				
Parameter	Lag 1	Lag 5	Lag 10	Lag 50
Intercept	0.1262	−0.0030	−0.0114	0.0008
female	0.0780	−0.0230	−0.0070	−0.0041
ghq	0.6868	0.1340	−0.0123	−0.0180

Geweke Diagnostics		
Parameter	z	Pr > |z|
Intercept	−1.9130	0.0557
female	−0.0936	0.9254
Ghq	2.0280	0.0426

Effective Sample Sizes			
		Autocorrelation	
Parameter	ESS	Time	Efficiency
Intercept	6902.8	1.4487	0.6903
female	8650.6	1.1560	0.8651
ghq	2098.7	4.7649	0.2099

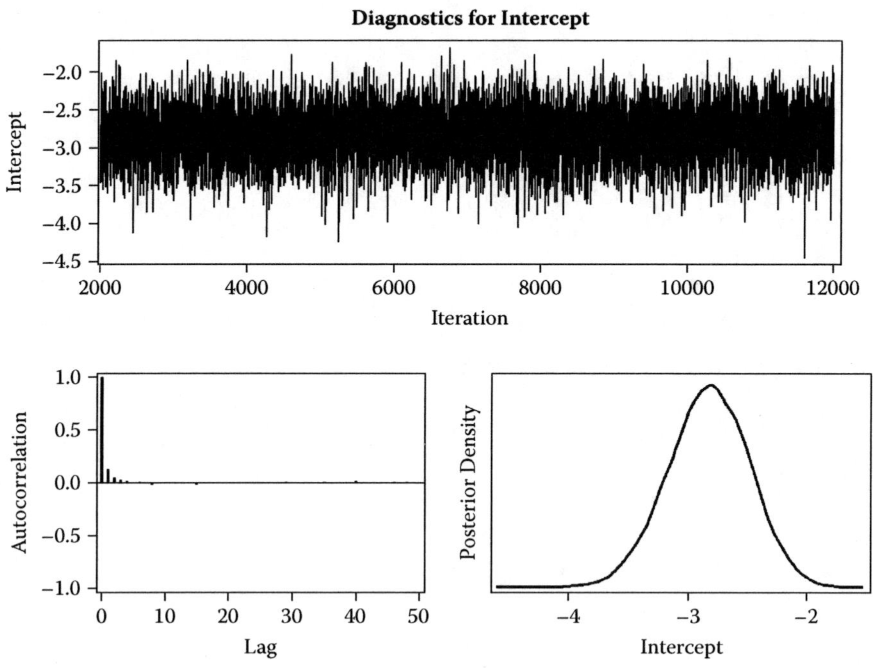

Diagnostics for Intercept
Intercept
-2.0
-2.5
-3.0
-3.5
-4.0
-4.5
2000 4000 6000 8000 10000 12000
Iteration
Autocorrelation
1.0
0.5
0.0
-0.5
-1.0
0 10 20 30 40 50
Lag
Posterior Density
-4 -3 -2
Intercept

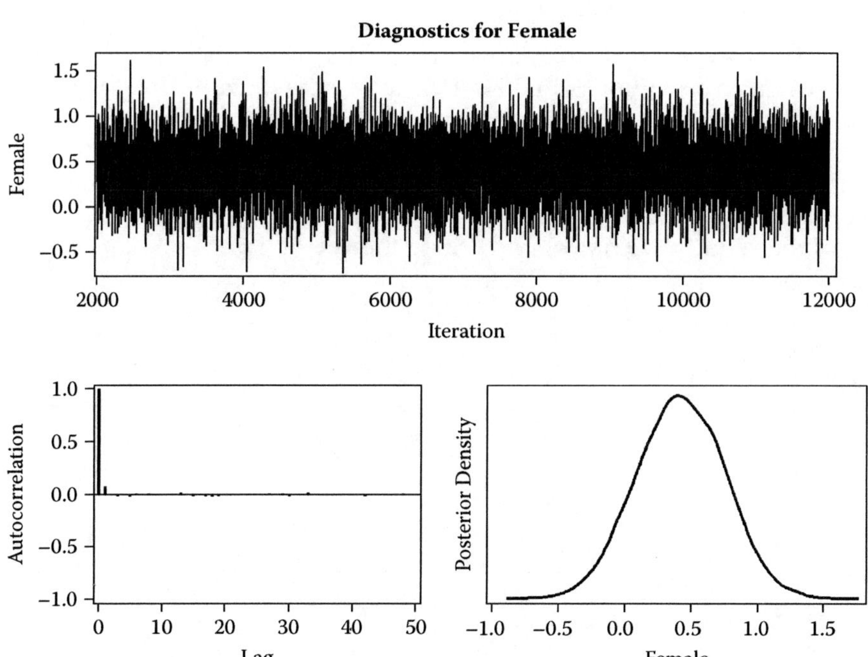

Diagnostics for Female
Female
1.5
1.0
0.5
0.0
-0.5
2000 4000 6000 8000 10000 12000
Iteration
Autocorrelation
1.0
0.5
0.0
-0.5
-1.0
0 10 20 30 40 50
Lag
Posterior Density
-1.0 -0.5 0.0 0.5 1.0 1.5
Female

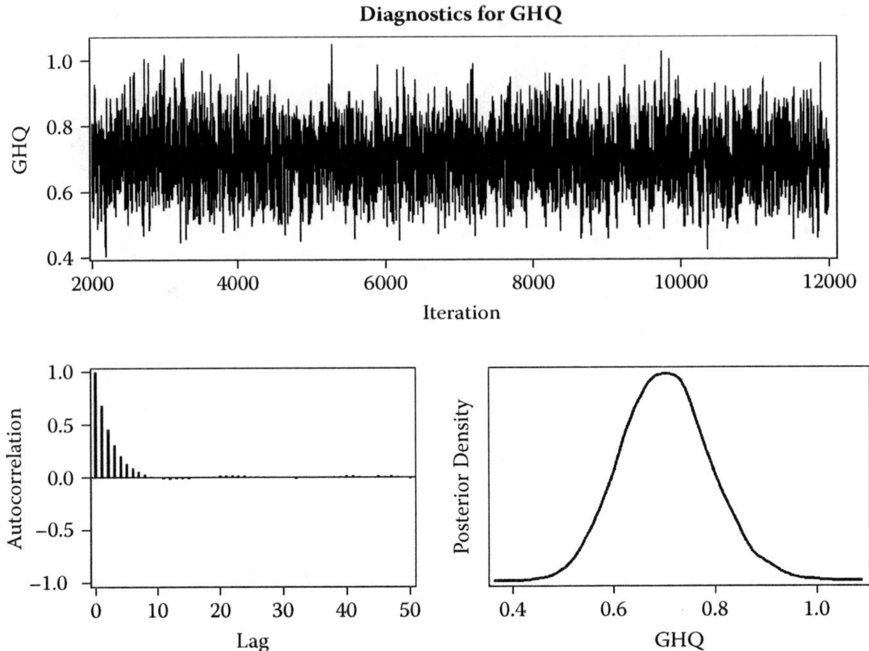

17.6.2 Cardiac Surgery in Babies

Our second example of the application of Bayesian statistics involves an example taken from Spiegelhalter et al. (1996). The data in this case are the number of cardiac surgery operations in babies performed in 12 UK hospitals and the number of operations in each hospital that resulted in the death of the baby. The data are shown in Table 17.3. (These data are comprehensively analysed in Spiegelhalter et al. 1996 using WinBUGS; here we replicate two of the WinBUGS analyses described there, using SAS.)

The data can be read in as follows:

```
data paeds;
input hospital $ operations deaths;
id=_n_;
datalines;
A  47  0
B 148 18
C 119  8
D 810 46
E 211  8
F 196 13
G 148  9
H 215 31
```

```
I 207 14
J  97  8
K 256 29
L 360 24
;
```

For a small data set like this, we can use instream data and separate the values with spaces so that list input can be used. We will need a numeric identifier later, so this is created using the automatic SAS variable _n_.

We will fit two Bayesian models to the data: one fixed effects and one involving random effects. In the fixed-effects model, we assume that the number of deaths in a particular hospital, r_i, has a binomial distribution with parameters (n_i, p_i) and that p_i has a beta distribution with $\alpha = \beta = 1$ as its prior. The required SAS code to fit the fixed-effects model is

```
proc mcmc data=paeds seed=123 nbi=1000 nmc=10000
stats(percent=2.5 97.5);
 array pr[12];
 parms pr1-pr12;
 prior pr1-pr12 ~ beta(1,1);
 model deaths~binomial(operations,pr[id]);
ods output postsummaries=fixsum geweke=fgew;
run;
```

Proc mcmc is a general purpose procedure for fitting Bayesian models via MCMC simulation. In version 9.3 of SAS, relatively few procedures have Bayesian capabilities. For models not covered by these proc mcmc may be used.

The proc statement used here, in addition to specifying the data set and the random seed, illustrates some of the most important options. The nbi option specifies the number of burn-in iterations and nmc the number of main iterations. The default for each of these is 1000. We increased the main iterations to 10,000 following the WinBUGS analysis. The stats option specifies the statistics to be calculated from the posterior samples (the mean is included by default).

TABLE 17.3

Cardiac Operations in 12 Hospitals

Hospital	A	B	C	D	E	F	G	H	I	J	K	L
No. of operations	47	148	119	810	211	196	148	215	207	97	256	360
No. of deaths	0	18	8	46	8	13	9	31	14	8	29	24

Source: Gilks, W. R., Richardson, S., and Spiegelhalter, D. J. (Eds.). 1996. *Markov Chain Monte Carlo in Practice*. London: Chapman and Hall.

A typical `proc mcmc` step will consist of one or more `parms` statements, `prior` statements, a `model` statement, and some programming statements. The `parms` statement declares the parameters to be estimated and, optionally, gives them starting values. The `prior` statement declares the prior distributions of the parameters and the model statement specifies the conditional distribution of the data given the parameters (i.e., the likelihood function). In this case, we also have an `array` statement, which is similar to the data step `array` statement. The form here is equivalent to `array pr[12] pr1-pr12;`.

In this model, we wish to estimate, for each of the 12 hospitals, the probability that an operation will result in death and the variables `pr1-pr12` are for the 12 probabilities. As they are to be estimated by the procedure, they are declared on the `parms` statement. Starting values could also be given on the `parms` statement, although this is usually not necessary. The `prior` statement declares them to have a beta distribution with both parameters of the distribution being one. On the `prior` statement, the tilde character (~) separates the list of parameters from their distribution. The `model` statement declares that the outcome (the numbers of deaths) follows a binomial distribution dependent on the number of operations and the hospital-specific probability of death. Using the `pr` array with the hospital `id` as the subscript ensures that separate probabilities are estimated. The `ods output` statement saves the posterior summaries and Geweke statistics to data sets for later use.

To begin, we will look at the Geweke tests that assess the convergence of the MCMC process; these are given in Table 17.4. A number of these are

TABLE 17.4

Geweke Statistics for the Fixed-Effects Model
Fitted to the Data on Cardiac Surgery in
Babies

Geweke Diagnostics		
Parameter	**z**	**Pr >|z|**
pr1	1.2268	0.2199
pr2	1.6058	0.1083
pr3	−0.5262	0.5988
pr4	−1.6383	0.1014
pr5	−2.5808	0.0099
pr6	−0.1475	0.8828
pr7	−0.0189	0.9849
pr8	−2.6682	0.0076
pr9	1.8439	0.0652
pr10	5.6501	<.0001
pr11	1.2075	0.2272
pr12	0.3037	0.7613

significant at the 5% level, indicating that the number of iterations allowed has not resulted in convergence.

We will now run the model again with 2000 burn-in iterations and then 20,000 main iterations. But before looking at the results, we will describe how to fit the random-effects model; here, we assume that the logits of the probability of death for the hospitals follow a normal distribution with a population mean and variance to be estimated. However, we want to have the results on the original scale, so we back-transform them within the proc mcmc step with some programming statements. The appropriate code is

```
proc mcmc data=paeds seed=123 nbi=2000 nmc=20000 monitor=(pr)
stats(percent=2.5 97.5);
   array pr[12];
   parms mu sigma;
   prior mu ~normal(0,v=100000);
   prior sigma~gamma(.001,is=.001);
   random bi ~ normal(mu,sd=sigma)  subject=id;
   pi=logistic(bi);
   model deaths~binomial(operations,p=pi);
   pr[id] = pi;
ods output postsummaries=randsum geweke=rgew;
run;
```

The first difference to note from the previous example is the use of the monitor= option on the proc statement. This lists the variables for which we want output to be generated. The default output includes the parameters estimated by the model, but only those and not, for instance, any additional variables calculated. The monitor option can be used to extend or restrict the output generated. Here we do both. We would like the back-transformed estimates, so the array that will contain these is listed in parentheses. The population mean, mu, and standard deviation, sigma, of the random effects are parameters to be estimated and thus are mentioned in the parms and prior statements. They would normally be included in the output, but as they are not mentioned in the monitor option, they are excluded.

The random statement specifies that random effects are to be estimated—one for each hospital (subject=id)—and that these are normally distributed with mean mu and standard deviation sigma. This generates 12 variables, bi1–bi12; to include these in the output, the random statement has its own monitor option. The following statement relates the probabilities to their logits (i.e., by the logistic function) and, after the model statement, the hospital-specific probability is stored in the appropriate element of the array.

To make comparison of the results for the two models simple, these results are combined into a single table as follows:

```
data results;
   set fixsum(in=in1) randsum;
   set fgew rgew;
```

```
  if in1 then Model='Fixed ';
     else Model='Random';
   mn=mean;
run;

proc tabulate data=results order=data f=8.3;
   class parameter model;
   var mn p25 p975 zscore pvalue;
   table parameter,
         model*((mn p25 p975 zscore )*sum=''
         pvalue*sum=''*f=pvalue6.3);
   label pvalue='p';
run;
```

For the four output data sets to be combined easily, they are all limited to the 12 probabilities, as ensured by the `monitor` option in the previous `mcmc` step. The mean is renamed to avoid confusion with the `mean` keyword in proc tabulate.

The results are shown in Table 17.5. Now the z-values of the Geweke statistics are all nonsignificant, indicating satisfactory convergence. The results from the fixed-effects and random-effects models can be compared graphically using the diagram shown in Figure 17.3.

To produce Figure 17.3, the summary statistics from the fixed- and random-effects models are combined as separate variables in a single observation per hospital, rather than as separate observations, as was done for the summary table. We also need the hospital identifier, so the original data file is combined with the summary statistics. This is done in a short data step with three `set` statements, although a single `merge` statement would have been equivalent. Where data sets are combined in this way without a common key, it is important to be sure that they are in the correct order and to check the results. The `rename` data set option is used to rename the summary variables.

The resulting data set is then sorted in order of the fixed-effect estimate. The sorted order is used for the y-value of the fixed effects and the random effects are to be plotted just below. The x0 variable is for plotting the hospital identifiers. In the `proc sgplot` step, separate `scatter` plot statements are used for the fixed and random estimates (means) and `highlow` plot statements to plot the intervals. The `xerrorlower` and `xerrorupper` options could have been used on the scatter statements, but the `highlow` plots produce a neater result. A third `scatter` statement is used to plot the hospital identifiers on the left. Finally, a reference line is added and the axes labelled:

```
data sumstats;
  set fixsum (rename=(mean=fmean p2_5=fp2_5 p97_5=fp97_5));
  set randsum(rename=(mean=rmean p2_5=rp2_5 p97_5=rp97_5));
  set paeds;
```

TABLE 17.5

Results for the Fixed- and Random-Effects Models Fitted to the Data on Cardiac Surgery on Babies, Using 2000 Burn-In Iterations and 20,000 Main Iterations

	Model									
	Fixed					Random				
	Mean	2.5%	97.5%	z	p	Mean	2.5%	97.5%	z	p
Parameter										
pr1	0.019	0.001	0.072	−0.510	0.610	0.052	0.017	0.093	−0.740	0.459
pr2	0.129	0.081	0.188	−1.414	0.157	0.103	0.067	0.148	−0.963	0.335
pr3	0.072	0.035	0.122	0.099	0.921	0.072	0.041	0.111	−0.278	0.781
pr4	0.058	0.043	0.075	−0.743	0.457	0.059	0.044	0.076	0.131	0.896
pr5	0.043	0.019	0.073	0.290	0.772	0.053	0.029	0.080	0.283	0.777
pr6	0.069	0.039	0.107	−0.251	0.802	0.068	0.041	0.098	1.605	0.109
pr7	0.067	0.033	0.114	0.860	0.390	0.066	0.039	0.101	0.471	0.638
pr8	0.148	0.105	0.201	0.677	0.498	0.122	0.082	0.173	−1.836	0.066
pr9	0.070	0.040	0.107	−0.688	0.491	0.070	0.045	0.101	0.902	0.367
pr10	0.095	0.045	0.159	0.276	0.782	0.078	0.042	0.123	0.800	0.423
pr11	0.116	0.080	0.158	1.669	0.095	0.102	0.071	0.140	−0.708	0.479
pr12	0.069	0.045	0.097	−1.626	0.104	0.068	0.048	0.092	−0.732	0.464

```
run;
proc sort data=sumstats out=sumstats;
  by fmean;
run;
data sumstats;
  set sumstats;
  fy=_n_;
  ry=fy-.3;
  x0=-.01;
run;
proc sgplot data=sumstats noautolegend;
  scatter x=fmean y=fy / markerattrs=(symbol=circlefilled);
  scatter x=rmean y=ry / markerattrs=(symbol=circle);
  highlow y=fy high=fp97_5 low=fp2_5 / lineattrs=(pattern=
  solid);
  highlow y=ry high=rp97_5 low=rp2_5;
  scatter x=x0 y=fy / markerchar=hospital;
  refline .073 / axis=x;
  yaxis display=(noticks novalues) label='Hospital';
  xaxis label='Proportion of deaths';
run;
```

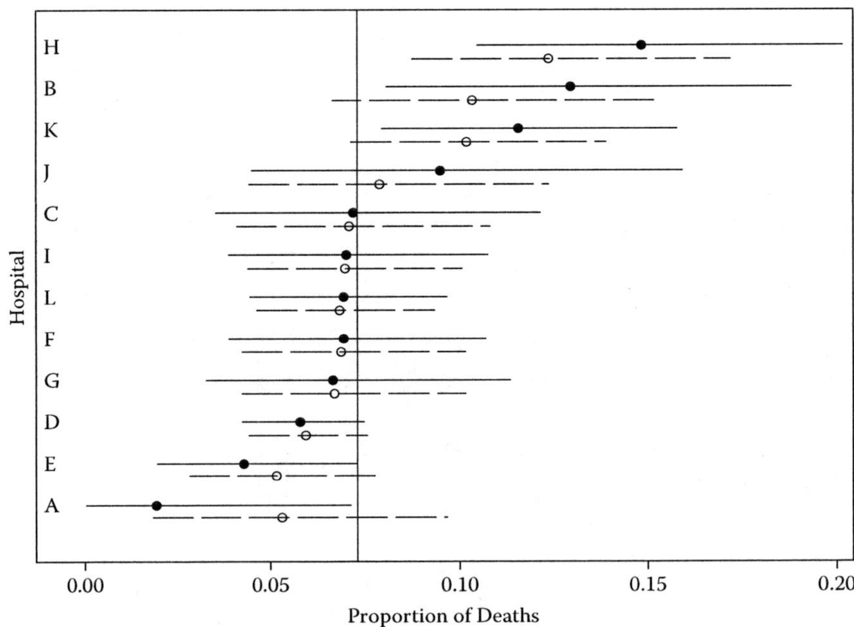

FIGURE 17.3

Comparison of estimates from fixed- and random-effects models (fixed effects are filled circles). (From Maxwell, S. E. and Delaney, H. D. 1990. *Designing Experiments and Analysing Data*. Belmont, CA: Wadsworth.)

The main point to note in Figure 17.3 is that the random effects tend to be closer to their overall mean than the fixed effects, particularly the more extreme ones. This 'shrinkage' effect is typical of random-effects models.

17.7 Summary

Hard-line opponents of Bayesian inference (the few that are left) reject the method because of the use of subjective prior distributions which, these opponents feel, have no place in scientific investigations in general and medical investigations in particular. And there are Bayesians who think that the only defence of using non-Bayesian methods is incompetence. But a more sensible, pragmatic view for the applied statistician is to avoid the extremes of both the hard-line frequentist and the overly enthusiastic Bayesian and focus on scientific modelling where there are pros and cons for both schools of thought.

Amongst the pros for the Bayesian approach are that it can incorporate prior knowledge (a con, of course, from the frequentist perspective), it can estimate much more complex models than can a frequentist approach, HPD intervals are more intuitive than CIs, and it has fewer problems when dealing with data containing missing data. Some of the cons are that Bayesian methods are perceived as more difficult to understand, it is computationally intensive, demonstrating the proper convergence of the MCMC sampling process is not always easy, and, lastly, the use of chosen prior distributions often needs to be defended. But in the twenty-first century, the use of Bayesian statistics has become widespread and even routine (almost); a conservative and (rightly) cautious body such as the US Food and Drug Administration (FDA) now welcomes Bayesian analysis of clinical trials. (Food and Drug Administration 2010) and is reported to have said that 'Bayesian statistical methods could trim costs and boost efficiency'.

In this chapter we have been able only to give a brief account of a large and growing area; readers are referred to Carlin and Louis (2008) and Hoff (2009) for a full account of Bayesian methods.

18

Missing Values

18.1 Introduction

Any well-designed study in medicine aims to draw a representative sample from the study population by following a sampling plan and a detailed protocol. But even the best laid plans can go a little wrong and, at the end of the study, some of the data that should have been collected are missing. In a sample survey, for example, some individuals may have refused to respond or have not been contactable, or some of the participants may have failed to answer particular items in a questionnaire. As we have already seen in Chapter 13, in longitudinal studies, data are often missing because subjects drop out prior to the end of the study.

Missing data can sometimes arise by design. For example, suppose one objective in a study of obesity is to estimate the distribution of a measure Y_1 of body fat in the population and correlate it with other factors. As Y_1 is expensive to measure, it can only be obtained for a limited sample, but a crude proxy measure, Y_2 (for example, body mass index), can be obtained for a much larger sample. A useful design is to measure Y_2 and a number of covariates for a large sample and Y_1, Y_2, and the same covariates for a smaller subsample. The subsample allows predictions of the missing values of Y_1 to be generated for the larger sample using one or other of the methods we shall discuss later in the chapter, thus yielding more efficient estimates than are possible from the subsample alone (this example is taken from Little 2005).

Ignoring the situation when missing data are deliberate by design, the most important approach to the potential problems that missing data can cause is for the investigator to do his or her very best to avoid missing values in the first case. But despite the very best efforts of the investigator, some of the intended data will often be missing after data collection. In any research study, the intent of any analysis is to make valid inferences regarding a population of interest. Missing data threaten this goal if they are missing in a manner which makes the sample different from the population from which it was drawn—that is, if the missing data create a *biased sample*. Therefore, it is important to respond to a missing data problem in a manner which, as far as possible, avoids this problem. It needs to be understood that, once data are missing, it is impossible not to treat them because *any* subsequent procedure applied to the data set represents a response in some form to the missing data problem.

In this chapter, a number of ways of dealing with missing values will be discussed; however, as pointed out by Little (2005), a basic (but often hidden) assumption with all these methods is that 'missingness' of a particular value hides a 'true' underlying value that is meaningful for analysis. This apparently obvious point is not always the case, however. For example, consider a longitudinal analysis of CD4 counts in a clinical trial with patients suffering from AIDS. For patients who leave the study because they move to a different location, it makes sense to consider the CD4 counts that would have been recorded had they remained in the study. For subjects who die during the course of the study, it is less clear whether it is reasonable to consider CD4 counts after time of death as missing values. In such a case, it may be preferable to treat death as a primary outcome and restrict analysis of CD4 counts to patients who are alive.

18.2 Patterns of Missing Data

It is useful at the outset to distinguish different *patterns* of missing data. The simplest way to do this is first to introduce an nxp matrix **Y** without missing values, the ith row of which, $\mathbf{y}_i' = [y_{i1}, y_{i2}, \ldots, y_{ip}]$, contains the values of all p variables for the ith subject and n is the number of subjects in the study. With missing values, the pattern is defined by the missing-data indicator matrix, **M**, which is also nxp and is such that $m_{ij} = 1$ if y_{ij} is missing and $m_{ij} = 0$ if y_{ij} is present. (The matrix **M** is sometimes called the *shadow matrix*; see Cook and Swayne 2007.)

One type of pattern is *univariate* nonresponse, in which missingness is confined to a single variable. Another type of pattern is *monotone* missing data, where the variables can be arranged so that $y_{ij+1}, y_{ij+2}, \ldots y_{ip}$ are missing for all subjects where y_{ij} is missing for all $j = 1, 2, \ldots p - 1$. This pattern arises commonly in longitudinal data subject to attrition where, once a subject drops, out no more data are observed for the subject. Some methods for handling missing data apply to any pattern, whereas others assume a special pattern.

18.3 Missing Data Mechanisms

The missing-data mechanism concerns the reasons why values are missing, in particular whether these reasons relate to recorded (nonmissing) values for a subject. A useful classification of mechanisms was first introduced by Rubin (1976). The type of mechanism involved has implications for which approaches to analysis are suitable and which are not. Rubin's suggested classification involves three types of missing-data mechanism: missing completely at random, missing at random, and nonignorable.

Missing completely at random (MCAR). The missing-data mechanism when missingness does not depend on the values of the data values in $\mathbf{Y}$, missing or observed (i.e., $f(\mathbf{M}|\mathbf{Y},\phi) = f(\mathbf{M}|\phi)$, where $f(\mathbf{M}|\mathbf{Y},\phi)$ is the conditional distribution of $\mathbf{M}$ given $\mathbf{Y}$ and ϕ is a vector of unknown parameters. Note that this assumption does not mean that the pattern itself is random, but only that missingness does not depend on either observed or unobserved data values. Consequently, the observed (nonmissing) values effectively constitute a simple random sample of the values for all subjects.

The classification of missing values as MCAR implies that Pr(missing |observed,unobserved) = Pr(missing). Possible examples include missing laboratory measurements because of a dropped test tube (if it was not dropped because of the knowledge of any measurement), the accidental death of a participant in a study, or a participant moving to another area. Intermittent missing values in a longitudinal data set, whereby a patient misses a clinic visit for transitory reasons ('went shopping instead' or the like) can reasonably be assumed to be MCAR. When data are MCAR, missing values are no different from nonmissing values in terms of the analysis to be performed, and the only real penalty in failing to account for the missing data is loss of power. But MCAR is a strong assumption because missing *does* usually depend on at least the observed/recorded values.

Missing at random (MAR). The missing at random missing-value mechanism occurs when the missingness depends only on observed values, $\mathbf{Y}_{obs}$, and not on values that are missing, $\mathbf{Y}_{miss}$. That is, $f(\mathbf{M}|\mathbf{Y},\phi) = f(\mathbf{M}|\mathbf{Y}_{obs},\phi)$, for all $\mathbf{Y}_{miss},\phi$. Here, missingness depends only on the observed data; the distribution of future values for a subject who drops out at a particular time is the same as the distribution of the future values of a subject who remains in at that time, if they have the same covariates and the same past history of outcome up to and including the specific time point. In classifying missing values as MAR, we imply that Pr(missing|observed,unobserved) = Pr(missing|observed). This type of missing value is also called *ignorable* because conclusions based on likelihood methods are not affected by MAR data.

Murray and Findlay (1988) provide an example of this type of missing value from a study of hypertensive drugs in which the outcome measure was diastolic blood pressure. The protocol of the study specified that a participant was to be removed from the study when his or her blood pressure got too high. Here, blood pressure at the time of dropout was observed before the participant dropped out, so although the missing-data mechanism is not MCAR because it depends on the values of blood pressure, it *is* MAR, because missingness depends only on the observed part of the data.

A further example of a MAR mechanism provided by Heitjan (1997) involves a study in which the response measure is body mass index (BMI). Suppose that the measure is missing because subjects who had high body mass index values at earlier visits avoided being measured at later visits out of embarrassment, regardless of whether they had gained or lost weight in the intervening period. The missing values here are MAR but *not* MCAR; consequently, methods applied to the data that assumed the latter might give misleading results (see later discussion). In this case, missing data depend on known values and thus are described fully by variables observed in the data set. Accounting for the values which 'cause' the missing data will produce unbiased results in an analysis.

Nonignorable (sometimes referred to as *informative*). The final type of dropout mechanism is one where the missingness depends on the unrecorded missing values. Observations are likely to be missing when the outcome values that would have been observed had the patient not dropped out are systematically higher or lower than usual (corresponding perhaps to the patient's condition becoming worse or improving). An example is a participant dropping out of a longitudinal study when his or her blood pressure became very high and this value was not observed, or when pain becomes intolerable and the associated pain value is not recorded. And in the BMI example, if subjects were more likely to avoid being measured if they had put on extra weight since the last visit, then the data are nonignorably missing.

Dealing with data containing missing values that result from this type of missing-data mechanism is difficult. The correct analyses for such data must estimate the dependence of the missingness probability on the missing values. Models and software that attempt this are available (see, for example, Diggle and Kenward 1994) but their use is not routine. In addition, it must be remembered that the associated parameter estimates can be unreliable.

18.4 Exploring Missingness

Before considering how to deal with the missing value problem, it is usually helpful to explore the distribution of missing values and to try to determine whether they appear to occur randomly or whether there is any indication that there is some relationship between the occurrence of missing values on one variable and the recorded values for some other variable or variables. In this section, we shall illustrate some possible approaches to exploring missingness using the data shown in Table 18.1. These data, which relate to air

TABLE 18.1

Air Pollution in 41 US Cities

City	SO$_2$	Temp	Manu	Pop	Wind	Precip	Days
Phoenix	10	70.3	213	582	6	7.05	36
Little Rock	13	61.0	91	132		48.52	
San Francisco		56.7	453	716	8.7	20.66	67
Denver	17	51.9	454	515	9	12.95	86
Hartford	56	49.1	412	158		43.37	127
Wilmington	36	54.0		80		40.25	114
Washington	29	57.3	434	757	9.3	38.89	111
Jacksonville	14	68.4	136	529	8.8	54.47	116
Miami	10	75.5	207	335	9.0	59.8	128
Atlanta	24	61.5	368	497	9.1	48.34	115
Chicago	110	50.6	3344	3369	10.4	34.44	122
Indianapolis	28	52.3	361	746	9.7	38.74	121
Des Moines		49	104	201		30.85	
Wichita		56.6		277	12.7	30.58	82
Louisville	30	55.6	291	593	8.3	43.11	123
New Orleans	9	68.3	204	361	8.4	56.77	113
Baltimore	47	55	625	905	9.6	41.31	111
Detroit	35	49.9	1064	1513	10.1	30.96	129
Minneapolis	29	43.5	699	744	10.6	25.94	137
Kansas			381	507	10	37	99
St. Louis	56	55.9	775	622	9.5	35.89	105
Omaha	14	51.5	181	347	10.9	30.18	
Albuquerque	11	56.8	46	244	8.9	7.77	
Albany	46	47.6	44	116		33.36	
Buffalo	11	47.1		463	12.4	36.11	166
Cincinnati		54	462	453	7.1	39.04	132
Cleveland	65	49.7	1007	751	10.9	34.99	155
Columbus	26	51.5	266	540	8.6	37.01	134
Philadelphia	69	54.6	1692	1950	9.6	39.93	115
Pittsburgh	61	50.4	347	520	9.4	36.22	147
Providence		50	343	179	.	42.75	125
Memphis	10	61.6	337	624	9.2	49.1	105
Nashville	18	59.4	275	448	7.9	46	119
Dallas	9	66.2	641	844	10.9	35.94	78
Houston	10	68.9	721	1233	10.8	48.19	103
Salt Lake City	28	51	137	176		15.17	89
Norfolk	31	59.3	96	308	10.6	44.68	116
Richmond	26	57.8	197	299	7.6	42.59	115
Seattle	29	51.1	379	531	9.4	38.79	164

(Continued)

TABLE 18.1 (*Continued*)

Air Pollution in 41 US Cities

City	SO$_2$	Temp	Manu	Pop	Wind	Precip	Days
Charleston	31	55.2	35	71		40.75	
Milwaukee	16	45.7	569	717	11.8	29.07	123

Notes: SO$_2$: sulphur dioxide of air in micrograms per cubic metre; temp: average annual temperature in Fahrenheit; manu: number of manufacturing enterprises employing 20 or more workers; pop: population size in thousands; wind: average annual wind speed in miles per hour; precip: average annual precipitation in inches; days: average number of days with precipitation per year.

pollution in 41 US cities, are based on the complete data set given in Sokal and Rohlf (1981) and in Hand et al. (1994); a number of the observed values have been set to missing.

We begin by constructing the shadow matrix for the data using the following SAS code:

```
data usair;
  infile 'c:\amsus\data\usairmiss.dat' expandtabs;
  input city $16. so2 Temp Manu Pop Wind Precip Days;
run;

data usair;
  set usair;
  array xs {*} So2 Temp Manu Pop Wind Precip Days;
  array mx {*} m_so2 m_Temp m_Manu m_Pop m_Wind m_Precip
  m_Days;
  do i=1 to 7;
   if xs{i}=. then mx{i}=1;
             else mx{i}=0;
  end;
  nmvars=nmiss(of so2--days);
run;
proc print data=usair noobs;
 var city m_so2--m_days;
run;
```

The data are initially read in using list input, but with the format modified for `city`, as some of the city names are longer than the default of eight characters and can contain spaces. A second data step creates a set of seven indicator variables corresponding to the seven measured variables, which are assigned the value one if the measured variable is missing and zero if it is not. This is done with two arrays and an iterative do loop. The second `array` statement has the effect of creating the named variables. The `nmiss` function is also used to determine how many of the seven measured variables are missing for each city.

The resulting shadow matrix is shown in Table 18.2. In this binary matrix, one represents a missing value and zero a recorded value. It is easier to see

TABLE 18.2

Shadow Matrix for Air Pollution Data

City	m_so2	m_Temp	m_Manu	m_Pop	m_Wind	m_Precip	m_Days
Phoenix	0	0	0	0	0	0	0
Little Rock	0	0	0	0	1	0	1
San Francisco	1	0	0	0	0	0	0
Denver	0	0	0	0	0	0	0
Hartford	0	0	0	0	1	0	0
Wilmington	0	0	1	0	1	0	0
Washington	0	0	0	0	0	0	0
Jacksonville	0	0	0	0	0	0	0
Miami	0	0	0	0	0	0	0
Atlanta	0	0	0	0	0	0	0
Chicago	0	0	0	0	0	0	0
Indianapolis	0	0	0	0	0	0	0
Des Moines	1	0	0	0	1	0	1
Wichita	1	0	1	0	0	0	0
Louisville	0	0	0	0	0	0	0
New Orleans	0	0	0	0	0	0	0
Baltimore	0	0	0	0	0	0	0
Detroit	0	0	0	0	0	0	0
Minneapolis	0	0	0	0	0	0	0
Kansas	1	1	0	0	0	0	0
St. Louis	0	0	0	0	0	0	0
Omaha	0	0	0	0	0	0	1
Albuquerque	0	0	0	0	0	0	1
Albany	0	0	0	0	1	0	1
Buffalo	0	0	1	0	0	0	0
Cincinnati	1	0	0	0	0	0	0
Cleveland	0	0	0	0	0	0	0
Columbus	0	0	0	0	0	0	0
Philadelphia	0	0	0	0	0	0	0
Pittsburgh	0	0	0	0	0	0	0
Providence	1	0	0	0	1	0	0
Memphis	0	0	0	0	0	0	0
Nashville	0	0	0	0	0	0	0
Dallas	0	0	0	0	0	0	0
Houston	0	0	0	0	0	0	0
Salt Lake City	0	0	0	0	1	0	0
Norfolk	0	0	0	0	0	0	0
Richmond	0	0	0	0	0	0	0
Seattle	0	0	0	0	0	0	0
Charleston	0	0	0	0	1	0	1
Milwaukee	0	0	0	0	0	0	0

the positions of the missing values in this table and to consider their distribution apart from the data values.

In addition to the means of the observed values of each variable and the number of observations on which each mean is based, proc means can give the number of missing values. When specific statistics are requested on the proc means statement, only those will be output so that even the statistics which would otherwise be produced need to be specified explicitly, if required. We also use the maxdec option to limit the number of decimal places for the output:

```
proc means data=usair n nmiss mean std min max maxdec=2;
 var so2 -- Days;
run;
```

The resulting means, etc. are shown in Table 18.3. We shall return to these values later.

A variation on the shadow matrix can be produced directly from proc mi as follows:

```
proc mi data=usair nimpute=0;
var so2 -- Days;
run;
```

The resulting table is shown in Table 18.4. Here the frequencies of each pattern of missing values are given; for example, there are 26 cities with no missing value, 2 cities where days is missing, etc.

In longitudinal data where dropout occurs, Carpenter, Pocock, and Lamm (2002) suggest a relatively simple plot for assessing whether dropout is not completely at random. Values of the response variable for the subjects in each treatment group are plotted at each time point (including prerandomisation), differentiating those who do and those who do not attend their next scheduled visit on the plot between two categories

TABLE 18.3

Means of the Observed Values of the Data in Table 18.1

Variable	N	N Miss	Mean	Std Dev	Minimum	Maximum
SO$_2$	35	6	30.40	22.13	9.00	110.00
Temp	40	1	55.80	7.32	43.50	75.50
Manu	38	3	483.97	579.31	35.00	3344.00
Pop	41	0	608.61	579.11	71.00	3369.00
Wind	33	8	9.55	1.43	6.00	12.70
Precip	41	0	36.77	11.77	7.05	59.80
Days	35	6	115.09	25.87	36.00	166.00

TABLE 18.4

Missing Data Patterns

Group	SO$_2$	Temp	Manu	Pop	Wind	Precip	Days	Freq	Percent
1	X	X	X	X	X	X	X	26	63.41
2	X	X	X	X	X	X		2	4.88
3	X	X	X	X		X	X	2	4.88
4	X	X	X	X		X		3	7.32
5	X	X		X	X	X	X	1	2.44
6	X	X		X		X	X	1	2.44
7		X	X	X	X	X	X	2	4.88
8		X	X	X		X	X	1	2.44
9		X	X	X		X		1	2.44
10		X		X	X	X	X	1	2.44
11			X	X	X	X	X	1	2.44

of subject. Any clear difference between the distributions of values for 'attenders' and 'nonattenders' indicates that the missingness in the data is not MCAR. This type of plot can be illustrated on the 'Beat the Blues' data given in Chapter 13 (see Table 13.6). The following SAS code constructs the required plot:

```
data btb   (keep=sub--treatment BDIpre--BDI8m)
     btbl (keep=sub--treatment bdi time);
 infile 'c:\amsus\data\btb.dat' missover;
  array bdis {*} BDIpre BDI2m BDI3m BDI5m BDI8m;
  array t {*} t1-t5 (0 2 3 5 8);
  input sub drug$ Duration$ Treatment$ @;
 do i=1 to 5;
   input bdi @;
   bdis{i}=bdi;
   time=t{i}; * three lines added below;
   if time<8 and bdis{i+1}~=. then next=1;
   else next=0;
   nexttime=time-.1+next*.2;
   if bdi~=. then output btbl;
 end;
 output btb;
run;
proc sgpanel data=btbl;
   panelby treatment / rows=2 spacing=10;
   scatter y=bdi x=nexttime / group=next;
   colaxis label='time';
   where time<8;
run;
```

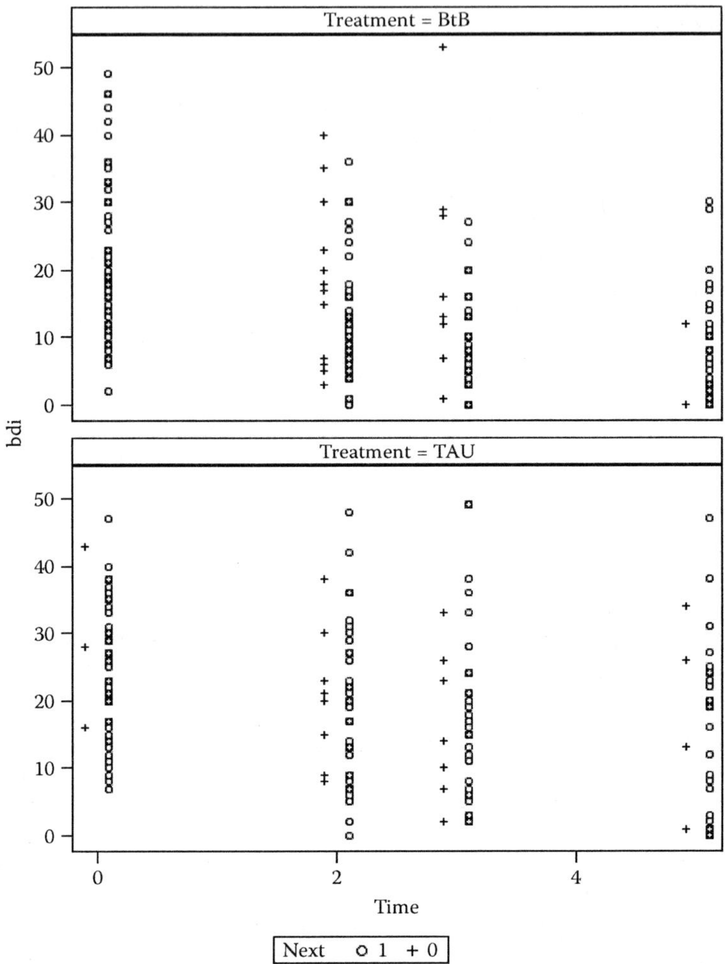

FIGURE 18.1
Distribution of BDI values for patients who do (circles) and do not (pluses) attend the next scheduled visit.

The data are read in as described in Chapter 13, with three lines added to calculate two new variables: `next` with values 1 or 0 to indicate whether the patient did or did not attend the following time point and `nexttime` to allow the depression scores to be plotted separately.

The resulting plot is shown in Figure 18.1. Comparing the distribution of BDI values for patients who do (circles) and do not (pluses) attend the next scheduled visit, there is no apparent difference. Thus, it is probably reasonable to assume dropout is completely random, which has implications for which types of analyses are appropriate for these data.

18.5 Dealing with Missing Values

There are three major approaches to dealing with missing values:

- Discard incomplete cases and analyse the remainder.
- Impute or fill in missing values and then analyse the filled-in data.
- Analyse the incomplete data by a method that does not require a complete (that is, rectangular) data set. This is the approach used when using maximum likelihood to estimate parameters in longitudinal data models as described in Chapter 14; this leads to valid inferences on the parameters in the model being applied when the missing-data mechanism is MAR.

In this chapter, the emphasis will be on imputation, but before describing the methods available, we need to say a little about the first approach in the preceding list.

A common approach to dealing with missing data in a study is *complete-case analysis,* where incomplete cases (cases with any missing value) are discarded and standard analysis methods applied to the remaining complete cases. In many statistical packages, this is the default approach. When the missing data are MCAR, the complete cases are a random subsample of the original sample and complete-case analysis provides valid inferences, but when there is a substantial proportion of incomplete cases, the method can be very inefficient and lead to a reduction of statistical power. If the missing data are not MCAR, then the complete cases are a biased sample and complete-case analysis can be misleading to a degree depending on the amount of missing data and the size of the departure from MCAR.

A simple alternative to complete-case analysis that is often used is *available-case analysis.* This is a method that uses all the cases available for estimating each quantity of interest. For example, all the cases that have recorded value for a pair of variables would be used to estimate the correlation between the variables. Clearly, available-case analysis makes more use of the available information in the data than the complete-case approach. But the method is not problem free; in our example, the sample base changes from correlation to correlation, and there is no guarantee that the resulting correlation matrix is positive definite. In addition, the available-case approach creates potential problems when the missing-data mechanism is not MCAR.

The possible serious drawbacks of using listwise deletion or complete case analysis are discussed in Schafer and Graham (2002).

18.6 Imputing Missing Values

An ancient (almost) and still often used technique for handling missing data is to impute (i.e., fill in) some value for each missing data point. This results in a complete data set so that standard methods of analysis can be applied. Perhaps the most frequently used method for obtaining the 'fill-in value' is to use the relevant sample mean obtained from the observed data. This is easy to apply but is poor because it is well known to lead, in general, to biased inferences. In addition, because the same value is being substituted for each missing observation, this approach artificially reduces the variance of the variable in question and also diminishes relationships with other variables.

An improvement is conditional mean imputation, in which each missing value is replaced by an estimate of its conditional mean given the values of the nonmissing values in the data, found via the prediction equation that results from the regression on the recorded values of a variable on the recorded values of the other variables in the data set. Although conditional mean imputation yields best predictions of the missing values in the sense of mean squared error, it leads to distorted estimates of quantities that are not linear in the data—for example, percentiles, variances, and correlations.

Other improved methods are available, but single imputation (i.e., imputing one value for each missing datum by whatever method) fails to satisfy statistical objectives concerning the validity of resulting inferences based on the filled-in data. Because a single imputed value cannot reflect any of the uncertainty about the true underlying value, analyses that treat imputed values just like observed values systematically underestimate uncertainty (see Barnard, Rubin, and Schenker 2005). Consequently, imputing a single value for each missing datum and then analysing the filled-in data using standard techniques for complete data will result in standard error estimates that are too small, confidence intervals that fail to attain their nominal coverage, and p-values that are too significant.

The problems of single imputation are largely overcome by the use of multiple imputation, which is an approach to the missing values problem that allows the investigator to obtain valid assessments of uncertainty. The basic idea of multiple imputation is to impute two or more times for the missing data using independent draws of the missing values from a distribution that is appropriate under assumptions made about the data and the missing-data mechanism. The resulting multiple data sets are then each analysed using the standard method appropriate for answering the questions of interest about the data. The analyses are then combined in a simple way that reflects the extra uncertainty due to having imputed rather than all the planned data being recorded. Multiple imputations can be created under a number of different models and details are given in Rubin and Schenker (1991). But the theoretical motivation for multiple imputation is Bayesian and the following brief account follows Barnard et al. (2005).

We begin by letting Q be the population quantity of interest. If all the data have been observed, then estimates of and inferences for Q would have been based on the complete-data posterior density $p(Q|\mathbf{Y}_{obs},\mathbf{Y}_{miss})$. But because $\mathbf{Y}_{miss}$ is not observed, inferences, etc. have to be based on the actual posterior density, $p(Q|\mathbf{Y}_{obs})$, which can be written as

$$p(Q\,|\,\mathbf{Y}_{obs}) = \int p(Q\,|\,\mathbf{Y}_{obs},\,\mathbf{Y}_{miss})p(\mathbf{Y}_{miss}\,|\,\mathbf{Y}_{obs})d\mathbf{Y}_{miss} \qquad (18.1)$$

The preceding equation shows that the actual posterior density of Q can be obtained by averaging the complete posterior density over the posterior predictive distribution of $\mathbf{Y}_{miss}$. In principle, multiple imputations are repeated independent draws from $p(Q|\mathbf{Y}_{miss},\mathbf{Y}_{obs})$. Thus, multiple imputation allows approximating (18.1) by separately analysing each data set completed by imputation and then combining the results of the separate analyses. Schafer (1997, Chapter 30) has developed algorithms that use the MCMC approach and allow multiple imputation when there are arbitrary patterns of missing data and the missing data mechanism is ignorable (i.e., MCAR or MAR).

The question of how many imputations (m) is an obvious one that needs to be considered. In most cases, a value for m between 3 and 10 is suggested. Intuitively, this seems rather small, but Rubin (1987) shows that the efficiency of an estimate based on m imputations is approximately $\left(1+\dfrac{\gamma}{m}\right)^{-1}$, where γ is the rate of missing information for the quantity being estimated. The efficiencies achieved for various values of m and rates of missing information are shown here:

	γ				
m	0.1	0.3	0.5	0.7	0.9
3	97	91	86	81	77
5	98	94	91	88	85
10	99	97	95	93	92
20	100	99	98	97	96

Unless the rate of missing information is very high, there is, in most cases, little advantage to producing and analysing more than a few imputed data sets. White, Royston, and Wood (2011) give a conservative rule of thumb that m should be set equal to the percentage of incomplete cases based on the argument that repeat analyses yield the same result.

18.7 Analysing Multiply Imputed Data

From the analysis of each data set, we need to look at the estimates of the quantity of interest and the standard errors of the estimates. We let $\hat{Q}_i$ be the estimate from the ith data set and S_i its corresponding standard error. The combined estimate of the quantity of interest is

$$\bar{Q} = \frac{1}{m} \sum_{i=1}^{m} \hat{Q}_i \qquad (18.2)$$

To find the combined standard error involves first calculating the *within-imputation variance*, $\bar{S}$

$$\bar{S} = \frac{1}{m} \sum_{i=1}^{m} S_i \qquad (18.3)$$

followed by the between-imputation variance, B

$$B = \frac{1}{m-1} \sum_{i=1}^{m} (\hat{Q}_i - \bar{Q})^2 \qquad (18.4)$$

The required total variance can now be found from

$$T = \bar{S} + \left(1 + \frac{1}{m}\right) B \qquad (18.5)$$

This total variance is made up of two components; the first, which preserves the natural variability, $\bar{S}$, is simply the average of the variance estimates for each imputed data set and is analogous to the variance that would be suitable if we did not need to account for missing data. The second component, B, estimates uncertainty caused by missing data by measuring how the point estimates vary from data set to data set.

The overall standard error is simply the square root of T. Significance test for Q and confidence intervals are found in the usual way from a Student's t-distribution with degrees of freedom given by

$$df = (m-1)\left(1 + \frac{m\bar{S}}{(m^{-1}+1)B}\right)^2 \qquad (18.6)$$

See Schafer (1997) for more details.

18.8 Some Examples of the Application of Multiple Imputation

There are a number of variations of multiple imputation available in SAS; the method of choice largely depends on the type of missing data patterns. For example, for monotone missing data, a parametric regression method that assumes multivariate normality is used. But in the examples in this section, we shall use the MCMC approach as it can be applied to data with an arbitrary pattern of missing values.

18.8.1 Air Pollution in US Cities

As a simple example of the application of multiple imputation, we shall determine the average sulphur dioxide level for the data in Table 18.1. We shall use 10 imputations. The required SAS code to generate the required imputations, find the estimate of the mean, and the variance of this estimate as given in (18.4) is as follows:

```
proc mi data=usair out=usimp nimpute=10 minimum=0 seed=123
noprint;
 var so2 -- Days;
 mcmc;
run;
proc means data=usimp;
 var so2;
 by _imputation_;
 output out=mimpout mean=so2 stderr=sso2;
run;
proc mianalyze data=mimpout edf=40;
   modeleffects so2;
   stderr sso2;
run;
```

In addition to describing the pattern of missing data, as we saw previously, proc mi creates multiply imputed data sets. This example illustrates some of the most commonly used options. The out option names the data set that contains the imputed data. This data set also contains the variable _imputation_, which identifies the separate imputations. The nimpute option specifies the number of imputations to be made. With nimpute=0, proc mi can be used simply to describe the pattern of missing values in the data, as in the earlier example. The minimum option sets a minimum for the imputed values. In the case of the air pollution data, negative values for any of the variables would not be possible, so we have set a minimum value of zero for all of them. If we wished to set a different minimum for each variable, we would list these on the minimum option in the same order as the corresponding variables are listed on the var statement.

To impose minima for some variables and not others, a dot is included in the list for variables that are not to be restricted. Maximum values could also be imposed on the imputations in the same way with the `maximum` option. The `seed` option to set the random number seed is useful if we want the results to be reproducible. As we are now only interested in the imputed data, the `noprint` option is used to suppress the output. The MCMC method for arbitrary missing data patterns is invoked by including the `mcmc` statement.

The `proc means` step calculates the mean `so2` value and its standard error for each imputation and outputs these to a data set, `mimpout`. Then, `proc mianalyze` is used to apply Rubin's rules in order to combine the results from the separate imputations. The `edf` option is used to specify the degrees of freedom ($N-1$ in this case). The effects to be summarised are specified with the `modeleffects` statement, which is the mean `so2` value, also named `so2`, and the `stderr` statement specifies the variable that contains its standard error.

The means of sulphur dioxide concentration for each of the 10 imputed data sets are shown in Table 18.5 and the relevant variances, etc. are given in Table 18.6. Here the mean from the observed values, 30.40, is quite similar to the mean from using multiple imputation, 31.13. The relative increase in variance is simply the proportion of the total variance in the imputed data that is due to the between-imputation variance—namely, in this example, .44/11.6, about 4%; this is the proportion of the uncertainty due to the missing data.

The main interest in the air pollution data is using multiple regression to find which of the six explanatory variables are predictive of sulphur dioxide concentration. The SAS code for using multiple regression with multiple imputation of the missing values is as follows:

```
proc reg data=usimp outest=rout covout noprint;
   model so2=Temp -- Days;
   by _imputation_;
run;

proc mianalyze data=rout edf=34;
 modeleffects intercept Temp Manu Pop Wind Precip Days;
run;
```

`Proc reg` is used to analyse the imputed data set. The `outest` option saves the parameter estimates to the `rout` data set and the `covout` option includes the covariance matrix of the parameter estimates in the same data set. The printed output is not needed, so the `noprint` option is included. The `by` statement ensures that each imputation is analysed separately.

`Proc mianalyze` reads the parameter estimates and their covariance matrix from the `rout` data set, applies Rubin's rules, and outputs the results for those effects listed on the `modeleffects` statement. If any of the effects were categorical, they would also need to be listed on a `class` statement. In this case, the `edf` option on the proc statement specifies the degrees of freedom as 34—that is, $N = 41$ minus the seven effects. The results are shown in Table 18.7.

TABLE 18.5

Mean Sulphur Dioxide Values for 10 Imputed Samples

Analysis Variable: SO$_2$				
Imputation Number	N obs	Mean	Minimum	Maximum
1	41	31.69	9.00	110.00
2	41	32.31	9.00	110.00
3	41	31.30	9.00	110.00
4	41	30.40	9.00	110.00
5	41	30.47	9.00	110.00
6	41	30.74	9.00	110.00
7	41	30.43	3.13	110.00
8	41	31.69	9.00	110.00
9	41	30.76	9.00	110.00
10	41	31.55	9.00	110.00

TABLE 18.6

Variance Information for Mean Sulphur Dioxide Concentration Calculated from 10 Imputed Samples

The MIANALYZE Procedure	
Model Information	
Data Set	WORK.MIMPOUT
Number of Imputations	10

Variance Information				
		Variance		
Parameter	Between	Within	Total	DF
SO$_2$	0.440735	11.120135	11.604944	36.289

Variance Information			
Parameter	Relative Increase in Variance	Fraction Missing Information	Relative Efficiency
SO$_2$	0.043597	0.042147	0.995803

Parameter Estimates					
Parameter	Estimate	Std Error	95% Confidence Limits		DF
SO$_2$	31.134246	3.406603	24.22724	38.04125	36.289

Parameter Estimates					
Parameter	Minimum	Maximum	Theta0	*t* for H0: Parameter = Theta0	Pr > |t|
SO$_2$	30.404072	32.310421	0	9.14	<.0001

TABLE 18.7

Results of a Multiple Regression Analysis of the Air Pollution Data Using Multiple Imputation to Deal with the Missing Values

The MIANALYZE Procedure	
Model Information	
Data Set	WORK.ROUT
Number of Imputations	10

Variance Information				
	Variance			
Parameter	Between	Within	Total	DF
Intercept	611.408115	1250.572511	1923.121438	16.286
Temp	0.079461	0.224372	0.311779	19.254
Manu	0.000028009	0.000135	0.000166	23.78
Pop	0.000032980	0.000123	0.000159	21.722
Wind	0.941273	1.993658	3.029058	16.605
Precip	0.031276	0.077970	0.112374	18.107
Days	0.010854	0.015956	0.027895	13.385

Variance Information			
Parameter	Relative Increase in Variance	Fraction Missing Information	Relative Efficiency
Intercept	0.537793	0.366699	0.964627
Temp	0.389565	0.292599	0.971572
Manu	0.228697	0.192324	0.981131
Pop	0.295110	0.236623	0.976885
Wind	0.519347	0.358271	0.965412
Precip	0.441241	0.320167	0.968977
Days	0.748252	0.449945	0.956943

Parameter Estimates					
Parameter	Estimate	Std Error	95% Confidence Limits		DF
Intercept	123.791333	43.853409	30.95871	216.6240	16.286
Temp	−1.252874	0.558372	−2.42052	−0.0852	19.254
Manu	0.057770	0.012866	0.03120	0.0843	23.78
Pop	−0.032227	0.012618	−0.05841	−0.0060	21.722
Wind	−4.214070	1.740419	−7.89270	−0.5354	16.605
Precip	0.395652	0.335222	−0.30832	1.0996	18.107
Days	−0.038813	0.167019	−0.39858	0.3210	13.385

Parameter Estimates					
Parameter	Minimum	Maximum	Theta0	t for H0: Parameter = Theta0	Pr > |t|
Intercept	91.238007	178.146640	0	2.82	0.0121
Temp	−1.839059	−0.820414	0	−2.24	0.0368

TABLE 18.7 (*Continued*)

Results of a Multiple Regression Analysis of the Air Pollution Data Using
Multiple Imputation to Deal with the Missing Values

		Parameter Estimates				
Parameter	Minimum	Maximum	Theta0	*t* for H0: Parameter = theta0	Pr > |t|
Manu	0.049078	0.067748	0	4.49	0.0002
Pop	−0.042961	−0.022748	0	−2.55	0.0182
Wind	−6.206237	−2.905838	0	−2.42	0.0272
Precip	0.090262	0.691643	0	1.18	0.2532
Days	−0.256193	0.061823	0	−0.23	0.8198

TABLE 18.8

Results from a Multiple Regression Analysis of the Air
Pollution Data Using Only the 26 Complete Cases

		Parameter Estimates			
Variable	DF	Parameter Estimate	Standard Error	t Value	Pr > |t|
Intercept	1	82.02175	54.57459	1.50	0.1493
Temp	1	−0.79096	0.66185	−1.20	0.2468
Manu	1	0.05135	0.01550	3.31	0.0037
Pop	1	−0.02363	0.01563	−1.51	0.1470
Wind	1	−4.30652	2.41199	−1.79	0.0902
Precip	1	0.20202	0.40875	0.49	0.6268
Days	1	0.13226	0.20452	0.65	0.5256

We can compare the results given in Table 18.7 with the results of applying
multiple regression to the air pollution data using only complete cases (of
which there are 26). The necessary SAS code is

```
proc reg data=usair;
  model so2=Temp -- Days;
run;
```

The results are shown in Table 18.8.

And in this example we can also get the multiple regression results from
the available *complete* data set as given in Hand et al. (1994) using the following SAS code:

```
data usairfull;
  infile 'c:\amsus\data\usairfull.dat' expandtabs;
  input city $16. so2 Temp Manu Pop Wind Precip Days;
run;
proc reg data=usairfull;
  model so2=Temp -- Days;
run;
```

TABLE 18.9

Results from Applying Multiple Regression Analysis to the
Complete Air Pollution Data

		Parameter Estimates			
Variable	DF	Parameter Estimate	Standard Error	t Value	Pr > |t|
Intercept	1	111.72848	47.31810	2.36	0.0241
Temp	1	−1.26794	0.62118	−2.04	0.0491
Manu	1	0.06492	0.01575	4.12	0.0002
Pop	1	−0.03928	0.01513	−2.60	0.0138
Wind	1	−3.18137	1.81502	−1.75	0.0887
Precip	1	0.51236	0.36276	1.41	0.1669
Days	1	−0.05205	0.16201	−0.32	0.7500

The results are shown in Table 18.9.

Comparing the three different sets of parameter estimates, etc., we see that there are interesting differences. With the complete case analysis, only the number of manufacturing enterprises is found to be significantly predictive of sulphur dioxide concentration. Using multiple imputation, temperature, manufacturing, population size, and wind speed are found to be significant predictors of SO_2 concentration using the simple t-tests (see Chapter 8 for warnings about using these tests for selecting variables). The analysis of the complete data set finds temperature, manufacturing, and population size to be significant. In general terms, the results from multiple imputation are more similar to those from the complete data set than are the results from the complete-case analysis. (Wood, White, and Royston 2008 describe some methods that can be used for variable selection with multiply imputed data.)

18.8.2 Growth of Danish Boys

In this section, we will look at a 10% random sample from a set of data used to construct the 1997 Dutch growth references for boys. In Table 18.10, the recorded observations for 10 boys are given; in the complete data set, there are observations on 373 boys, aged 9–18.

To begin, we can count the number of missing values for each variable in the data using the following code:

```
data boys;
   infile 'c:\amsus\data\boysgrowth.dat';
   input id age height weight bmi tanner phair tv;
   ageyrs=int(age);
run;

proc means data=boys n nmiss mean min max maxdec=2;
 var height weight bmi tanner phair tv;
run;
```

TABLE 18.10

Growth Observations on 10 Boys

ID	Age	Height	Weight	BMI	Tanner	Phair	TV
3323	9.004	151.2	48.2	21.08	2	1	2
3327	9.021	141.4	29.4	14.7	1	1	2
3329	9.021	132.7	30	17.03			
3334	9.034	139.6	33.8	17.34			
3357	9.119	140	28	14.28	1	1	2
3388	9.201	125.8	22	13.9	1	1	3
3398	9.234	139.8	35.6	18.21	2	1	2
3409	9.27	140.4	32	16.23	2	1	1
3416	9.303	142.2	31.6	15.62	1	1	3
3422	9.316	147.4	31.4	14.45	1	1	2

Notes: Age in years; height in centimetres; weight in kilograms; BMI: body mass index; Tanner stage 1–5; phair = pubic hair (1–6); Tv = testicular volume (millilitres). For more details about the data, see Fredriks, A. M. et al. 2000. *Archives of Disease in Childhood* 82:107–112.

TABLE 18.11

The Number of Missing Values for Each Variable in the Danish Boys' Growth Data

Variable	N	N Miss	Mean	Minimum	Maximum
Height	372	1	167.07	125.80	196.70
Weight	372	1	54.43	22.00	113.00
BMI	372	1	19.01	13.69	31.34
Tanner	220	153	3.00	1.00	5.00
Phair	220	153	3.21	1.00	6.00
Tv	203	170	11.16	1.00	25.00

The results are shown in Table 18.11. There are a large number of missing values for some variables; for example, 153 values of the Tanner variable are missing.

For more detail about the number of missing values for the Tanner pubertal stage variable, we can count the number of missing values at each year of age; the necessary code is

```
proc means data=boys n nmiss mean min max maxdec=2;
 var tanner;
 class ageyrs;
run;
```

The results are shown in Table 18.12. The majority of missing values for the Tanner variable occur for the older boys.

TABLE 18.12

Number of Missing Values According to Age for the Tanner
Pubertal Stage in the Danish Boys' Growth Data

				Analysis Variable : tanner		
Age	N obs	N	N Miss	Mean	Minimum	Maximum
9	16	14	2	1.21	1.00	2.00
10	28	21	7	1.43	1.00	2.00
11	30	23	7	1.26	1.00	2.00
12	28	21	7	1.52	1.00	3.00
13	38	24	14	2.46	1.00	4.00
14	48	25	23	3.20	2.00	5.00
15	56	28	28	4.25	3.00	5.00
16	50	31	19	4.42	2.00	5.00
17	32	14	18	4.71	4.00	5.00
18	29	11	18	4.91	4.00	5.00
19	18	8	10	4.75	4.00	5.00

Let us now look at the distributions of the observed Tanner scores at each
age graphically, using proc sgpanel:

```
proc sgpanel data=boys;
 panelby ageyrs / columns=2 rows=5;
 histogram tanner;
run;
```

The resulting histograms are shown in Figure 18.2. As we would expect, the
distributions differ at the different ages.

Now we will impute the missing values for *all* the variables in the data,
although our particular interest here will be the imputed values on the
Tanner variable to compare their distributions for differently aged boys with
the corresponding distributions of observed values shown in Figure 18.2. But
the imputation model must include all the variables that are going to be in
any model fitted to the data, so even age, which does not have missing data,
should be included, in case missing values are dependent on age, as is likely.

We can impute the missing values for all the variables as follows:

```
proc mi data=boys nimpute=20 out=impboys seed=123
               min=. . 1 1 0 .
               max=. . 5 6 . .
               round=. . 1 1 . . ;
 var height weight tanner phair tv age;
 mcmc;
run;
```

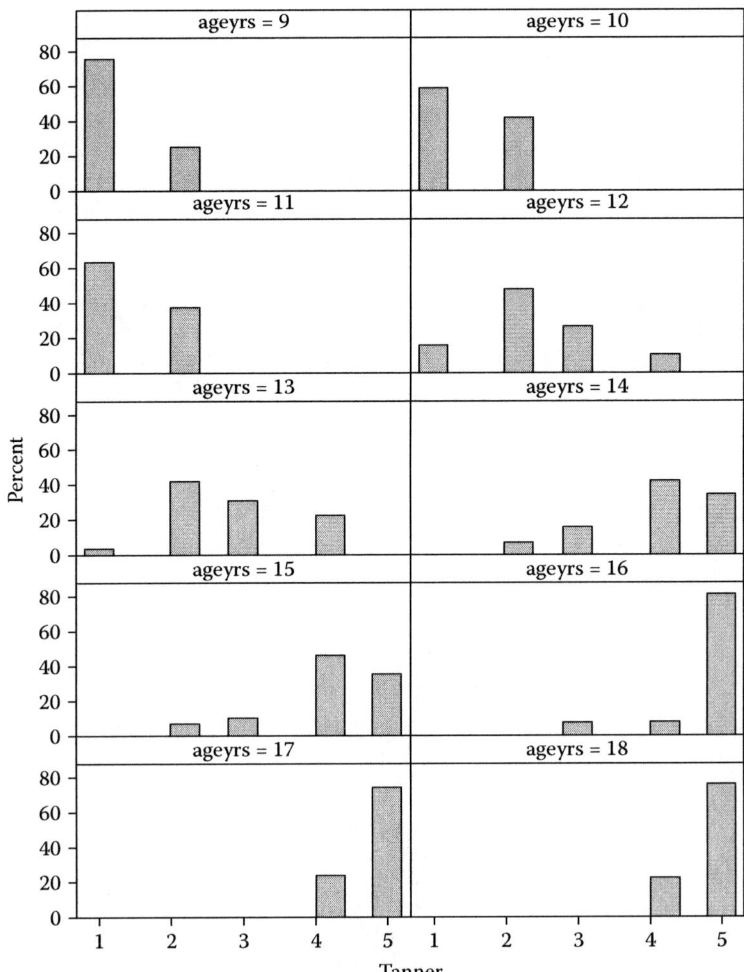

FIGURE 18.2
Distributions of observed Tanner score by age.

As the Tanner score is limited to values one to five and the pubic hair rating to one to six, we specify corresponding minima and maxima and round the values to integers via the `min`, `max`, and `round` options. For each option, the values apply to the variable in the corresponding position on the `var` statement. Values represented by periods do not have their imputed values constrained. (We should say here that constraining the imputed values as we have done in this example for two of the variables is not universally recommended. For some statisticians, 'impossible' imputed values are not a problem because they argue that those values are being imputed to satisfy the overall distribution; consequently, particular imputed values

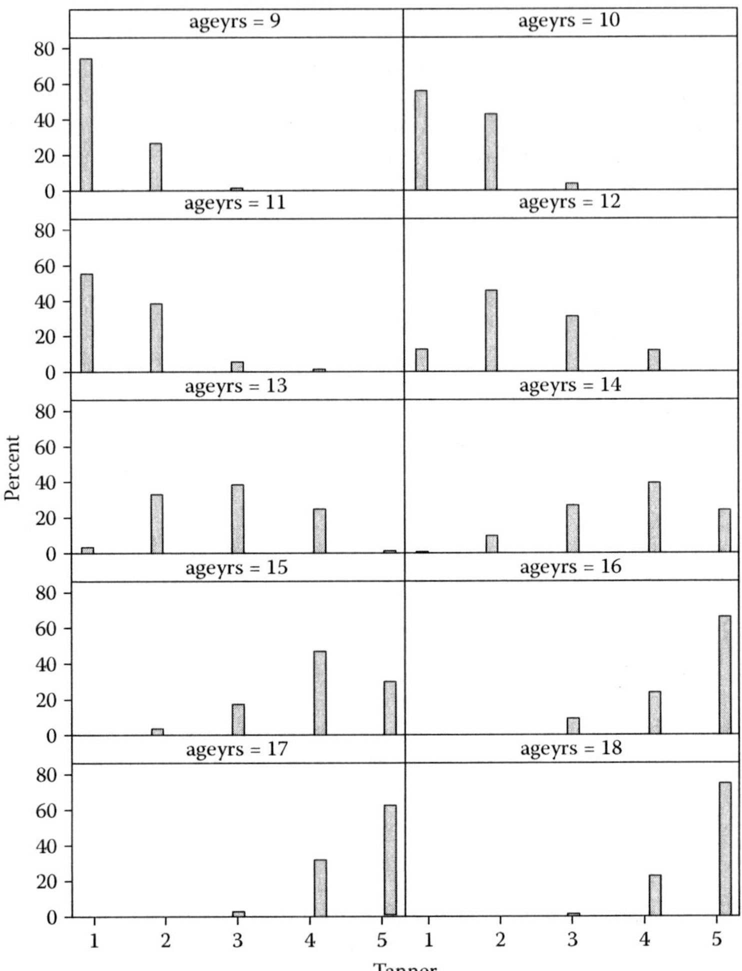

FIGURE 18.3
Distributions of imputed Tanner scores by age.

are unimportant and it is only the aggregated estimates that are of any concern.)

We can now examine the distribution of the imputed values for the Tanner variable by age as before:

```
proc sgpanel data=impboys;
 panelby ageyrs / rows=5;
 histogram tanner;
run;
```

The result is Figure 18.3.

Comparing these results with those in Figure 18.2, we can see that the shapes of the distributions match closely, despite relatively large proportions of missing data having been imputed at the older ages.

After the imputation, a variety of complete-data analyses might be applied to the data depending on the aims of most interest. See van Buuren (2007) for examples of what might be done.

18.9 Summary

Missing values are an ever present possibility in medical studies, although everything possible should be done to avoid them. But when data contain missing values, multiple imputation can be used to provide valid inferences for parameter estimates form the incomplete data. If carefully handled, multiple imputation can cope with missing data in all types of variables. In this chapter, we have given only a brief account of dealing with missing values; a detailed account is available in the issue of *Statistical Methods in Medical Research* entitled 'Multiple Imputation: Current Perspectives' (Volume 16, Number 3, 2007).

References

Adelusi, B. 1977. Carcinoma of the cervix uteri in Ibadan coital characteristics. *International Journal of Gynaecology and Obstetrics* 15:5–11.

Agresti, A. 1996. *Introduction to Categorical Data Analysis.* New York: Wiley.

Aitkin, M. 1978. The analysis of unbalanced cross classifications. *Journal of the Royal Statistical Society, Series A* 141:195–223.

Altman, D. G. 1991. *Practical Statistics for Medical Research.* London: CRC/Chapman & Hall.

Altman, D. G., and Bland, J. M. 1995. Absence of evidence is not evidence of absence. *British Medical Journal* 326:1267.

Altman, D. G., and De Stavola, B. L. 1994. Practical problems in fitting proportional hazards model to data with updated measurements of the covariates. *Statistics in Medicine* 13:301–341.

Amess, J. A., Burman, J. F., Rees, G. M., et al. 1978. Megaloblastic haemopoiesis in patients receiving nitrous oxide. *Lancet* ii:339–342.

Andersen, B. 1990. *Methodological Errors in Medical Research.* Oxford, England: Blackwell.

Bailey, K. R. 1987. Inter-study differences; how should they influence the interpretation of results? *Statistics in Medicine* 6:351–360.

Barnard, J., Rubin, D. B., and Schenker, N. 1998. Multiple imputation methods. In *Encyclopaedia of Biostatistics,* 2nd ed., ed. P. Armitage and T. Colton. Chichester, England: Wiley.

Beck, A. T., Steer, A., and Brown, G. K. 1996. *Beck Depression Inventory Manual.* San Antonio, TX: The Psychological Corporation.

Begg, T. B., and Hearns, J. B. 1966. Components in blood viscosity. The relative contributions of haematocrit, plasma fibrinogen and other proteins. *Clinical Science* 31:87–93.

Bernado, J. M., and Smith, A. F. M. 1994. *Bayesian Theory.* Chichester, England: Wiley.

Bland, M. 2011. Correlation. In *Encyclopaedic Companion to Medical Satistics,* 2nd ed., ed. B. S. Everitt and C. R. Palmer. Chichester, England: Wiley.

Bradford Hill, A. 1962. *Statistical Methods in Clinical and Preventive Medicine.* Edinburgh: Livingstone.

Breslow, N. E., and Day, N. E. 1987. *Statistical Methods in Cancer Research, Volume II. The Design and Analysis of Cohort Studies.* Oxford, England: Oxford University Press.

Brown, K. S. 2005. Analysis of covariance. In *Encyclopaedia of Biostatistics,* 2nd ed., ed. P. Armitage and T. Colton. Chichester, England: Wiley.

Burman, P. 1996. Model fitting via testing. *Statistica Sinica* 6:589–601.

Carlin, B. P., and Louis, T. A. 2008. *Bayesian Methods for Data Analysis.* Boca Raton, FL: Chapman & Hall/CRC.

Carpenter, J., Pocock, S. J., and Lamm, C. J. 2002. Coping with missing data in clinical trials: A model-based approach to asthma trials. *Statistics in Medicine* 21:1043–1066.

Chalmers, T., Celano, P., Sacks, H. S., and Smith, H., Jr. 1983. Bias in treatment assignment in controlled clinical trials. *New England Journal of Medicine* 309:1358–1361.

Chalmers, T. C., and Lau, J. 1993. Meta-analysis stimulus for change in clinical trials. *Statistical Methods in Medical Research* 2:161–172.

Chaloner, K. 1996. Elicitation of prior distributions. In *Bayesian Biostatistics*, ed. D. A Berry and D. K Stangl. New York: Marcel Dekker.

Chaloner, K., and Verdinelli, I. 1995. Bayesian experimental design: A review. *Statistical Science* 10:273–304.

Chambers, J. M., and Hastie, T. J. 1993. *Statistical Models in S.* New York: CRC/ Chapman & Hall.

Chatterjee, S., and Price, B. 2000. *Regression Analysis by Example,* 3rd ed. New York: Wiley.

Cleveland, W. S. 1979. Robust locally weighted regression and smoothing scatter plots. *Journal of the American Statistical Association* 74:829–836.

Cohen, J. 1960. A coefficient of agreement for nominal scales. *Educational and Psychological Measurement* 20:37–46.

Colditz, G. A., Brewer, T. F., Berkey, C. S., Wilson, M. E., Burdick, E., Fineberg, H. V., and Mosteller, F. 1994. Efficacy of BCG vaccine in the prevention of tuberculosis. Meta-analysis of published literature. *Journal of the American Medical Association* 271:698–702.

Collett, D. 2003a. *Modelling Binary Data,* 2nd ed. London: Chapman & Hall/CRC Press.

———. 2003b. *Modelling Survival Data in Medical Research,* 2nd ed. London: Chapman & Hall/CRC Press.

Cook, D., and Swayne, D. F. 2007. *Interactive and Dynamic Graphics for Data Analysis.* New York: Springer.

Cook, R. D., and Weisberg, S. 1982. *Residuals and Influence in Regression.* London: CRC/Chapman & Hall.

Cox, D., and Snell, E. L. 1968. A general definition of residuals. *Journal of the Royal Statistical Society, Series B* 30:248–275.

Cox, D. R. 1972. Regression models and life tables. *Journal of the Royal Statistical Society Series B* 34:187–200.

Cullen, B. F., and van Belle, G. 1975. Lymphocyte transformation and changes in leukocyte count: Effects of anaesthesia and operation. *Anaesthesiology* 43:577–583.

Daly, D., Hand, D. J., Jones, M. C., Lunn, A. D., and McConway, K. J. 1995. *Elements of Statistics.* Reading, MA: Addison–Wesley, The Open University.

Davis, C. S. 1991. Semiparametric and nonparametric methods for the analysis of repeated measurements with applications to clinical trials. *Statistics in Medicine* 16:1959–1980.

———. 2002. *Statistical Methods for the Analysis of Repeated Measurements.* New York: Springer.

Demets, D. L. 1987. Methods for combining randomised clinical trials: Strengths and limitations. *Statistics in Medicine* 6:341–350.

DerSimonian, R., and Laird, N. 1986. Meta-analysis in clinical trials. *Controlled Clinical Trials* 7:177–188.

de Vet, H. C. W., Terwee, C. B., Mokkink, L. B., and Knol, D. L. 2011. *Measurement in Medicine.* Cambridge, England: Cambridge University Press.

Diggle, P. J., and Kenward, M. G. 1994. Informative drop-out in longitudinal analysis (with discussion). *Applied Statistics* 43:49–93.

Diggle, P. L., Liang, K., and Zeger, S. L. 2002. *Analysis of Longitudinal Data,* 2nd ed. Oxford, England: Oxford University Press.

Dizney, H., and Groman, L. 1967. Predictive validity and differential achievement in three MLA comparative foreign language tests. *Educational and Psychological Measurement* 27:1127–1130.

Dobson, A. J., and Barnett, A. 2008. *An Introduction to Generalized Linear Models,* 2nd ed. London: Chapman & Hall.

Doll, R., and Hill, A. B. 1950. Smoking and carcinoma of the lung: Preliminary report. *British Medical Journal* 2:739–748.

———. 1954. The mortality of doctors in relation to their smoking habits. *British Medical Journal* 1:1451–1455.

———. 1956. Lung cancer and other causes of death in relation to smoking. *British Medical Journal* 2:1071–1081.

Draper, N. R., and Smith, H. 1998. *Applied Regression Analysis.* New York: Wiley.

Dunn, G. 2004. *Statistical Evaluation of Measurement Errors.* London: Arnold.

Duval, S., and Tweedie, R. L. 2000. A nonparametric 'trim and fill' method of accounting for publication bias in meta-analysis. *Journal of the American Statistical Association* 95:89–98.

Easterbrook, P. J., Berlin, J. A., Gopalan, R., and Matthews, D. R. 1991. Publication bias in research. *Lancet* 337:867–872.

Emerson, J. D. 1994. Combining estimates of the odds ratio: The state of the art. *Statistical Methods in Medical Research* 3:157–178.

Everitt, B. S. 1992. *The Analysis of Contingency Tables,* 2nd ed. London: CRC/Chapman & Hall.

———. 1994. *Statistical Methods for Medical Investigations,* 2nd ed. London: Arnold.

———. 2002. *Modern Medical Statistics.* London: Arnold.

———. 2011. High-dimensional data. In *Encyclopaedic Companion to Medical Statistics,* 2nd ed., ed. B. S. Everitt and C. Palmer. Chichester, England: Wiley.

Everitt, B. S., Landau, S., Leese, M., and Stahl, D. 2011. *Cluster Analysis,* 5th ed. Chichester, England: Wiley.

Everitt, B. S., and Pickles, A. 2004. *Statistical Aspects of the Design and Analysis of Clinical Trials.* London: Imperial College Press.

Everitt, B. S., and Skrondal, A. 2010. *Cambridge Dictionary of Statistics,* 4th ed. Cambridge, England: Cambridge University Press.

Everitt, B. S., and Wessely, S. 2008. *Clinical Trials in Psychiatry,* 2nd ed. Chichester, England: Wiley.

Eysenck, H. 1978. An exercise in mega silliness. *American Psychologist* 33:517.

Faraggi, D., and Reisser, B. 2011. Receiver operating characteristic (ROC) curve. In *Encyclopaedic Companion to Medical Statistics,* 2nd ed., ed. B. S. Everitt and C. Palmer. Chichester, England: Wiley.

Fisher, R. A. 1970. *Statistical Methods for Research Workers,* 14th ed. New York: Macmillan.

Fitzmaurice, G. M., Laird, N. M., and Ware, J. H. 2004. *Applied Longitudinal Analysis.* New York: Wiley.

Fleiss, J. L. 1999. *The Design and Analysis of Clinical Experiments.* New York: Wiley.

Fleming, T., and Harrington, D. 1991. *Counting Processes and Survival Analysis.* New York: Wiley.

Food and Drug Administration. 2010. Guidance for the use of Bayesian statistics in medical device clinical trials.

Fredricks, A. M., van Buuren, S., Wit, J. M., and Verloove-Vanhorick, S. P. 2000. Body index measurements in 1996–1997 compared with 1980. *Archives of Disease in Childhood* 82:107–112.

Freiman J. A., Chalmers, T. C., and Smith, H. 1978. The importance of beta, the type II error and sample size in the design and interpretation of the randomized control trial: Surgery of 'negative' trials. *New England Journal of Medicine* 299:690–694.

Friedman, L. M., Furberg, C. D., and De Mets, D. L. 1985. *Fundamentals of Clinical Trials,* 2nd ed. Littleton, MA: PSB Publishing.

Frison, L., and Pocock, S. J. 1992. Repeated measures in clinical trials: Analysis using mean summary statistics and its implications for design. *Statistics in Medicine* 11:1685–1704.

Gardner, M. J., and Altman, D. G. 1986. Confidence intervals rather than p-values: Estimation rather than hypothesis testing. *British Medical Journal* 292:746.

Gelman, A. 1996. Inference and monitoring convergence. In *Markov Chain Monte Carlo in Practice,* ed. W. R. Gilks, S. Richardson, and D. J. Spiegelhalter. London: Chapman & Hall.

Geweke, J. 1992. Evaluating the accuracy of sampling-based approaches to calculating posterior moments. In *Bayesian Statistics 4,* ed. J. M. Bernado, J. O. Berger, A. P. Dawid, and A. F. M. Smith. Oxford, England: Clarendon Press.

Gilks, W. R., Richardson, S., and Spiegelhalter, D. J. 1996. Introducing Markov chain Monte Carlo. In *Markov Chain Monte Carlo in Practice,* ed. W. R. Gilks, S. Richardson, and D. J. Spiegelhalter. London: Chapman & Hall.

Glaseby, C. A., and Horgan, G. W. 1996. *Image Analysis for the Biological Sciences.* Chichester, England: Wiley.

Glass, G. 1976. Primary care, secondary and meta-analysis of research. *Education Research* 5:3–8.

Goldberg, D. 1972. *The Detection of Psychiatric Illness by Questionnaire.* Oxford, England: Oxford University Press, Oxford.

Gotzsche, P. C., and Lange, B. 1991. Comparison of search strategies for recalling double-blind trials from MEDLINE. *Danish Medical Bulletin* 38:476–478.

Greenwald, A. G. 1975. Consequences of prejudice against the null hypothesis. *Psychological Bulletin* 82:1–20.

Greenwood, M., and Yule, C. V. 1920. An inquiry into the nature of frequency distributions representative of multiple happenings, with particular reference to the occurrence of multiple attacks of disease or repeated accidents. *Journal of the Royal Statistical Society, Series A* 89:255–279.

Hand, D. J., Daly, F., Lunn, A. D., McConway, K. J., and Ostrowski, E. 1994. *Handbook of Small Data Sets.* London: Chapman & Hall.

Hastie, T. J., and Tibshirani, R. J. 1990. *Generalised Additive Models.* London: CRC/ Chapman & Hall.

Hastings, W. K. 1970. Monte Carlo sampling methods using Markov chains and their applications. *Biometrika* 57:97–109.

Heitjan, D. F. 1997. Annotation: What can be done about missing data? Approaches to imputation. *American Journal of Public Health* 87:548–550.

Hocking, R. R. 1976. The analysis and selection of variables in linear regression. *Biometrics* 32:1–49.

Hoff, P. D. 2009. *A First Course in Bayesian Statistical Methods.* New York: Springer.

Hommel, E., Parving, H., Mathiesen, E., Edsberg, B., Nielsen, M. D., and Giese, F. 1986. Effect of captopril on kidney function in insulin-dependent diabetic patients with neuropathy. *British Medical Journal* 293:467–470.

Hopewell, S., Clarke, M., Lusher, A., Lefebvre, C., and Westby, M. 2002. A comparison of hand-searching versus MEDLINE searching to identify reports of randomized controlled trials. *Statistics in Medicine* 21:1625–1634.

Hosmer, D. W., and Lemeshow, S. 1999. *Applied Survival Analysis*. New York: Wiley.

———. 2000. *Applied Logistic Regression,* 2nd ed. New York: Wiley.

———. 2005. Logistic regression, conditional. In *Encyclopaedia of Biostatistics,* 2nd ed., ed. P. Armitage and T. Colton. Chichester, England: Wiley.

Howell, D. C. 1992. *Statistical Methods for Psychologists.* Belmont, CA: Duxbury Press.

Joyce, J., Rabe-Hesketh, S., and Wessely, S. 1998. Reviewing the reviews; the example of chronic fatigue syndrome. *Journal of the American Medical Association* 280:264–266.

Juni, P., Witschi, A., Bloch, R., and Egger, M. 1999. The hazards of scoring the quality of clinical trials for meta-analysis. *Journal of the American Medical Association* 282:54–60.

Kafadar, K. 2011. Microarray experiments. In *Encyclopaedic Companion to Medical Statistics,* 2nd ed., ed. B. S. Everitt and C. Palmer. Chichester, England: Wiley.

Kalbfleisch, J. D., and Prentice, J. L. 1973. Marginal likelihood based on Cox's regression and life model. *Biometrika* 60:267–278.

———. 1980. *The Statistical Analysis of Failure Time Data.* New York: Wiley.

Kinsey, A. C., Wardell, B. P., and Martin, C. E. 1948. *Sexual Behavior in the Human Male.* Philadelphia, PA: W. B. Saunders.

Kinsey, A. C., Wardell, B. P., Martin, C. E., and Gebhard, P. H. 1953. *Sexual Behavior in the Human Female.* Philadelphia, PA: W. B. Saunders.

Kirsch, I., and Sapirstein, G. 1998. Listening to Prozac but hearing placebo: A meta-analysis of antidepressant medication. *Prevention and Treatment* 1: Article 0002a (http://journals.apa.org/prevention/volume 1/pre0010002a.html).

Kleijnen, J. 1997. Current controversies in the application of meta-analysis (with special reference to oncological treatments). A commentary. *Pharmacy World & Science* 19:117–118.

Kleinblaum, D. G., Kupper, L. L., and Muller, K. E. 1988. *Applied Regression Analysis and Other Multivariate Methods,* 2nd ed. Boston: PWS-Kent Publishing.

Kontula, K., Anderrson, L. C., Paavonen, T., Myllyla, G., Terrenharr, L., and Vuopio, P. 1980. Glucocorticord receptors and glucocorticord sensitivity of human leukaemia cells. *International Journal of Cancer* 26:177–783.

Krzanowski, W., and Hand, D. J. 2009. *ROC Curves for Continuous Data.* London: Chapman & Hall/CRC.

Lakatos, E. 1988. Sample sizes based on the log-rank statistic in complex clinical trials. *Biometrics* 44:229–241.

Landis, J. R., and Koch, G. C. 1977. The measurement of observer agreement for categorical data. *Biometrics* 33:159–174.

Larner, M. 1996. Mass and its relationship to physical measurements. Department of Mathematics, University of Queensland.

Leatham, A. J., and Brooks, S. A. 1987. Predictive value of lectin binding on breast-cancer recurrence and survival. *Lancet* i:1054.

Lee, E. T. 1992. *Statistical Methods for Survival Data Analysis.* New York: Wiley.

Le Fanu, J. 1999. *The Rise and Fall of Modern Medicine.* London: Abacus.

Liang, K. Y., and Zeger, S. L. 1986. Longitudinal data analysis using generalized linear models. *Biometrika* 73:13–22.

Lin, D. Y., Wei, L. J., and Ying, Z. 1993. Checking the Cox model with cumulative sums of Martingale-based residuals. *Biometrika* 80:557–572.

Little, R. J. 2005. Missing data. In *Encyclopaedia of Biostatistics*, 2nd ed., ed. P. Armitage and T. Colton. Chichester, England: Wiley.

Liu, G. 2005. Sample sizes in epidemiological studies. In *Encyclopaedia of Biostatistics*, 2nd ed., ed. P. Armitage and T. Colton. Chichester, England: Wiley.

Longford, N. T. 1993. *Random Coefficient Model.* Oxford, England: Oxford University Press.

Mallows, C. L. 1973. Some comments on C_p. *Technometrics* 15:661–675.

———. 1995. More comments on C_p. *Technometrics* 37:362–372.

Mantel, N., and Haenszel, W. 1959. Statistical aspects of the analysis of data from retrospective studies of disease. *Journal of the National Cancer Institute* 22:719–748.

Martin, M. A., and Welsh, A. H. 2005. Graphical displays. In *Encyclopaedia of Biostatistics*, 2nd ed., ed. P. Armitage and T. Colton. Chichester, England: Wiley.

Matthews, J. N. S. 1993. A refinement to the analysis of serial data using summary measures. *Statistics in Medicine* 12:27–37.

———. 2005. Summary measure analysis of longitudinal data. In *Encyclopaedia of Biostatistics*, 2nd ed., ed. P. Armitage and T. Colton. Chichester, England: Wiley.

Matthews, J. N. S., Altman, D. G., Campbell, M. J., and Royston, P. 1990. Analysis of serial measurements in medical research. *British Medical Journal* 300:230–235.

Maxwell, S. E., and Delaney, H. D. 1990. *Designing Experiments and Analysing Data.* Belmont, CA: Wadsworth.

McCullagh, P., and Nelder, J. A. 1989. *Generalised Linear Models,* 2nd ed. London: CRC/Chapman & Hall.

McMichael, A. J. 2010. Book review of *Smoking Kills: The Revolutionary Life of Richard Doll. International Journal of Epidemiology* 39:1123–1126.

McNemar, Q. 1947. Note on the sampling error of the difference between correlated proportions or percentages. *Psychometrika* 12:153–157.

Mehta, C. R., and Patel, N. R. 1986. A hybrid algorithm for Fisher's exact test on unordered $r \times c$ contingency tables. *Communications in Statistics* 15:387–403.

Metropolis, N., Rosenbluth, A. W., Rosenbluth, M. N., Teller, A. H., and Teller, E. 1953. Equations of state calculations by fast computing machine. *Journal of Chemical Physics* 21:1087–1091.

Moher, D., Jadad, A. R., Nichol, G., Penman, M., Tugwell, P., and Walsh, S. 1995. Assessing the quality of randomized controlled trials: An annotated bibliography of scales and checklists. *Controlled Clinical Trials* 16:62–73.

Moore, D. S. 1998. Statistics among the liberal arts. *Journal of the American Statistical Association* 93 (444): 1253–1259.

Mulrow, C. 1987. The medical review article: State of the art. *Annals of Internal Medicine* 106:485–488.

Murray, G. D., and Findlay, J. G. 1988. Correcting for the bias caused by drop-outs in hypertension trials. *Statistics in Medicine* 7:941–946.

Nelder, J. A. 1977. A reformulation of linear models. *Journal of the Royal Statistical Society, Series A* 140:48–63.

Nelder, J. A., and Wedderburn, R. W. M. 1972. Generalised linear models. *Journal of the Royal Statistical Society, Series A* 135:370–384.

Niel-Weise, B. S., Stijnen, T., and van den Broek, P. J. 2007. Anti-infective-treated central venous catheters: A systematic review of randomized controlled trials. *Intensive Care Medicine* 33:2058–2068.

Oakes, M. 1986. *Statistical Inference: A Commentary for the Social and Behavioural Sciences.* Chichester, England: Wiley.

———. 1993. The logic and role of meta-analysis in clinical research. *Statistical Methods in Medical Research* 2:147–160.

Ogundipe, L. O., Boardman, A. P., and Masterson, A. 1999. Randomization in clinical trials. *British Journal of Psychiatry* 175:581–584.

Oldham, P. D. 1962. A note on the analysis of repeated measurements of the same subjects. *Journal of Chronic Disease* 15:969–977.

Pan, W. 2001. Akaike's information criterion in generalised estimating equations. *Biometrics* 57:120–125.

Piantadosi, S. 1997. *Clinical Trials: A Methodologic Perspective.* New York: Wiley.

Pickering, G. W. 1949. The place of the experimental method in medicine. *Proceedings of the Royal Society of Medicine* 42:229–234.

Pickles, A. 2005. Generalized estimating equations. In *Encyclopaedia of Biostatistics,* 2nd ed., ed. P. Armitage and T. Colton. Chichester, England: Wiley.

Pocock, S. J. 1983. *Clinical Trials.* Chichester, England: Wiley.

———. 1992. When to stop a clinical trial. *British Medical Journal* 305:235–240.

———. 1996. Clinical trials: A statistician's perspective. In *Advances in Biometry,* ed. P. Armitage and H. A. David. Chichester, England: Wiley.

Pocock, S. J., Assmann, S. E., Enos, L. E., and Kasten. L. E. 2002. Subgroup analysis, covariate adjustment and baseline comparisons in clinical trial reporting: Current practice and problems. *Statistics in Medicine* 21:2917–2930.

Prentice, R. L. 2005. Cohort studies. In *Encyclopaedia of Biostatistics,* 2nd ed., ed. P. Armitage and T. Colton. Chichester, England: Wiley.

Proudfoot, J., Goldberg, D., Mann, A., Everitt, B. S., Marks, I., and Gray, J. 2003. Computerised, interactive, multimedia cognitive behavioural therapy for anxiety and depression in general practice. *Psychological Medicine* 33:217–227.

Rifland, A. B., Canale, V., and New, M. I. 1976. Antipyrine clearance in homozygenous beta-thalassemia. *Clinical Pharmaceuticals and Therapeutics* 20:476–483.

Roberts, G. 1996. Markov chain concepts related to sampling algorithms. In *Markov Chain Monte Carlo in Practice,* ed. W. R. Gilks, S. Richardson, and D. J. Spiegelhalter. London: Chapman & Hall.

Rosenberger, W. F., and Lachin, J. M. 2002. *Randomization in Clinical Trials: Theory and Practice.* New York: Wiley.

Rosenman, R. H., Brand, R. J., Jenkins, C. D., Friedman, M., Strauss, R., and Wurm, M. 1975. Coronary heart disease in the Western Collaborative Study: Final follow-up experience of 8.5 years. *Journal of the American Medical Association* 233:872–877.

Rubin, D. B. 1976. Inference and missing data. *Biometrika* 63:581–592.

———. 1987. *Multiple Imputation for Nonresponse in Surveys.* New York: Wiley.

Rubin, D. B., and Schenker, N. 1991. Multiple imputation in healthcare databases: An overview and some applications. *Statistics in Medicine* 10:585–598.

Sackett, D. L. 1979. Bias in analytic research. *Journal of Chronic Disorders* 32:51–63.

Sacks, H., Berrier, J., Reitman, D., Ancona-Berk, V. A., and Chalmers, T. C. 1987. Meta-analyses of randomised controlled trials. *New England Journal of Medicine* 316:450–455.

Sauerbrei, W., and Royston, P. 1999. Building multivariable prognostic and diagnostic models: Transformation of the predictors by using fractional polynomials. *Journal of the Royal Statistical Society, Series A* 162:71–94.

Schafer, J. L. 1997. *Analysis of Incomplete Multivariate Data.* London: Chapman & Hall.

Schafer, J. L., and Graham, J. W. 2002. Missing data: Our view of the state of the art. *Psychological Methods* 7:147–177.

Scheffe, H. 1953. A method for judging all contrasts in the analysis of variance. *Biometrika* 40:87–104.

Schlesselman, J. J. 1982. *Case-Control Studies: Design, Conduct, Analysis.* Oxford, England: Oxford University Press.

Schoenfeld, D. A. 1983. Sample-size formulae for the proportional-hazards regression model. *Biometrics* 39:499–503.

Schulz, K., Chalmers, I., Hayes, R., and Altman, R. G. 1995. Empirical evidence of bias: Dimensions of methodological quality associated with estimates of treatments effects in controlled trials. *Journal of the American Medical Association* 273:408–412.

Schulz, K., and Grimes, D. 2002. Allocation concealment in randomised trials: Defending against deciphering. *Lancet* 359:614–618.

Schumacher, M., Basert, G., Bojar, H., Hubner, K., Olschewski, M., Sauerbrei, W., Schmoor, C., Meumann, R. L. A., and Rauschecker, H. F. for the German Breast Cancer Study Group. 1994. Randomized 2 × 2 trial evaluating hormonal treatment and the duration of chemotherapy in node-positive breast cancer patients. *Journal of Clinical Oncology* 12:2086–2093.

Schuman, H., and Kalton, G. 1985. Survey methods. In *Handbook of Social Psychology*, vol. 1, ed. G. Lindzey and E. Aronson. Reading, MA: Addison–Wesley.

Scott, N. W., McPherson, G. C., Ramsay, C. R., and Campbell, M. K. 2002. The method of minimization for allocation to clinical trials: A review, *Controlled Clinical Trials* 23:662–674.

Seeber, G. U. H. 1989. On the regression analysis of tumour recurrence rates. *Statistics in Medicine* 8:1363–1369.

Senie, R. T., Rosen, P. P., Lesser, M. L., and Kinne, D. W. 1981. Breast self-examination and medical examination related to breast cancer stage. *American Journal of Public Health* 71:583–590.

Senn, S. 1997. *Statistical Issues in Drug Development.* Chichester, England: Wiley.

———. 2006. Change from baseline and analysis of covariance revisited. *Statistics in Medicine* 25:4334–4344.

Sibbald, B., and Roland, M. 1998. Why are randomised controlled trials important? *British Medical Journal* 316:201.

Silagy, C. 2003. Nicotine replacement therapy for smoking cessation (Cochrane Review). In *The Cochrane Library, issue 4,* Chichester, England: Wiley.

Silverman, B. W. 1986. *Density Estimation in Statistics and Data Analysis.* London: CRC/Chapman & Hall.

Simon, R. 1991. A decade of progress in statistical methodology for clinical trials. *Statistics in Medicine* 10:1789–1817.

Simon, S. D. 2001. Is the randomized clinical trial the gold standard of research? *Journal of Andrology* 22:38–43.

Smith, M. L. 1980. Publication bias and meta-analysis. *Evaluating Education* 4:22–24.

Socket, E. B., Daneman, D., Clarson, C., and Ehrich, R. M. 1987. Factors affecting and patterns of residual insulin secretion during the first year of type I (insulin dependent) diabetes mellitus in children. *Diabetes* 30:453–459.

Sokal, R. R., and Rohlf, R. J. 1981. *Biometry,* 2nd ed. San Francisco: W. H. Freeman.

Spiegelhalter, D. J., Abrams, K. R., and Myles, J. P. 2003. *Bayesian Approaches to Clinical Trials and Health-Care Evaluation.* Chichester, England: Wiley.

Spiegelhalter, D. J., Thomas, A., Best, N., and Gilks, W. 1996. BUGS 0.5 examples, vol. 1. MRC Biostatistics Unit, Cambridge, England.

Sterlin, T. D. 1959. Publication decisions and their possible effects on inferences drawn from tests of significance—or vice versa. *Journal of the American Statistical Association* 54:30–34.

Stijnen, T., Hamza, T. H., and Ozdemir, P. 2010. Random-effects meta-analysis of event outcome in the framework of the generalized linear mixed model with applications in sparse data. *Statistics in Medicine* 29:3046–3067.

Sudman, S., and Bradburn, N. 1982. *Asking Questions.* San Francisco: Jossey–Bass.

Sutton, A. J., Abrams, K. R., Jones, D. R., and Sheldon, T. A. 2000. *Methods for Meta-Analysis in Medical Research.* Chichester, England: Wiley.

Sweeting, M. J., Sutton, A. J., and Lambert, P. C. 2004. What to add to nothing? Use and avoidance of continuity corrections in meta-analysis of sparse data. *Statistics in Medicine* 23:1351–1375.

Thall, P. F., and Vail, S. C. 1990. Some covariance models for longitudinal count data with overdispersion. *Biometrics* 46:657–671.

Therneau, T. M., and Grambsch, P. M. 2000. *Modelling Survival Data: Extending the Cox Model.* New York: Springer.

Therneau, T. M., Grambsch, P. M., and Fleming, T. R. 1990. Martingale hazard regression models and the analysis of censored survival data. *Biometrika* 77:147–160.

Thompson, S. G. 1998. Meta-analysis of clinical trials. In *Encyclopaedia of Biostatistics,* 2nd ed., ed. P. Armitage and T. Colton. Chichester, England: Wiley.

Thourangeau, R., Rips, L. J., and Rasinski, K. 2000. *The Psychology of Survey Response.* New York: Cambridge University Press.

Tufte, E. R. 1983. *The Visual Display of Quantitative Information.* Cheshire, CT: Graphics Press.

Turner, S. W., Toone, B. K., and Brett-Jones, J. R. 1986. Computerized tomographic scan changes in early schizophrenia—Preliminary findings. *Psychological Medicine* 16:219–225.

van Buuren, S. 2007. Multiple imputation of discrete and continuous data by fully conditional specification. *Statistical Methods in Medical Research* 16:219–242.

Vaupel, J. W., Manton, K. G., and Stallard, E. 1979. The impact of heterogeneity in individual frailty on the dynamics of mortality. *Demography* 16:439–454.

Vellman, P. F., and Wilkinson, L. 1993. Nominal, ordinal, interval and ratio typologies are misleading. *American Statistician* 47:65–72.

Wacholder, S., and Hartge, P. 2005. Case-control studies. In *Encyclopaedia of Biostatistics,* 2nd ed., ed. P. Armitage and T. Colton. Chichester, England: Wiley.

White, I. R., Royston, P., and Wood, A. M. 2010. Multiple imputation using chained equations: Issues and guidance for practice. *Statistics in Medicine* 30:377–399.

Williams, C. J., Davies, C., Ravel, M., Middleton, J., Luken, J., and Stone, B. 1989. Comparison of antiemetic treatment 24 hours before or concurrently with cytotoxic chemotherapy. *British Medical Journal* 298:430–431.

Wittes, S. 2001. Randomized treatment assignment. In *Biostatistics in Clinical Trials,* ed. C. Redmond and T. Colton. Chichester, England: Wiley.

Wood, A. M., White, I. R., and Royston, P. 2008. How should variable selection be performed with multiply imputed data? *Statistics in Medicine* 27:3227–3246.

Woodward, M. 2011. Epidemiology. In *Encyclopaedic Companion to Medical Statistics,* 2nd ed., ed. B. S. Everitt and C. Palmer. Chichester, England: Wiley.

Yates, F. 1982. Regression models for repeated measurements. *Biometrics* 38:850–853.

Ye, Y., and Kaskutas, L. A. 2009. Using propensity scores to adjust for selection bias when assessing the effectiveness of Alcoholics Anonymous in observational studies. *Drug and Alcohol Dependence* 104:56–64.

Zeger, S. L., and Liang, K. Y. 1986. Longitudinal data analysis for discrete and continuous outcomes. *Biometrics* 42:121–130.

Zerbe, G. O. 1979. Randomization analysis of the completely randomised design extended to growth and response curves. *Journal of the American Statistical Association* 74:215–221.

Index

TABLE 1—The Frequency of Self Examination in Relation to Selected Variables

	(350 Patients) Monthly		(488 Patients) Occasionally		(378 Patients) Never	
Age Group at Diagnosis[1]	N	%	N	%	N	%
<45 years	91	39	90	39	51	22
45–59	150	30	200	40	155	31
60 +	109	23	198	41	172	36
Menstrual Status[2]						
Pre	117	36	121	37	88	27
Peri	82	30	107	40	79	30
Post	151	24	260	42	211	34
Education Level[3]						
<High School	65	24	120	44	85	32
HS or Vocational	123	27	194	42	146	32
College or higher	162	34	174	36	147	30
Family History[4]						
Present	131	34	139	36	115	30
Absent	219	26	349	42	263	32
Prior Benign Breast Disease						
Biopsy Proven[5]	86	40	75	35	54	25
Clinical Only[6]	96	33	119	41	76	26
None	168	24	294	41	248	35
Hypertension						
History	80	22	162	44	126	34
No History	270	32	326	38	252	30
Marital Status[6]						
Never Married	25	25	43	43	34	32
Currently Married	255	32	306	39	224	29
Previously Married	70	21	139	42	120	36

[1] $P < .001$, $\gamma = .19$
[2] $P < .005$, $\gamma = .5$
[3] $P < .04$, $\gamma = -.08$
[4] $P < .02$
[5] $P < .001$
[6] $P < .003$
[7] $P < .02$, $\gamma = -.15$